Basic Current Procedural Terminology and HCPCS Coding

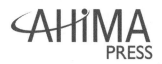

ISBN: 978-1-58426-682-2
AHIMA Product No.: AC200619

AHIMA Staff:
Chelsea Brotherton, MA, Assistant Editor
Colton Gigot, MA, Production Development Editor
Megan Grennan, Managing Editor

Cover image: © exdez, iStockphoto

American Health Information Management Association
233 North Michigan Avenue, 21st Floor
Chicago, Illinois 60601-5809
ahima.org

Basic Current Procedural Terminology and HCPCS Coding

Gail I. Smith, MA, RHIA, CCS-P

2019

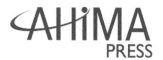

AHIMA PRESS

Brief Table of Contents

Online Resources
   AHIMA Code of Ethics
   AHIMA Standards of Ethical Coding
   Evaluation and Management Documentation Guidelines
   Glossary
   Web Resources for CPT and HCPCS Coding

Detailed Table of Contents

8   Evaluation and Management Documentation Requirements   233

9   Medicine   259

10   Anesthesia   287

11   HCPCS Level II   293

12   CPT and Reimbursement   303

13   Computer-Assisted Coding   315

About the Author

Gail I. Smith, MA, RHIA, CCS-P, is president of Gail I. Smith Consulting in Estero, Florida. Prior to launching an independent consulting business in 2011, Ms. Smith was an associate professor and director of the Health Information Management (HIM) program at the University of Cincinnati. Before joining the University of Cincinnati, she served as the director of the HIM program at Cincinnati State Technical and Community College for 18 years. Before a career in education, Smith held management positions in two Cincinnati hospitals. On a part-time basis, Ms. Smith served as a coding consultant for more than 30 years. Her projects include developing content for courses and workshops, delivering presentations, and performing coding and documentation reviews. Ms. Smith is an AHIMA-approved ICD-10-CM/PCS trainer.

Ms. Smith served as president of the Ohio Health Information Management Association and received the Professional Achievement Award in 1996 and Distinguished Member Award in 2005. Ms. Smith also served on the Board of Directors of the American Health Information Management Association from 2003 to 2006.

Ms. Smith received her bachelor's degree in HIM from The Ohio State University and her master's degree in education from The College of Mt. St. Joseph in Cincinnati, Ohio.

Preface

This textbook provides basic training and practice in the application of procedural codes from the *Current Procedural Terminology* (CPT) and the *Healthcare Common Procedure Coding System* (HCPCS). CPT is published by the American Medical Association (AMA). Updated annually on January 1, CPT is a proprietary terminology created and maintained by the AMA. Its purpose is to provide a uniform language for describing and reporting the professional services performed by physicians. HCPCS is maintained by the Centers for Medicare and Medicaid Services (CMS). Its purpose is to provide a system for reporting the medical services received by Medicare beneficiaries. HCPCS is made up of two parts: Level I is composed entirely of the current version of CPT; HCPCS Level II provides codes to represent medical services that are not covered by the CPT system, for example, medical supplies and services performed by healthcare professionals who are not physicians.

Like previous editions, the 2019 edition of *Basic Current Procedural Terminology and HCPCS Coding* is intended for students who have limited knowledge of, or experience in CPT/HCPCS coding, and also as a resource and review guide for professionals. The instructional materials in this workbook are not specific to any particular practice setting, and they apply to both hospital-based and office-based coding. The exercises provide hands-on experience in coding some of the more common procedures and services performed by physicians and other healthcare professionals.

Many healthcare facilities and providers develop their own systematic methods for assigning CPT codes to frequently performed diagnostic procedures. For this reason, this workbook provides only minimal practice in assigning CPT/HCPCS codes for diagnostic procedures.

The CPT/HCPCS coding process requires coders to apply analytic skills in combination with a practical knowledge of medical science. To become effective coding professionals, students must be able to apply their knowledge of medical terminology, anatomy and physiology, pathophysiology, pharmacology, and medical-surgical techniques. This workbook assumes that students will already have a basic understanding of these subject areas.

The primary objectives of this workbook include the following:

- To provide a basic introduction to the format of CPT codes as well as CPT coding conventions
- To demonstrate how to translate surgical procedures to CPT nomenclature
- To identify ways to ensure accurate code assignment through the application of coding guidelines from the AMA and CMS
- To delineate the documentation necessary for code assignment

Specifically, Chapter 1, Introduction to Clinical Coding, discusses the purpose of CPT/HCPCS codes. It also addresses diagnostic coding and the Medicare requirements for claims submission.

Chapter 2, Application of the CPT System, introduces the CPT coding conventions and explains the application of CPT codes for healthcare reimbursement. Exercises are included for use with the *CPT® QuickRef* app and/or *CPT Assistant*. Exercises will demonstrate the power of using resources to explore *CPT Assistant* guidance and coding vignettes. The *CPT® QuickRef* app is available for purchase with *the CPT® 2019 Professional Edition* code book at https://my.ahima.org/search/books.

Chapter 3, Modifiers, provides an overview of the purpose and use of CPT and HCPCS Level II modifiers.

Chapter 4, Surgery, reviews the coding guidelines associated with the surgical procedures performed to treat illnesses and injuries of the various anatomical systems. It emphasizes the surgical procedures that are performed most commonly in the ambulatory setting (hospital and physician's office). Over 15 new full-color images have been added to this edition. Most of the surgical images are incorporated into the content with scenarios linked to the procedure and corresponding CPT codes. Visualization of surgical procedures helps students to abstract complex operative report documentation, leading the way for translation into CPT nomenclature. Content has been added to highlight coding of skin biopsies, a significant CPT update for 2019.

Chapter 5, Radiology, discusses the claims process for radiology services performed by physicians and hospital-based outpatient providers. The chapter also discusses the principles of radiology code reporting.

Chapter 6, Pathology and Laboratory Services, addresses the code assignment process for common laboratory tests and procedures performed, supervised, or interpreted by pathologists and other physicians.

Chapter 7, Evaluation and Management Services, provides a concise explanation of the evaluation and management section of CPT. The chapter also provides practice exercises designed to address the complexities of assigning evaluation and management (E/M) codes. So that students may scaffold their learning of this complex subject, the fundamentals of E/M coding, including format and organization, are presented in chapter 7, and a new chapter 8 is dedicated to E/M documentation requirements.

Chapter 8, Evaluation and Management Documentation Requirements, provides details about the documentation requirements to support coding decisions.

Chapter 9, Medicine, provides a general overview of the procedures and services described in the medicine chapter of the CPT codebook.

Chapter 10, Anesthesia, introduces the codes used by the physicians who provide or supervise anesthesia services.

Chapter 11, HCPCS Level II, reviews the format and usage of HCPCS National Codes and modifiers.

Chapter 12, CPT and Reimbursement, has been significantly revised. The focus of this chapter has transitioned to how CPT code assignments impact reimbursement and emphasizes the importance of an accurate coding assignment. After a discussion of the Medicare Outpatient Code Editor and editing software tools, students will practice "looking up" pricing of HCPCS codes for case studies that contain errors. This exercise permits students to use auditing skills and discover the impact of coding errors in one reimbursement methodology.

Chapter 13, Computer-Assisted Coding, allows students to practice skills required for using CAC software.

The 2019 edition of *Basic Current Procedural Terminology and HCPCS Coding* has been expanded and updated in several ways. As in previous editions, review exercises are interspersed in each chapter. Appendix A includes references and bibliography. Appendix B of *Basic Current Procedural Terminology and HCPCS Coding* includes operative reports. The answers to these operative reports are only available to approved faculty of educational programs. Appendix C includes an answer key to the odd-numbered exercises in the book. These answers provide a self-assessment tool for students. A complete answer key, including answers to appendix B operative reports, is available in the supplementary materials for instructors.

This book must be used with the 2019 edition of *Current Procedural Terminology* (CPT 2019) (code changes effective January 1, 2019), published by the AMA. The HCPCS Level II codes included in this publication were current as of October 1, 2018. The most current version of the HCPCS Level II codes can be found on the CMS website.

Students beginning a CPT course of study should have several additional references to help them assign codes. Suggested references and recommended readings that may be helpful to students are listed in the online student resources for this book.

Chapter 8 of this publication is based on the E/M documentation guidelines developed jointly by the AMA and CMS. For additional information on these guidelines or to check for additional revisions, students and educators should visit the CMS website.

Downloadable resources for students include the full evaluation and management documentation guidelines, a glossary of key terms, a list of web resources, the AHIMA Code of Ethics, and the AHIMA Standards of Ethical Coding. See the inside front cover of this book for details.

AHIMA provides supplementary materials for educators who use this workbook in their classes. Materials include lesson plans, keys to all exercises and operative reports in appendix B, PowerPoint slides, and other educational resources. All answer keys are available to approved instructors in online format from the AHIMA Press website. If you have any questions regarding the instructor materials, contact AHIMA Customer Relations at (800) 335-5535 or submit a customer support request at the AHIMA website.

Acknowledgments

AHIMA wishes to acknowledge

Rita A. Scichilone, MHSA, RHIA, CCS, CCS-P, CHC;
Toula Nicholas, RHIT, CCS, CCS-P;
and the late Rita Finnegan, RHIA, CCS

who served as authors of previous editions of Basic *CPT/HCPCS Coding*, as well as the many internal and external reviewers who have contributed throughout the years to this publication, including Lauree E. Handlon, MHA, MS, RHIA, CCS, CPC-H, FAHIMA. The author wishes to thank Teri Jorwic, MPH, RHIA, CCS, CCS-P and Ann Zeisset, RHIT, CCS, CCS-P for their contribution to this publication.

Introduction to Clinical Coding

1

Learning Objectives

- Differentiate between CPT, ICD-10-CM, and ICD-10-PCS.
- Identify the purposes and uses of CPT.
- Distinguish between CPT and National codes.
- Define medical necessity.
- Successfully link a diagnosis to the appropriate procedure for professional claims.

Several medical terminologies and classification systems are used to document and report information related to healthcare services in the United States. *Current Procedural Terminology* (CPT) is a coding system designed to numerically describe medical procedures and services. *The International Classification of Diseases, Clinical Modification*, currently in its tenth revision (ICD-10-CM), is used to describe and report the illnesses, conditions, and injuries of patients who require medical services.

The *International Classification of Diseases, Procedure Coding System (ICD-10-PCS)*, provides a system for coding medical procedures performed in the *inpatient* departments of hospitals. In addition to CPT, *Healthcare Common Procedure Coding System* (HCPCS), is a standardized coding system developed by the federal government that is used primarily to identify products, supplies an services not included in CPT. (Table 1.1 provides a summary).

> ICD-10-CM answers the question: WHY did the patient seek healthcare services?
> CPT answers the question: WHAT services were performed?

Table 1.1. Reporting codes by setting

Healthcare Setting	Report Diagnosis Codes	Report Procedure Codes
Physician Offices	ICD-10-CM	CPT and HCPCS
Hospital Outpatient Services	ICD-10-CM	CPT and HCPCS
Hospital Inpatient Services	ICD-10-CM	ICD-10-PCS

As an example for reporting codes, refer to figure 1.1, which is an excerpt from the paper billing form for use by physician offices. In this illustration, assume a patient was seen for a growth on the skin of the foot. The physician documented that the following procedure was performed: shaving of a 0.5 centimeter epidermal lesion of the foot. For billing purposes, Field 21.1 would contain the ICD-10-CM diagnosis code of L98.9 for lesion of the skin, which explains the *reason for the encounter*. The *services provided* would be listed in Field 24D, with CPT code 11305 (shaving). Payers could deny or question the bill if the services do not coincide with the diagnosis that it is linked to. In the illustration, column 24E identifies the diagnosis (skin lesion) that supports the procedure performed (shaving).

Figure 1.1. Reporting codes for physician's claim

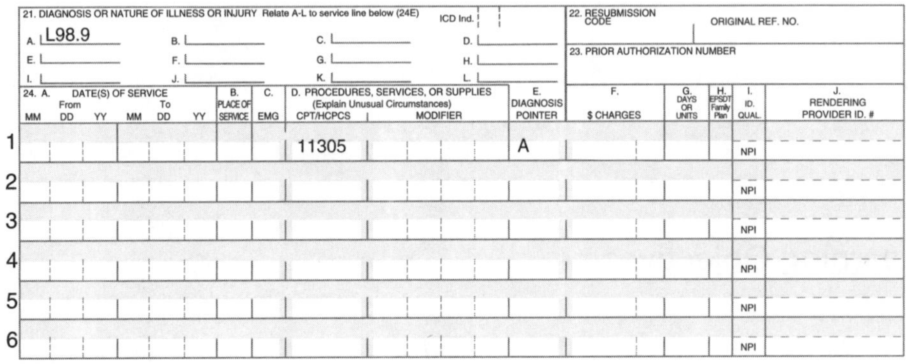

21. DIAGNOSIS OR NATURE OF ILLNESS OR INJURY Relate A-L to service line below (24E) ICD Ind.
A. L98.9 B. C. D.
E. F. G. H.
I. J. K. L.
22. RESUBMISSION CODE ORIGINAL REF. NO.
23. PRIOR AUTHORIZATION NUMBER

24. A. DATE(S) OF SERVICE From MM DD YY To MM DD YY	B. PLACE OF SERVICE	C. EMG	D. PROCEDURES, SERVICES, OR SUPPLIES (Explain Unusual Circumstances) CPT/HCPCS MODIFIER	E. DIAGNOSIS POINTER	F. $ CHARGES	G. DAYS OR UNITS	H. EPSDT Family Plan	I. ID. QUAL.	J. RENDERING PROVIDER ID. #
1			11305	A				NPI	
2								NPI	
3								NPI	
4								NPI	
5								NPI	
6								NPI	

Current Procedural Terminology

CPT, published by the AMA, provides a system for describing and reporting the professional services furnished to patients by physicians and hospital outpatient services.

CPT was initially developed in 1966 and was designed to meet the reporting and communication needs of physicians. The system was adopted for application to the Medicare reimbursement system in 1983. Since that time, CPT has been widely used as the standard for outpatient and ambulatory care procedural coding and reimbursement.

The information represented by CPT codes is also used for several purposes other than reimbursement, including:

- Trending and planning outpatient and ambulatory services
- Benchmarking activities that compare and contrast the services provided by similar non-acute care programs
- Assessing and improving the quality of patient services

The CPT code book includes several additional appendices and an index of procedures. CPT code books and codes are updated annually, with additions, revisions, and deletions becoming effective on January 1 of each year. A new edition of the CPT code book is published annually, and the new edition should be purchased every year to ensure accurate coding. Healthcare providers are expected to begin using the newest edition for encounters on January 1 of each year.

CPT Category I

The CPT code book includes a general introduction followed by six main sections that together make up the list of Category I CPT codes:

Evaluation and Management
Anesthesia
Surgery
Radiology
Pathology and Laboratory
Medicine

Specific coding guidelines are provided for each of the main sections.

The Category I codes in each of the main sections are further broken down into subsections and subcategories according to the type of service provided and the body system or disorder involved. For example, code 76641—Ultrasound, breast, unilateral, real time with image documentation, including axilla when performed; complete—appears in the radiology section under the subsection entitled Diagnostic Ultrasound and the subcategory Chest.

> The AMA does not publish a separate document or book of guidelines; they are all embedded within the code book itself.

Subcategory →

Chest

76641   Ultrasound, breast, unilateral, real time with image
        documentation, including axilla when performed; complete

Similar procedures are grouped to form ranges of codes. For example, the range of codes from 19300 through 19307 represents the various types of mastectomy procedures in the subsection covering the integumentary system in the surgery section. The codes in each of the six main sections (or Category I) of the CPT code book are composed of five digits and are primarily arranged in numerical order within each section. Several coding sections are not in numerical order (for example, 23071). This type of formatting is explained in chapter 2.

CPT Supplementary Codes

CPT also provides three types of supplementary codes: Category II codes, Category III codes, and modifiers. Each of these code sets is listed and explained in a separate section. The Category II and III sections are located after the medicine codes in the code book. The list of modifiers and the coding guidelines for modifiers are included in appendix A of CPT 2019.

CPT Category II Codes

Category II provides supplementary tracking codes that are designed for use in performance assessment and quality improvement activities. CPT Category II codes are composed of five characters: four numbers and an alphabetic fifth character, capital letter F. Code 1000F, for example, describes a specific aspect of patient history: assessments of patient tobacco use. The following is an example of a Category II code under the Physical Examination subsection:

> Category II and III codes are located behind the Medicine section of CPT.

Physical Examination

Physical examination codes describe aspects of physical examination or clinical assessment.

2000F   Blood pressure measured (CKD) (DM)

The use of Category II codes is triggered by clinical criteria such as the documentation of the diagnosis of coronary artery disease or hypertension for use of 2000F. The assignment of Category II CPT codes is optional. However, some payers may require the codes for adjudication of claims. For example, a payer may require Category II code 3008F (Body mass index, documented) when submitting a CPT code for reporting nutritional therapy. Because the Category II codes describe clinical aspects, there is not a billable charge associated with the code. Category II supplementary codes are implemented and released as needed throughout the year. These updates can be obtained by accessing the AMA website and entering the term "Category II codes" into the site's search engine.

CPT Category III Codes

CPT Category III includes temporary codes that represent emerging medical technologies, services, and procedures that have not yet been approved for general use by the FDA and so are not otherwise covered by CPT codes. Category III codes give physicians and other healthcare providers and researchers a system for documenting the use of unconventional methods so that their efficacy and outcomes can be tracked. Like CPT Category II codes, Category III codes are composed of five characters: four numbers and an alphabetic fifth character, capital letter T.

Example:

Code 0085T Breath test for heart transplant rejection

Updated Category III codes are released semiannually on January 1 and July 1 via the AMA's CPT website. The complete list of temporary codes is published annually in the CPT code books.

CPT Modifiers

A third set of supplementary codes known as *modifiers* can be reported along with many of the Category I CPT codes. The two-character modifier codes are appended to Category I five-digit CPT codes to report additional information about any unusual circumstances under which a procedure was performed. The reporting of modifiers is meant to support the medical necessity of procedures that might not otherwise qualify for reimbursement.

Example:

Suppose that a surgeon successfully performed a percutaneous transluminal balloon angioplasty to remove a blockage from a patient's renal artery, but later that day it became evident that the artery had become occluded again. If the surgeon who performed the original procedure is not available, another surgeon on call would repeat the procedure to remove the blockage. Code 37246 would be reported by the first surgeon to identify the original angioplasty, and the second surgeon would report 37246–77 to identify the repeat angioplasty.

Most of the two-character modifiers for Category I codes are numerical. (Chapter 3 of this textbook includes a list of the CPT modifiers in CPT 2019.) However, there also are some alphanumeric modifiers to indicate the physical status of patients undergoing anesthesia. These modifiers begin with a capital letter P, as follows:

Anesthesia Modifiers:
P1 A normal healthy patient
P2 A patient with mild systemic disease
P3 A patient with severe systemic disease
P4 A patient with severe systemic disease that is a constant threat to life
P5 A moribund patient who is not expected to survive without the operation
P6 A declared brain-dead patient whose organs are being removed for donor
    purposes

(Chapter 2 of this textbook provides additional guidelines for applying CPT codes, and chapter 3 discusses modifiers in more detail.)

Healthcare Common Procedure Coding System (HCPCS)

Healthcare Common Procedure Coding System (HCPCS) was developed by the U.S. Department of Health and Human Services (HHS) to identify services typically reimbursed by Medicare and Medicaid but do not appear in CPT. For example, HCPCS provides codes for ambulance services, durable medical equipment and supplies.

An example of an HCPCS
National Code: L8614
Cochlear implant system

HCPCS codes enable providers and suppliers to accurately communicate information about the services they provide. Analysis of HCPCS data also helps Medicare carriers to establish financial controls that prevent expense escalation. Finally, the information from coded claims facilitates uniform application of Medicare and Medicaid coverage and reimbursement policies.

HCPCS is often described as having two levels to describe healthcare services: Level I is based on the current edition of CPT and Level II is HCPCS.

HCPCS Level I (CPT)

Copyrighted and published by the American Medical Association (AMA), Level I of HCPCS consists of five-digit Category I CPT codes. Level I HCPCS (CPT) codes are used by physicians to report services such as hospital visits, surgical procedures, radiological procedures, supervisory services, and other medical services. Hospitals also use Level I codes to report hospital-based outpatient services, such as laboratory and radiological procedures and ambulatory services, to Medicare and other third-party payers. Level I codes represent approximately 80 percent of the HCPCS codes submitted for reimbursement each year.

Example:

> If a patient is admitted to the hospital for an emergency open appendectomy, the hospital would report, to the payer, CPT code 44950. The reimbursement would be based on costs associated with that procedure being performed at the hospital, such as use of the operating room, equipment, drugs, and hospital staff (nursing and surgical assistants). In addition, the surgeon would also report the same code (44950) to the payer and would be reimbursed for the surgical services of actually performing the procedure.

HCPCS Level II (National Codes)

HCPCS Level II codes were developed by CMS for use in reporting medical services not covered in CPT. Medicare, Medicaid, and private health insurers use HCPCS codes and modifiers for claims processing. Level II codes are provided for injectable drugs, ambulance services, prosthetic devices, and selected provider services.

Level II codes are made up of five characters: The first character is a capital alphabetic letter, and the following four characters are numbers. Examples of HCPCS Level II codes include the following:

> A4550   Surgical trays
> E1625   Water softening system, for hemodialysis
> J0475   Injection, Baclofen, 10 mg

Example:

> If a patient required an intramuscular injection of an antibiotic, the correct CPT code would be 96372 (Therapeutic; prophylactic, or diagnostic injection). The CPT code identifies the service (injection) but does not identify the substance (drug) in the injection. An additional HCPCS code would identify the actual drug, such as: *J0561-Penicillin g benzathine, 100,000 units.*

HCPCS Level II codes are updated for use January 1 and the files are available for free on the CMS website and contain an update or errata for the code set. Several commercial publishing companies distribute the HCPCS Level II National Codes in book form, adding enhancements such as indexes and cross-references to make them more user-friendly than the government-issued lists. (HCPCS Level II codes are discussed in more detail in chapter 10.) Table 1.2 highlights the differences between Level I and Level II codes. An overview of the HCPCS system is provided in figure 1.2.

Table 1.2. HCPCS coding system

Level	Coding Set	Development and Maintained by	Common Uses
I	CPT	American Medical Association	Identify surgical procedures, office visits, laboratory services
II	HCPCS	Centers for Medicare and Medicaid Services (CMS)	Injectable drugs, devices, supplies, equipment

For simplification purposes, this textbook will refer to Level I codes as CPT and Level II codes as HCPCS codes.

International Classification of Diseases, Tenth Revision, Clinical Modification (ICD-10-CM)

The *International Classification of Diseases, Tenth Revision, Clinical Modification* (ICD-10-CM), is based on an international classification system originally developed and maintained by the World Health Organization (WHO). The purpose of the international version of the ICD is the classification and reporting of morbidity data (illnesses and injuries) and mortality data (fatalities) from around the world. In the United States, the National Center for Health Statistics (NCHS) has developed a clinical modification of the classification, thus it is referred to as ICD-10-CM (CM indicating the modification).

Figure 1.2. Overview of HCPCS coding system

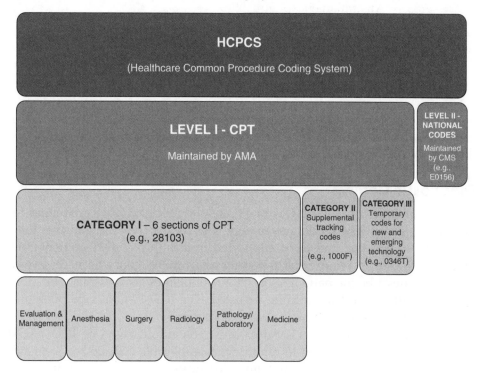

ICD-10-CM diagnosis codes are required for Medicare and private third-party payers to support medical necessity of procedures and services. By definition, medical necessity is the determination that a service or procedure rendered is reasonable and necessary for the diagnosis or treatment of an illness or injury.

ICD-10-CM is divided into two main sections: an Alphabetic Index of Diseases and Injuries and a Tabular List of codes. The codes are organized into chapters such as chapter 1, which is titled Certain Infectious and Parasitic Disease.

Like CPT and HCPCS, ICD-10-CM codes are reevaluated and appropriate revisions are implemented on a regular basis.

ICD-10-CM Diagnostic Codes

ICD-10-CM diagnostic codes represent the reasons *why* patients require and seek medical care. Each alphanumerical code represents a specific symptom, condition, injury, or disease. ICD-10-CM diagnostic codes in the main classification (codes A00-Z99.89) consist of a minimum of three characters and a maximum of seven characters. The first three numbers represent a family of codes, and additional numbers may follow a decimal point after the three-number code to provide information that is more specific. The following illustration provides a snapshot of the classification system for Mosquito-borne viral encephalitis.

Example:

A83	Mosquito-borne viral encephalitis
A83.0	Japanese encephalitis
A83.1	Western equine encephalitis
A83.2	Eastern equine encephalitis
A83.3	St Louis encephalitis
A83.4	Australian encephalitis
A83.5	California encephalitis
A83.6	Rocio virus disease
A83.8	Other mosquito-borne viral encephalitis
A83.9	Mosquito-borne viral encephalitis, unspecified

Note that A83 introduces the family of codes, but it is not a valid code for submission on the claim form. Because there is a selection of codes subcategorized under A83, a more specific code must be selected.

Diagnostic Coding

The Central Office on ICD-10-CM maintains the official coding guidelines for diagnostic coding. The guidelines require ICD-10-CM code assignments to be as specific as possible and to be supported by health record documentation. The guidelines also require the reporting of as many codes as necessary to completely describe the patient's condition. Guidelines also establish the order in which multiple codes are to be reported. The ICD-10-CM code book also provides detailed advice on assigning codes correctly.

Every claim for outpatient services must contain at least one ICD-10-CM code, but care must be taken to report every applicable code in the sequence specified in the official coding guidelines. Medicare and most other third-party payers reject claims that report incomplete ICD-10-CM codes.

Coding professionals must thoroughly understand and carefully follow the *Official ICD-10-CM Coding Guidelines for Outpatient Services* (reference the CDC website) published by the National Center for Health Statistics (NCHS). Official ICD-10-CM coding advice is also published by the American Hospital Association (AHA) in its quarterly publication, *Coding Clinic*. The official coding guidelines for ICD-10-CM are available from the National Center for Health Statistics as well as from the CMS website.

The following example illustrates correct and incorrect ICD-10-CM code assignments for a patient with a diagnosis of Type II diabetes with no mention of complications:

Example:

E11.9	Type 2 diabetes mellitus without complications	**Correct**
E11	Type 2 diabetes mellitus *(this 3-character code introduces the category for diabetes but a more specific code must be selected based on documentation)*	**Incorrect**
E11.0	Type 2 diabetes mellitus with hyperosmolarity *(this code is incomplete and requires a 5th character of either E11.00 or E11.01 based on the patient's diagnosis)*	**Incorrect**

Basic ICD-10-CM/PCS Coding, 2019 Edition, by Lou Ann Schraffenberger, MBA, RHIA, CCS, CCS-P and Brooke N. Palkie, EdD, RHIA provides a more detailed discussion of the basics of ICD-10-CM/PCS coding.

ICD-10-PCS Procedural Classification System

ICD-10-PCS is the procedural system developed for use to report inpatient procedures according to the principles of a classification. The 7-character alpha-numeric code systematically classifies characteristics of procedures such as body part and surgical approach. The following table provides a side-by-side comparison of CPT and ICD-10-PCS for a laparoscopic cholecystectomy (removing the gallbladder).

> CPT is a nomenclature (naming) system, and ICD-10-PCS is a classification system (systematic arrangement).

CPT Procedure Code	ICD-10-PCS Procedure Code
47562 Laparoscopy, surgical; cholecystectomy	0FT44ZZ Resection of gallbladder, percutaneous endoscopic approach

Documentation for Reimbursement

Health record documentation continues to play a pivotal role in the accurate and complete collection of health services data. The documentation records pertinent facts, findings, and observations about an individual's health history, including past and current illnesses, examinations, tests, treatments, and outcomes. By chronologically documenting the patient's care, the health record becomes an important element in the provision of high-quality healthcare and serves as the source document for code assignment.

The following general principles of health record documentation, developed jointly by the AMA and CMS, apply to the records maintained for all types of medical and surgical services:

- The health record should be complete and legible.
- The documentation of each patient encounter should include:
  - The reason for the encounter and the patient's relevant history, physical examination findings, and prior diagnostic test results
  - A patient assessment, clinical impression, or diagnosis
  - A plan for care
  - The date of the encounter and the identity of the observer
- The rationale for ordering diagnostic and other ancillary services should be documented or easily inferred.

- Past and present diagnoses should be accessible to the treating and consulting physicians.
- Appropriate health risk factors should be identified.
- The patient's progress and response to treatment and any revision in the treatment plan and diagnoses should be documented.
- The CPT and ICD-10-CM codes reported on health insurance claim forms or billing statements should be supported by documentation in the health record.

Additional documentation guidelines pertinent to evaluation and management (E/M) services are discussed in chapter 7.

The Medicare Program

The Social Security Act of 1965 and its subsequent amendments established the federal regulations that govern Medicare. The Medicare program is organized into two separate sections: Part A, which pays for the cost of hospital and facility care, and Part B, which covers the physician services and durable medical equipment that are not paid for under Part A. Medicare regulations require the collection of several types of coded information on reimbursement claims for services provided to Medicare beneficiaries:

- ICD-10-CM diagnostic and ICD-10-PCS procedural codes for <u>inpatient</u> hospital services
- ICD-10-CM diagnostic codes and CPT/HCPCS procedural codes for hospital <u>outpatient</u> services, including laboratory and radiology procedures
- ICD-10-CM diagnostic codes and CPT/HCPCS procedural codes (regardless of the service location) for medical services provided by physicians and allied health professionals (psychologists, nurse practitioners, social workers, licensed therapists, and dietitians)

Figure 1.3. illustrates the uses of ICD-10-CM/PCS and CPT/HCPCS by type of healthcare service.

Figure 1.3.   Uses of coding

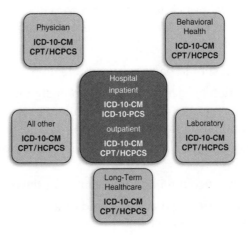

Health Insurance Portability and Accountability Act (HIPAA) Administrative Simplification

The intent of the federal government's simplification mandate is to streamline and standardize the electronic filing and processing of health insurance claims, to save money, and to provide better service to providers, insurers, and patients.

HIPAA Transaction and Code Set Standards

Before the implementation of HIPAA transaction and code set standards, healthcare providers and health plans used various formats when performing daily electronic transactions, which led to confusion. HIPAA requirements specify that all electronic data interchange formats be standardized. These standards apply to any health plan, clearinghouse, and any healthcare providers that transmit health information in electronic form in connection with defined transactions. HIPAA also requires the standardization of the reporting of medical procedures with industry-established and -maintained codes. These are codes used by healthcare providers to identify what procedures, services, and diagnoses pertain to any specific encounter. The following code sets have been approved for use by HIPAA:

- International Classification of Diseases, Tenth Edition, Clinical Modification (ICD-10-CM)
- International Classification of Diseases, 10th Revision, Procedure Coding System (ICD-10-PCS)
- Current Procedural Terminology (CPT)
- Healthcare Common Procedure Coding System (HCPCS)
- Current Dental Terminology (CDT)
- National Drug Codes (NDC)

Claims Submission

Except in limited situations, claim forms must be submitted electronically. Electronic claims must follow the standards developed by the Accredited Standards Committee and mandated by HIPAA.

For learning purposes, this textbook will reference the paper claim form for several exercises that link the diagnoses and procedure codes. These exercises will use an excerpt of the claim form to practice linking CPT codes to diagnosis codes (ICD-10-CM) to support medical necessity.

CMS-1500 Claim Form

The CMS-1500 Health Insurance Claim Form shown in figure 1.4 is the standard paper billing document used for physician claims. These data elements are translated into the electronic format; however, for the purposes of relating coding and reimbursement, note Field 21 that identifies the ICD-10-CM codes. Field 24D contains fields for both CPT/HCPCS codes and modifiers. Field 24E links the diagnosis codes to the related CPT/HCPCS codes by placing an alphabetic character to show which diagnostic code is related to the procedure.

Figure 1.4. Sample CMS-1500 form

HEALTH INSURANCE CLAIM FORM

APPROVED BY NATIONAL UNIFORM CLAIM COMMITTEE (NUCC) 02/12

CARRIER

| | PICA | | | | | | PICA | |

1. MEDICARE (Medicare#) MEDICAID (Medicaid#) TRICARE (ID#/DoD#) CHAMPVA (Member ID#) GROUP HEALTH PLAN (ID#) FECA BLK LUNG (ID#) OTHER (ID#)

1a. INSURED'S I.D. NUMBER (For Program in Item 1)

2. PATIENT'S NAME (Last Name, First Name, Middle Initial)

3. PATIENT'S BIRTH DATE MM DD YY SEX M F

4. INSURED'S NAME (Last Name, First Name, Middle Initial)

5. PATIENT'S ADDRESS (No., Street)

6. PATIENT RELATIONSHIP TO INSURED Self Spouse Child Other

7. INSURED'S ADDRESS (No., Street)

CITY STATE

8. RESERVED FOR NUCC USE

CITY STATE

ZIP CODE TELEPHONE (Include Area Code) ( )

ZIP CODE TELEPHONE (Include Area Code) ( )

9. OTHER INSURED'S NAME (Last Name, First Name, Middle Initial)

10. IS PATIENT'S CONDITION RELATED TO:

11. INSURED'S POLICY GROUP OR FECA NUMBER

a. OTHER INSURED'S POLICY OR GROUP NUMBER

a. EMPLOYMENT? (Current or Previous) YES NO

a. INSURED'S DATE OF BIRTH MM DD YY SEX M F

b. RESERVED FOR NUCC USE

b. AUTO ACCIDENT? YES NO PLACE (State)

b. OTHER CLAIM ID (Designated by NUCC)

c. RESERVED FOR NUCC USE

c. OTHER ACCIDENT? YES NO

c. INSURANCE PLAN NAME OR PROGRAM NAME

d. INSURANCE PLAN NAME OR PROGRAM NAME

10d. CLAIM CODES (Designated by NUCC)

d. IS THERE ANOTHER HEALTH BENEFIT PLAN? YES NO If yes, complete items 9, 9a, and 9d.

READ BACK OF FORM BEFORE COMPLETING & SIGNING THIS FORM.
12. PATIENT'S OR AUTHORIZED PERSON'S SIGNATURE I authorize the release of any medical or other information necessary to process this claim. I also request payment of government benefits either to myself or to the party who accepts assignment below.

SIGNED _____ DATE _____

13. INSURED'S OR AUTHORIZED PERSON'S SIGNATURE I authorize payment of medical benefits to the undersigned physician or supplier for services described below.

SIGNED _____

PATIENT AND INSURED INFORMATION

14. DATE OF CURRENT ILLNESS, INJURY, or PREGNANCY (LMP) MM DD YY QUAL.

15. OTHER DATE QUAL. MM DD YY

16. DATES PATIENT UNABLE TO WORK IN CURRENT OCCUPATION MM DD YY FROM TO MM DD YY

17. NAME OF REFERRING PROVIDER OR OTHER SOURCE 17a. 17b. NPI

18. HOSPITALIZATION DATES RELATED TO CURRENT SERVICES MM DD YY FROM TO MM DD YY

19. ADDITIONAL CLAIM INFORMATION (Designated by NUCC)

20. OUTSIDE LAB? YES NO $ CHARGES

21. DIAGNOSIS OR NATURE OF ILLNESS OR INJURY Relate A-L to service line below (24E) ICD Ind.
A. B. C. D.
E. F. G. H.
I. J. K. L.

22. RESUBMISSION CODE ORIGINAL REF. NO.

23. PRIOR AUTHORIZATION NUMBER

24. A. DATE(S) OF SERVICE From To MM DD YY MM DD YY	B. PLACE OF SERVICE	C. EMG	D. PROCEDURES, SERVICES, OR SUPPLIES (Explain Unusual Circumstances) CPT/HCPCS MODIFIER	E. DIAGNOSIS POINTER	F. $ CHARGES	G. DAYS OR UNITS	H. EPSDT Family Plan	I. ID. QUAL.	J. RENDERING PROVIDER ID. #
1									NPI
2									NPI
3									NPI
4									NPI
5									NPI
6									NPI

25. FEDERAL TAX I.D. NUMBER SSN EIN

26. PATIENT'S ACCOUNT NO.

27. ACCEPT ASSIGNMENT? (For govt. claims, see back) YES NO

28. TOTAL CHARGE $

29. AMOUNT PAID $

30. Rsvd for NUCC Use

31. SIGNATURE OF PHYSICIAN OR SUPPLIER INCLUDING DEGREES OR CREDENTIALS (I certify that the statements on the reverse apply to this bill and are made a part thereof.)

SIGNED _____ DATE _____

32. SERVICE FACILITY LOCATION INFORMATION
a. NPI b.

33. BILLING PROVIDER INFO & PH # ( )
a. NPI b.

PHYSICIAN OR SUPPLIER INFORMATION

NUCC Instruction Manual available at: www.nucc.org **PLEASE PRINT OR TYPE** APPROVED OMB-0938-1197 FORM 1500 (02-12)

Medical Necessity

Codes on claim forms should tell the story about the patient's care and the need for services. The diagnosis codes explain why the patient needs healthcare services and the CPT/HCPCS procedure codes describe the services that are performed. The relationship between diagnosis and procedure codes is described as meeting medical necessity. Coding professionals must be sure that any association of ICD-10-CM diagnostic codes with CPT/HCPCS procedure codes is logical and appropriate.

Example:

Patient's chief complaint is lower leg pain. The physician orders a lower leg x-ray and an electrocardiogram (EKG). The lower leg pain is linked with the x-ray, but there is no logical symptom or diagnosis to link with the EKG. Review of the health record may reveal an existing condition, such as premature ventricular contractions, or a symptom, such as tachycardia. Documentation must support the procedure or service provided; otherwise, the claim will be denied.

Linking the appropriate ICD-10-CM diagnosis to the correct CPT code supports medical necessity. Medical necessity answers the following question for those paying the claim: *Was the service provided logical for the diagnosis reported?*

Medicare and many commercial third-party payers establish coverage limits for certain services. Reimbursement claims for services with coverage limits (for example, inpatient psychiatric care) must include sufficient diagnostic information to support the medical necessity of the services provided. This diagnostic information is communicated in the form of ICD-10-CM codes.

Medicare policies include two types of coverage limits: national coverage decisions (NCDs) and local coverage determinations (LCDs). These policies include decisions on items and services that are reasonable and necessary for the diagnosis or treatment of an illness or injury. For example, a Medicare policy may deny coverage for cosmetic surgical procedures. CMS establishes contractual arrangements with Medicare Administrative Contractors (MACs) who process Medicare claims in local geographic regions. These contractors are responsible for making coverage decisions for Medicare beneficiaries, and the contractors base their decisions on established national coverage requirements for specific medical supplies and services. For cases that are not covered by existing national policies, contractors may make LCDs at their own discretion. A list of the Medicare coverage policies can be found on the CMS website. The following policy is an example of an LCD:

Example:

CPT code 43235, Esophagogastroduodenoscopy, flexible, transoral; diagnostic, including collection of specimen(s) by brushing or washing, when performed (separate procedure), is covered by Medicare only with an appropriate ICD-10-CM diagnosis code submitted on the claim, such as (abbreviated list for illustration):
  B37.81   Candidal esophagitis
  C15.3   Malignant neoplasm of upper third of esophagus
  C16.4   Malignant neoplasm of pylorus

CMS-1450 Claim Form (UB-04)

Data elements from the CMS-1450 form (UB-04) (figure 1.5), is used primarily by hospitals for both outpatient and inpatient services. These data elements are

Figure 1.5. Sample UB-04 (CMS-1450) form

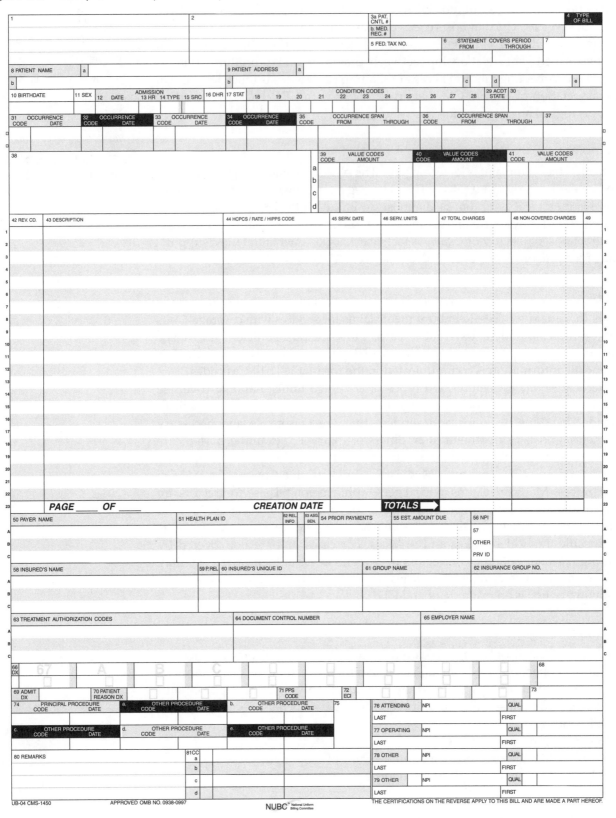

part of the fields for electronic claim submission for Medicare Part A services. Further information on UB-04 can be found at the website of the National Uniform Billing Committee.

Completion and coding instructions can be found in the Medicare Claims Processing Manual. UB-04 has been revised to accommodate ICD-10-CM/PCS codes.

Chapter 1 Review

Answers to odd-numbered questions can be found in appendix C of this book. The answers to even-numbered questions are located in the instructor materials and are available to approved instructors.

Review each of the following questions and write the appropriate answers in the spaces provided.

1. What organization(s) are responsible for updating CPT codes?

   _____

2. What organization is responsible for maintaining HCPCS Level II codes?

   _____

3. What code set describes the diagnosis code to support medical necessity?

   _____

4. On December 3, 2018, Dr. Smith saw a Medicare patient with a diagnosis of rectal abscess in Central Hospital. She performed an incision and drainage in the outpatient surgery department.

   a. Which coding system would be used to capture the diagnosis of rectal abscess?

   b. Which coding system would Central Hospital use to bill for the surgical services?

   c. Which coding system would Dr. Smith use to report her surgical services?

5. Place a check mark in front of all of diagnoses that would logically support medical necessity for CPT code 92550 Tympanometry and reflex threshold measurements.

   ___ D33.3   Benign neoplasm of cranial nerves

   ___ G10   Huntington's Disease

   ___ G83.84 Todd's paralysis (postepileptic)

   ___ H82.3   Vertiginous syndromes in diseases classified elsewhere, bilateral

   ___ H83.12 Labyrinthine fistula, left ear

   ___ H65.06 Acute serous otitis media, recurrent, bilateral

6. Which of the following CPT codes would be linked to the diagnosis B80 Enterobiasis?

a. 86612 Antibody; Blastomyces

b. 86666 Antibody; Ehrlichia

c. 87172 Pinworm exam

d. 87197 Serum bactericidal titer (Schlichter test)

7. A patient was seen in a physician's office for excision of a 0.5-cm facial nevus (CPT [HCPCS Level I] code 11440). The ICD-10-CM diagnostic code for the benign lesion is D22.30. During this encounter, the physician also evaluated the patient's hyperglycemia (ICD-10-CM code R73.9). A glucose tolerance test (HCPCS Level I (CPT) code 82951) was performed. Using figure 1.6, an excerpt from the CMS-1500 form provided in figure 1.4, link the appropriate ICD-10-CM codes found in block 21 with HCPCS Level I (CPT) codes found in block 24D. In column 24E, select the appropriate letter (A or B) to indicate which diagnostic code is related to the procedure.

Figure 1.6. Excerpt of CMS-1500

21. DIAGNOSIS OR NATURE OF ILLNESS OR INJURY Relate A-L to service line below (24E) ICD Ind.

A.	B.	C.	D.
E.	F.	G.	H.
I.	J.	K.	L.

	24. A. DATE(S) OF SERVICE From MM	DD	YY	To MM	DD	YY	B. PLACE OF SERVICE	C. EMG	D. PROCEDURES, SERVICES, OR SUPPLIES (Explain Unusual Circumstances) CPT/HCPCS	MODIFIER	E. DIAGNOSIS POINTER
1											
2											

8. Look up the patient's ICD-10-CM diagnosis code and CPT procedure or service codes that appear on the following claim form. What is the patient's reason for the treatment and service provided?

21. DIAGNOSIS OR NATURE OF ILLNESS OR INJURY Relate A-L to service line below (24E) ICD Ind.

A. H25.9	B.	C.	D.
E.	F.	G.	H.
I.	J.	K.	L.

	24. A. DATE(S) OF SERVICE From MM	DD	YY	To MM	DD	YY	B. PLACE OF SERVICE	C. EMG	D. PROCEDURES, SERVICES, OR SUPPLIES (Explain Unusual Circumstances) CPT/HCPCS	MODIFIER	E. DIAGNOSIS POINTER
1									66984	LT	A
2											

Application of the CPT System

2

Learning Objectives

- Describe the general organization of CPT.
- Define the common symbols used in the CPT code book.
- Explain the use of unlisted codes.
- Interpret conventions and characteristics of CPT.

- Successfully apply the general rules and guidelines for coding assignments.
- Given an operative report, successfully abstract pertinent clinical information.
- Reference official coding guidance (*CPT Assistant*) to support an accurate coding assignment.

The American Medical Association (AMA) developed *Current Procedural Terminology* (CPT) to provide a uniform language that could be used to accurately designate medical, surgical, and diagnostic services. The CPT coding system is an effective means of facilitating communication among physicians, patients, and third-party payers nationwide. The first edition was published in 1966, and now is updated yearly to reflect advances in the field of medicine.

The AMA's CPT Editorial Panel, consisting of physicians and representatives from professional organizations, is responsible for the annual revision and modification of the code book. The panel is assisted in this task by the CPT Advisory Committee, which is composed of physicians nominated by the National Medical Specialty Societies, and by the AMA Healthcare Professionals Advisory Committee, which is composed of other healthcare professionals.

Organization of CPT

To be included in the CPT code book, a procedure or service must meet the following conditions:
   (1) It must be commonly performed by many physicians across the country, and
   (2) it must be consistent with contemporary medical practice.

An example of a CPT code for cosmetic purposes is 69090 Ear Piercing.

Consequently, a procedure's inclusion in, or exclusion from, the CPT code book does not imply that the AMA does or does not endorse it. Nor does it mean that the procedure is or is not covered for reimbursement by insurance plans. For example, although codes exist in CPT to describe cosmetic surgery, most insurance carriers do not provide reimbursement for such procedures. Thus, patients would pay for such services out of pocket. Reimbursement rules and guidelines are not always consistent with CPT coding rules and guidelines. Just as insurance policies for healthcare services vary, so do the reporting requirements involving codes.

The listing of procedures or services and their codes by subsections does not restrict use of these codes to certain specialty groups. For example, when describing a service that has been rendered, a surgeon may use codes from any section, not just those from the surgery section. Similarly, a family practice physician may use a code from the surgery section to describe office procedures or maternity care.

Each main section in the CPT code book is divided into subsections, subcategories, headings, and procedures/services, as follows:

Surgery	Section
Integumentary system	Subsection
Skin, subcutaneous, and accessory structures	Subcategory
Incision and drainage	Heading
Incision and drainage of pilonidal cyst, simple	Procedure

The subsections, subcategories, and headings may identify any of the following:

- Services
- Procedures or therapies
- Examinations or tests
- Body systems
- Anatomic sites

Figure 2.1 provides an example of the hierarchy for CPT code 47100 Biopsy of liver (wedge).

Figure 2.1. Organization of CPT digestive system

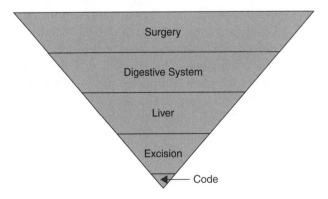

Exercise 2.1 Organization of CPT

Answers to odd-numbered questions can be found in appendix C of this book. The answers to even-numbered questions are located in the instructor materials and are available to approved instructors.

Identify the location of the following codes: CPT (Category I), section and subsection, or Category II, or Category III codes.

1. 00918 _____

2. 76604 _____

3. 80155 _____

4. 4013F _____

5. 99221 _____

6. 92986 _____

7. 45388 _____

8. 0511T _____

9. 59000 _____

10. 99218 _____

11. 78012 _____

12. 88307 _____

Conventions and Characteristics of CPT

The CPT code book follows several conventions, including the use of the following symbols:

- Semicolon ;
- Bullet •
- Triangle ▲
- Facing triangles ►◄

- Plus symbol +
- Null symbol ⊘
- Pending symbol ⌁
- Out-of-numerical sequence code #
- Telemedicine ★

CPT 2019 introduced a new symbol exclusive to Proprietary Laboratory Analyses (PLA) codes (after 89398). When more than one PLA test has an identical descriptor, the codes will use this symbol (⧎).

The meanings of these symbols are explained in an introduction section at the beginning of the CPT book.

Semicolons

The format of the CPT code book is designed to provide descriptions of procedures that can stand alone without additional explanation. To conserve space, many descriptions refer to a common portion of the procedure listed in a preceding entry rather than repeating the procedure in its entirety. When this occurs, the incomplete procedural description or descriptions are indented under the main entry, and the common portion of the main entry is followed by a semicolon (;). This signifies that the main entry applies to, and is part of, all indented entries that follow with their codes. The indented entries can yield different kinds of information, as illustrated in the following examples:

- The indented information may provide diagnostic data.

49520	Repair recurrent inguinal hernia, any age; reducible
49521	incarcerated or strangulated

The common portion of the description for code 49520 (the part before the semicolon) should be considered part of code 49521. Therefore, the full description of code 49521 reads: Repair recurrent inguinal hernia, any age; incarcerated or strangulated.

- The indented entries may describe alternate anatomical sites.

27705	Osteotomy; tibia
27707	fibula
27709	tibia and fibula
27712	multiple, with realignment on intramedullary rod (for example, Sofield-type procedure)

The full description of code 27707 reads: Osteotomy; fibula.

- The indented entries may designate specific procedures.

44150	Colectomy, total, abdominal, without proctectomy; with ileostomy or ileoproctostomy
44151	with continent ileostomy

The full description of code 44151 reads: Colectomy, total, abdominal, without proctectomy; with continent ileostomy.

Bullets and Triangles

CPT uses bullets (•) and triangles (▲) to identify changes in the current code book. A bullet before a code identifies that code as a new addition, and a triangle before a code identifies a revision to the narrative description accompanying that code. Appendix B of the CPT code book contains a comprehensive list of all revisions, including deletions and additions in code order. The following entry is an example of a new code found in CPT 2019:

> • 10005   Fine needle aspiration biopsy, including ultrasound guidance; first lesion

The next is an example of a code that has been changed in CPT 2019:

> ▲61641   Balloon dilatation of intracranial vasospasm, percutaneous; each additional vessel in same vascular territory (List separately in addition to code for primary procedure)

Facing Triangles

The facing triangles symbol (▶◀) is used to indicate the beginning and ending of new or revised text within the guidelines and instruction notes. The coding professional should carefully review the information identified within facing triangles to ensure correct code assignment. An example of new text found in CPT 2019 can be found beneath code 11107.

> ▶(Report 11107 in conjunction with 11106)◀

Plus Symbols

When a procedure is commonly carried out with another procedure, it may be designated as an add-on code. Therefore, it should not be used alone. CPT identifies add-on codes with plus symbols. For example:

> 11000 Debridement of extensive eczematous or infected skin; up to 10% of body surface
> +11001 each additional 10 percent of body surface, or part thereof (list separately in addition to code for primary procedure)

The plus symbol (+) indicates that 11001 is an add-on code and must be used with code 11000. It may not be reported alone. Notes reinforce the correct use of add-on codes. For example, after code 11001, the following instructional note appears:
(Use 11001 in conjunction with code 11000)
Appendix D of CPT 2019 contains a complete list of add-on codes.

Null Symbol

The null symbol (⊘) indicates codes that may not be appended with modifier 51, Multiple Procedures. Modifier 51 is used to inform payers that two or more procedures are being reported on the same day. When appended to a CPT code, it communicates to the payer to apply the multiple procedure payment formula.

For example, code 17004, Destruction (such as, laser surgery, electrosurgery, cryosurgery, chemosurgery, surgical curettement), premalignant lesions (such as, actinic keratoses), 15 or more lesions may not be used with modifier 51. Appendix E of CPT 2019 provides a complete list of codes that are exempt from the use of modifier 51 (for a more detailed discussion of modifiers, see chapter 3).

Pending Symbol

The pending symbol (𝑵) indicates that the CPT code is for a vaccine that is pending approval from the Food and Drug Administration (FDA). For example:

> 𝑵 90666   Influenza virus vaccine, pandemic formulation, split virus, preservation free, for intramuscular use

Appendix K of CPT 2019 contains a list of codes identifying products that are pending FDA approval.

Resequenced Symbol

The resequenced symbol (#) emphasizes that the CPT codes do not appear in numeric sequence. Resequencing codes allow for CPT codes to be relocated without unnecessarily deleting codes. Appendix N of the CPT code book provides a list of codes that are out of numerical sequence. Note that code 46320 (Excision of thrombosed hemorrhoid, external) was relocated to the hemorrhoidectomy section after code 46230).

Telemedicine

A star before a CPT code (★) indicates that the services may be reported for synchronous telemedicine services.

Category I, II, and III Codes

The AMA continues to focus on enhancing the functionality of CPT nomenclature. As part of this initiative, CPT has been expanded to include the needs of data reporting and data collection without significantly changing the current structure and payment focus of CPT. As a result, three categories of CPT codes have been established.

Category I Codes (CPT)

Category I codes include the traditional, five-digit numeric codes that identify procedures and services. Code 11104 Punch biopsy of skin (including simple closure, when performed); single lesion—is an example of a Category I CPT code.

Exercise 2.2   CPT Conventions

Answers to odd-numbered questions can be found in appendix C of this book. The answers to even-numbered questions are located in the instructor materials and are available to approved instructors.

Review each of the following questions and write the appropriate answers in the spaces provided.

1. Can code 15003 be used alone?

2. The reporting of CPT codes 28150 and 28150 indicates the removal of how many toes?

3. Is code 33275 identified as a code with a new descriptor or a revised descriptor?

4. What is the full description for code 53215?

5. Is code 77022 identified as a code with a new descriptor or a revised descriptor?

6. What is the full description of code 35535?

7. Can code 31500 be appended with modifier 51?

8. Review the range of CPT codes 42820 through 42836. What is the correct code assignment for a 4-year-old who had a tonsillectomy and adenoidectomy?

9. Review the range of CPT codes 40810 through 40816. What is the correct code assignment for an excision of a mucosal lesion of the vestibule of the mouth with a complex repair?

10. Review the range of CPT codes 13100 through 13102. What is the correct code assignment for a 7.7 cm complex wound repair of the chest?

Category II Codes

Category II codes include alphanumeric codes that are used for tracking purposes to represent performance measurements. Use of these codes enables organizations to monitor internal performance for key measures throughout the year. Category II codes are located in a section after the Medicine codes in the CPT code book. The use of tracking codes for performance measurement facilitates data collection and minimizes administrative burden. The five-digit alphanumeric codes can be identified by adding the letter *F* at the end of the code. Code 4000F—Tobacco use cessation intervention, counseling—is an example of a Category II code.

The use of Category II codes is optional. The tracking codes are reviewed as part of healthcare quality tracking by the AMA, the Joint Commission, and the National Committee for Quality Assurance (NCQA), among others. Appendix H—Alphabetical Clinical Topics Listing of the code book has been relocated to the AMA website.

Category III Codes

Category III codes are temporary codes used to represent emerging technology services and procedures. These codes were developed to allow researchers to track the use of emerging technology services. Data collection of Category III codes can assist with the following:

- Clinical efficacy
- Utilization
- Outcomes
- Avoid the use of unlisted CPT codes

The codes are included in a section of the code book that falls after the Category II codes and the Medicine section.

> Note that all of the Category III code descriptions have a "sunset date" by which a decision should be made to make the code a Category I (CPT) or not.

Category III codes are assigned an alphanumeric identifier (for example, 0071T). After they have been approved by the CPT Editorial Panel, new Category III codes are added on a semiannual (twice-yearly) basis and made available through the AMA website. Category III codes are archived when they have not been moved to the Category I section after five years unless it can be demonstrated that the codes are still useful. For example, 0388T (Transcatheter removal of permanent leadless pacemaker, ventricular) appeared in the 2018 edition of CPT, but the procedure was assigned code 33275 in 2019. Therefore, 0388T was deleted from the list of Category III codes. Payment for Category III services and procedures depends on the reimbursement policies of individual payers.

Unlisted Procedures

> Laparoscopic total pancreatectomy would be assigned 48999 for unlisted. There is an open approach (48155), but it is not laparoscopic.

Because of rapid advances in medical research and technology, new services or procedures may be performed before codes have been added to the CPT system to represent them. In these rare instances, an unlisted code should be reported along with a written report describing the procedure or service. The operative report is usually sufficient when reporting an unlisted surgical code. The introduction to each section of the CPT code book includes a complete list of the unlisted service or procedure codes available for that section. Unlisted codes for various subsections can be found in the alphabetic index of the CPT code book under the main heading Unlisted Services and Procedures. Before any unlisted code is assigned, the coding professional should review HCPCS

Level II (National) codes to confirm that CMS has not developed a specific code for the procedure or service in question. CPT Category III codes, which are developed specifically for reporting new technology, should also be reviewed. CPT guidelines support the use of a Category III code instead of a Category I unlisted code.

Appendixes

The following is a summary of two of the most commonly referenced appendixes located after the Category III codes in CPT. New coding professionals should peruse the appendixes for content.

Appendix A—Modifiers

Appendix A provides a complete list of modifiers for use with CPT Level I and HCPCS Level II (National) codes. Chapter 3 of this book will highlight the use of modifiers.

Appendix B—Summary of Additions, Deletions, and Revisions

Every year, CPT undergoes a revision process. The summary of this work is provided in Appendix B.

Notes

Coding professionals using the CPT code book should pay special attention to the notes located at various levels within the text. The instructional notes guide the selection and use of CPT codes. Although computer software programs help with editing and inappropriate use of codes, coding professionals should read and apply the notes that appear within the book. Notes may appear at the beginning of a heading, within parentheses before or after a code, or within parentheses in the code description.

Notes placed at the beginning of a heading provide additional information about the services or procedures that follow. For example:

- Integral components of a service or procedure

Example:

A note under the heading Endoscopy before code 31231 states that a surgical sinus endoscopy always includes a sinusotomy (when appropriate) and a diagnostic endoscopy.

- Definitions of terms and codes

Example:

Under the heading Shaving of Epidermal or Dermal Lesions before code 11300 a note defines shaving as "the sharp removal by transverse incision or horizontal slicing to remove epidermal and dermal lesions without a full-thickness dermal excision." This includes local anesthesia, chemical or electrocauterization of the wound. The wound does not require suture closure.

- Directions to assign additional codes

Reading the notes and carefully highlighting key points is important. For example, in CPT 2019 there is a detailed note before code 11102 that helps to differentiate between the biopsy procedure codes.

Example:

Under the heading Coronary Artery Bypass–Combined Arterial-Venous Grafting before code 33517 the note reminds the coding professional that two codes are required to identify coronary artery bypass grafting using both arterial and venous grafts.

Notes that appear before or after individual codes provide additional coding guidelines. For example:

- Alternative codes

Example:

The note appearing after code 11772 directs the coding professional to see 10080 or 10081 for an incision of a pilonidal cyst.

- Deleted codes

Example:

The note appearing after code 0345T advises the coding professional that code0346T has been deleted and to see 76981, 76982, 78983.

- Add-on codes

Example:

The note appearing after code 19001 instructs the coding professional not to assign code 19001 as a single code. It must be used with code 19000.

- Other instructional information

Example:

The note appearing after code 64611 instructs the coding professional to use modifier 52 if fewer than four salivary glands are injected.

Notes also appear within the text of some codes to provide additional explanation.

Example:

Within code 10040, the coding professional is provided with the examples such as removal of multiple milia.

Coding Tips

The Professional Edition of CPT 2019 includes "Coding Tips" to provide guidance in appropriate code selection. For example, preceding code 11000 is the following tip:

Coding Tip

Use of Depth and Surface Area for Reporting Debridement of Wounds

When performing debridement of a single wound, report depth using the deepest level of tissue removed. In multiple wounds, sum the surface area of those wounds that are at the same depth, but do not combine sums from different depths.

Alphabetic Index

At the back of the CPT code book, an index provides a list of specific codes organized by main entries such as:

Replantation
Report Preparation
Reposition
Repositioning
Reproductive tissue
Reprogramming
Resection

The main entries are printed in boldface type and arranged in alphabetic order. The main entries are based on:

- Procedures, services, or examinations such as coccygectomy, mastopexy, preventive medicine, physical therapy, nuclear medicine, and organ or disease-oriented panel

- Organs or other anatomic sites such as bladder, blood vessels, ethmoid, ganglion, muscle, and sweat glands

- Conditions or diagnoses such as abrasion, hematoma, heel spur, meningioma, mumps, omphalocele, and septal defect

- Synonyms, eponyms, or abbreviations such as Ewart procedure, FAST, LHR, Pereyra procedure, Pomeroy's operation, TLC screen, and HLA typing

- Some of the main entries include subterms that provide additional information that must be reviewed before a code can be selected. For example, note the excerpt below:

Laryngoscopy	
Direct	31515–31571
Aspiration	31515
Biopsy	31535, 31536
Diagnostic	31525, 31526

The CPT alphabetic index also uses cross-references to help coding professionals identify the most appropriate code. *See* cross-references appear most frequently with eponyms, synonyms, and abbreviations and refer coding professionals to other main terms. For example, the entry for AHG includes a cross-reference that refers the coding professional to the main entry for clotting factor.

See cross-references can also direct the coding professional to another main term, but only when the information sought did not follow the first main term. For example:

Sweat Test	82435
See Chloride, Blood	

These examples illustrate the importance of referring to the additional main entries as directed by the cross-references to ensure the highest level of specificity in code selection.

> The surgeon may not describe the procedure in the exact term to look up in the Alphabetic Index. Coding professionals will find themselves needing to use alternative terms. It is always best to research a procedure that is unfamiliar.

The alphabetic index offers at least one code under each entry, although in some cases more than one code or a range of codes is provided. Every code and its description must be reviewed carefully to ensure accurate code assignment and appropriate payment.

Consider the following example:

Mastectomy	
Gynecomastia	19300
Modified Radica	119307
Partial	19301, 19302
Radical	19303–19306
Simple, Complete	19303
Subcutaneous	19304
with Axillary Lymphadenectomy	19302

When coding a partial mastectomy, the coding professional must review the descriptions for both 19301 and 19302 before assigning a final code.

Use of the Alphabetic Index

The first step in locating a code in the alphabetic index is to find the procedure or service performed, such as jejunostomy or peritoneocentesis. If the service or procedure is not listed, the coding professional should locate the organ or anatomic site involved; the condition or diagnosis; or the synonym or eponym, such as phalanx, Epstein-Barr virus, or Dandy operation. The subterms should be reviewed and any cross-references followed. Each code listed in the index should be noted and each description reviewed until a match is established.

Becoming familiar with the CPT code book will expedite the coding process. For example, a comprehensive knowledge of the code book would show that correct codes often are found under several main terms.

Consider a breast biopsy procedure. A review of the Alphabetic Index will reveal entries under *Biopsy, breast*, as well as under the main term *Breast, biopsy*.

A Word of Caution

Experienced coders may use the index to locate the general section for a list of potential codes.

However, coding professionals should not rely solely on the Alphabetic Index for assigning the correct CPT code. If you cannot locate an Alphabetic Index entry, it does not mean there is not a correct CPT code. In some circumstances, the Alphabetic Index can be misleading; therefore, the final decision is based on the CPT code description. For example, if the operative report documentation describes a surgical debridement of necrotized fasciitis of the abdominal wall (no mention of mesh), note the following entry from the Alphabetic Index:

Debridement
Skin
Subcutaneous Tissue
Necrotized 49568

Verifying the code description for 49568 reveals "Implantation of mesh or other prosthesis for open incisional or ventral hernia repair or mesh for closure of debridement for necrotizing soft tissue infection." This code is obviously incorrect; the correct CPT code is 11005.

Appendix C of this textbook provides answers to the odd-numbered questions along with *one* Index pathway, not all possible index entries. New coders should be aware that this coding pathway helps to discover the organization of CPT. It does not imply that using the Alphabetic Index is the only method for locating a correct code.

CPT Translation

The physician documented the following procedure: closure of vesicostomy. There is no entry in the CPT Index under Closure, vesicostomy.

Problem Solving: Research the procedure. What is a vesicostomy? What are alternative medical terms to describe this procedure?

Answer: Vesicostomy is a surgical opening in the bladder to outside the body. Cysto- is a medical term for bladder. Search in the Index under Closure, Cystostomy for code 51880.

Tips for Locating Codes When Alphabetic Index Is Not Helpful

- Research the procedure and alternative medical terms (do not code what you do not understand).
- Go to the general CPT anatomic/procedure section and pursue the coding
- descriptions.
- Research *CPT Assistant (more about CPT Assistant at the end of this chapter)*.
- Reference websites of professional associations. For example, the American Urological Association has articles and a coding question and answer section.

General Rules for CPT Coding

Here are some general rules to consider when applying CPT codes:

- Analyze the note or procedural statement provided by the physician or other healthcare provider, and/or included in the health record.
- Translate the physician's documentation to determine the procedure, test, or service to be coded.
- For guidance, locate the main term in the index by checking under the procedure, anatomic site, condition, synonym, eponym, service, or abbreviation as necessary.
- Review and select the subterms indented below the main term.
- Note the code number(s) found opposite the selected main term or subterm:
  - If a single code number is provided, locate the code in the body of the CPT code book. Verify the code and its description against the procedural statement to make sure they match.
  - If two or more codes separated by a comma are shown, locate each code in the body of the CPT code book. Read the description of each code before selecting the appropriate one to match the procedural statement.

- If a range of codes is shown, locate that range in the body of the CPT code book. Review the description of each entry before selecting a code. The code description should always match the procedural statement.
- If applicable, follow cross-references.
- **Never code directly from the index.**
- Read all notes that apply to the code selected. They can appear at the beginning of a section or subsection, directly under, or within the code description.
- Select the appropriate modifier, when applicable, to complete the code description. Modifiers may not always apply to hospital reporting of outpatient hospital procedures. Individual health plans may have specific guidelines for the use of modifiers and for the acceptance of Level II modifiers. For accurate reporting, the coding professional must be familiar with the specific reporting requirements for the circumstances.
- Continue coding all components of the procedure or service according to the directions in the CPT code book.

Exercise 2.3   Use of the Alphabetical Index

Answers to odd-numbered questions can be found in appendix C of this book. The answers to even-numbered questions are located in the instructor materials and are available to approved instructors.

Assign the appropriate CPT codes and provide the corresponding index entries for the following terms. In some cases, the CPT code may be found under different indexing terms.

1. Green operation

   Code: _____

   Index entry: _____

2. Repair of recurrent, incarcerated femoral hernia

   Code: _____

   Index entry: _____

3. Femoropopliteal bypass graft with the use of transplanted saphenous vein

   Code: _____

   Index entry: _____

4. Laparoscopic cholecystectomy with exploration of common bile duct

   Code: _____

   Index entry: _____

5. Incision and drainage of infected bursa of the hip

Code: _____

Index entry: _____

6. Anesthesia provided for repair of a ruptured Achilles tendon (assign only the code for the anesthesia services)

Code: _____

Index entry: _____

7. Direct diagnostic laryngoscopy with use of an operating microscope for 45-year-old patient

Code: _____

Index entry: _____

8. Intraoperative EEG performed during carotid endarterectomy procedure (*code only EEG*)

Code: _____

Index entry: _____

9. Paring of a single corn of the foot

Code: _____

Index entry: _____

10. Aspiration of excess fluid from the bursa of the elbow with ultrasound guidance (includes recording and reporting)

Code: _____

Index entry: _____

11. Biopsy of posterior third of tongue

Code: _____

Index entry: _____

12. Lysis of adhesions of prepuce, post-circumcision

Code: _____

Index entry: _____

13. Arthroscopic medial meniscectomy

Code: _____

Index entry: _____

14. Diagnostic MRI of the pelvis with contrast material

Code: _____

Index entry: _____

15. Removal of metal shaving from cornea with use of slit lamp

    Code: _____

    Index entry: _____

16. Endometrial cryoablation with ultrasound guidance

    Code: _____

    Index entry: _____

17. Beta-blocker therapy prescribed for hypertension

    Code: _____

    Index entry: _____

18. Excision of rectal tumor, TEMS (transanal endoscopic microsurgery) approach

    Code: _____

    Index entry: _____

19. Amniocentesis for fluid reduction

    Code: _____

    Index entry:

20. Surgical debridement through the fascia of the perineum due to Fournier's gangrene

    Code: _____

    Index entry: _____

Abstracting Documentation

This book provides two types of exercises: one-line procedure coding and operative narratives. The one-line procedures offer students the opportunity to use the index to locate the coding selection and apply the guidelines introduced in the chapter. Coding from operative notes found in office records, operative reports, and emergency department notes allows students to practice the skill of abstracting needed information to assign a code successfully. When reviewing the documentation in an operative report, students are encouraged to scan the report for procedures performed (action types of words: excision, incision, aspiration, endoscopy, and so forth) and associated diagnoses.

For example, note the contents of an operative report below with the highlighted action words.

Operative Report

Preoperative Diagnosis: Bladder tumor ⟶ | Reason for procedure |

Postoperative Diagnosis: Bladder tumor

Operation: Transurethral resection of a 3-cm bladder tumor ⟶ | Procedure performed |

Anesthesia: General

Specimens: Sessile bladder tumor and tumor base ⟶ | Tissue sent to laboratory |

Findings: A 3-cm high-grade appearing tumor, thought to be transitional cell carcinoma, right posterior bladder wall.

| Describes the beginning of the operative session— preparing the patient for the procedure. |

Indication: A 62-year-old patient with hematuria with bladder tumor identified on CT of the pelvis.

Description of procedure: The patient was brought to the operating room. General anesthesia was induced. The patient was placed in lithotomy and genitalia was prepped and draped in the usual manner. The patient was identified and the procedure was confirmed. Resectoscope passed. ⟶ | This is the operative approach | Tumor visualized, right posterior bladder wall, approximately 3 cm in greatest dimension. It is very sessile in nature, quite red and angry-appearing. There were some papillary areas. Overall the tumor had a very high-grade appearance to it. It was near, but did not involve the right ureteral orifice.

| Action word: resected |

| Action word: biopsies |

| The end of the operative report describes the closure of the operative session. |

The tumor was resected and the biopsy specimen sent for permanent section.

Separate biopsies were taken of the tumor base to rule out deep muscle invasion. The area was thoroughly cauterised with loop electrode. No bleeding was seen with the bladder decompressed. No other abnormalities were noted. Scope removed. The patient tolerated the procedure well.

After looking in the index and, subsequently, in the main body portion of the CPT code book to locate coding selections, it will be necessary to note the types of information that may influence the choice of codes and then to read the operative report again for information that will help determine the correct answer.

Exercise 2.4 CPT Coding Process

Answers to odd-numbered questions can be found in appendix C of this book. The answers to even-numbered questions are located in the instructor materials and are available to approved instructors.

Operative Report #1

Operative Report

Preoperative Diagnosis:	History of colon cancer ⟶ Reason for encounter
Postoperative Diagnosis:	Rectosigmoid polyp
Procedure:	Colonoscopy and polypectomy ⟶ Procedure performed
Indications:	The patient has had three previous resections of three different primary carcinomas of the colon. His last resection of carcinoma was in 2000. He has been doing well in general.
Premedications:	Demerol 50 mg IV and Versed 2.5 mg IV
Procedure:	The CF100-L video flexible colonoscope was passed without difficulty from the anus up through the anastomosis, which appears to be in the distal transverse colon. The instrument was advanced into the distal small bowel and then slowly withdrawn with good view obtained throughout. A small, 3-mm polyp near the rectosigmoid junction was removed with hot biopsy forceps and retrieved. Otherwise, the patient has a satisfactory postoperative appearance of the colon. It is shortened due to previous resections, but there is no other evidence of neoplasm. The instrument was completely withdrawn without other findings.

Read the preceding operative report. Then perform the steps in the coding process as listed below. Show your results in the spaces provided.

1. Scan the documentation to identify the procedure performed.

   _____

2. Search the index for Colonoscopy, Flexible, Removal, Polyp, and identify the code selection for the procedure.

   _____

3. Review the coding descriptions to determine what additional documentation is needed before you can accurately select a code.

   _____

4. Read the operative report again to determine the method of removal used.

   _____

5. Choose the code that reflects this documentation.

   _____

Operative Report #2

Operative Report

Preoperative
Diagnosis:
Subepidermal nodular lesion of the forearm Reason for
encounter

Operation: Excision of 2.0-cm lesion of the forearm

Procedure: Under local anesthesia, the 2.0-cm lesion was removed with
0.5-cm margins. The lesion was submitted to pathology.
Bleeding was controlled with electrocautery, and the wound
was closed with five vertical mattress sutures of 5-0 nylon.
Polysporin and dressing were applied to the wound.

Pathological
Diagnosis:
Well-organized basal cell carcinoma

Review the preceding operative report and note the pathological diagnosis.
Then perform the steps in the coding process as listed below. Record your results
in the spaces provided.

(Hint: Be sure to abstract the following information from the operative report:
size of lesion and margins; morphology, benign or malignant; location; and
method of removal.)

1. Scan the documentation and record the main procedure to be located in
   the alphabetic index.

   _____

2. Search the index for the main terms/subterms and record the code
   selections. What documentation is needed before a code selection is
   determined?

   _____

3. Review the code descriptions to determine what additional
   documentation is needed before you can accurately select a code.
   Coding guidance (listed before code 11400 of the *Professional Edition
   of CPT*, or published in *CPT Assistant*), states that the code selection
   is determined by measuring the greatest clinical diameter of the
   apparent lesion plus that margin required for complete excision
   (lesion diameter plus the most narrow margins required equals the
   excised diameter).

   _____

4. Read the operative report and pathological diagnosis again to determine
   the additional documentation to clarify the selection. Was the lesion
   benign or malignant?

   _____

5. Choose the code that reflects this documentation.

   _____

Operative Report #3

Operative Report

Preoperative Diagnosis: Umbilical hernia

Postoperative Diagnosis: Same

This is a 38-year-old man who presents with an umbilical hernia. He has been experiencing influenza-like symptoms, which he describes as crampy abdominal pain. Risks versus benefits including bleeding, infection, and the high recurrence rate because of his obesity were discussed. The patient states he understands and elects to proceed with surgery.

After adequate general endotracheal anesthesia had been induced, the patient was placed in the supine position, and prepped and draped in the usual sterile manner. A curvilinear incision was made just inferior to the umbilicus. This was extended down through adipose tissue to the level of the rectus fascia. The herniosac was amputated and sent to pathology. The fascia was then reapproximated transversely using interrupted 0 prolene sutures. The skin was reapproximated using 4-0 nylon. Sponge and needle counts were accurate. The patient tolerated the procedure well and left the operating room in stable condition.

Review the preceding operative report and abstract the information that is needed for a correct code assignment. Answer the following questions in the spaces provided.

1. What procedure was performed?

   _____

2. What code selections were listed in the index entry for the main terms describing the procedure?

   _____

3. What additional documentation is needed before an accurate code can be assigned?

   _____

4. What is the correct code for the procedure?

   _____

5. Should a CPT code also be assigned for the suturing of the wound at the conclusion of the procedure?

   _____

Identification of Operative Procedures for Coding

New coding professionals often have difficulty determining whether a procedure is an integral part of the main operative procedure or a separately identifiable procedure. For example, when a patient has a breast mass removed, a code for the wound closure would not be assigned because it is an integral part of the main procedure. The ability to discriminate between reportable and nonreportable procedures is a skill that must be developed and one that significantly affects accurate code selection. Coding professionals need to have surgical references and build a list of web resources to help them understand procedures and techniques. Some websites contain visual clips of how surgical procedures are performed. In addition to understanding surgical techniques, coding professionals must know when to assign additional codes and will find instructions on doing so in the CPT guidelines. Various types of notes and descriptions located throughout CPT guidelines are illustrated below.

Many CPT codes combine the main procedure with minor procedures that do not warrant additional codes. In these cases, the code description contains a note specifying the secondary procedures that are to be included in the primary code. In the example below, if the surgeon performs a transurethral electrosurgical resection of prostate (TURP) with vasectomy, the correct code assignment is 52601. Because the code description states that vasectomy is included in the code for the TURP procedure, the vasectomy is not assigned a separate code.

52601   Transurethral electrosurgical resection of prostate, including control of postoperative bleeding, complete (Vasectomy, meatotomy, cystourethroscopy, urethral calibration and/or dilation, and internal urethrotomy are included)

If the surgeon performs a total abdominal hysterectomy with salpingo-oophorectomy, the only code submitted would be 58150. The code description explains that no additional code would be submitted for the salpingo-oophorectomy.

58150   Total abdominal hysterectomy (corpus and cervix), with or without removal of tube(s), with or without removal of ovary(ies)

Some notes in the CPT code book offer guidance on multiple code assignment for an entire section. For example, look at the note before code 14000 in the Adjacent Tissue Transfer or Rearrangement portion of the integumentary system subsection of the surgery section. The second paragraph includes the following clause: "Excision (including lesion) and/or repair by adjacent tissue transfer or rearrangement." According to this note, when a surgeon removes a skin lesion and the defect is repaired with an adjacent tissue transfer, only the tissue transfer should be coded. The excision of lesion is not identified with an additional code.

Some notes provide instructions for use of add-on codes. For example, code 69990, Operating microscope, is reported only as an additional code. In some procedures, physicians utilize an operating microscope during the surgical episode. CPT provides specific instructions in the note before code 69990 to help the coding professional determine whether this add-on code is to be used with a particular primary procedure code.

Instruction is often given in the form of a note under a specific code, for example, the note under CPT code 63078 that instructs the coding professional not to report code 69990 in addition to codes 63075 through 63078.

Coding References

Both the American Medical Association (AMA) and the Centers for Medicare and Medicaid Services (CMS) are resources for CPT coding guidelines.

American Medical Association

The AMA is the primary, authoritative reference for CPT guidelines and changes. The AMA publishes *CPT Assistant*, a monthly newsletter that provides information on the correct application of CPT codes. The newsletter includes a question-and-answer section that provides answers to coding professionals' questions. The AMA also offers a subscription service for assistance with coding questions. Most large healthcare facilities subscribe to an online version of *CPT Assistant*.

CPT Changes: An Insider's View

The AMA publishes a book that reviews the yearly changes to CPT. This is not included in the standard *CPT Assistant* subscription and must be purchased separately.

CPT QuickRef App

The AMA has also released a mobile application that provides resources and access to *CPT Assistant*. The *CPT QuickRef* app allows users to quickly reference *CPT Assistant* topics that are noted beneath the CPT codes in the book format.

Example:

> 50234 Nephrectomy with total ureterectomy and bladder cuff; through same incision
> ➔ *CPT Assistant* Oct 01:8, Nov 02:3

Through the *CPT Assistant* subscription service or the *CPT QuickRef* app, you can locate two editions of *CPT Assistant* that have been written about this code (50234): October 2001 (page 8) and November 2002 (page 3).

Exercises 2.5, 2.6, and 2.7 require access to *CPT Assistant*. For these exercises, provide an answer and document the *CPT Assistant* edition that helped answer the coding question.

Exercise 2.5   *CPT Assistant* Coding Reference

Answers to odd-numbered questions can be found in appendix C of this book. The answers to even-numbered questions are located in the instructor materials and are available to approved instructors.

Exercise 2.4, Operative Report #1, asked you to analyze documentation and assign the correct code for a colonoscopy with a polypectomy procedure. For correct CPT assignment, you needed to know what method was used to remove the polyp. In the operative report for that exercise, the surgeon used hot biopsy forceps. For this exercise, assume that a surgeon removed the tiny polyp by using a cold biopsy forceps. The polyp was so small that it was completely removed during the biopsy.

1. What volume of *CPT Assistant* provides the information needed to arrive at this code assignment?

_____

2. What is the correct coding assignment for this procedure?

_____

Exercise 2.6 *CPT Assistant* Coding Reference

Answers to odd-numbered questions can be found in appendix C of this book. The answers to even-numbered questions are located in the instructor materials and are available to approved instructors.

In Exercise 2.4, 0perative Report #2, the surgeon excised a lesion of the forearm. Suppose that the surgeon took a biopsy of the lesion before removing it. (The following exercise requires reference to *CPT Assistant*.)

1. Should both the biopsy and the excision be coded or just the excision?

   _____

2. Which volume of *CPT Assistant* provided the information needed to answer this question?

   _____

Exercise 2.7 Coding References: *CPT QuickRef* App

Answers to odd-numbered questions can be found in appendix C of this book. The answers to even-numbered questions are located in the instructor materials and are available to approved instructors. For *CPT QuickRef* app users, the specific pathway is provided to answer the questions below. From the Dashboard, select *CPT Assistant*.

1. April 2016, Surgery: Integumentary (page 8). Does CPT code 42950 Pharyngoplasty include a free flap that was used to reconstruct both the neck and tongue defect?

   _____

2. July 2016, Surgery: Digestive System (page 8). The operative report stated that a very low level of electric current and infrared coagulation treatment was used to treat the internal hemorrhoids. Is 46930 the correct code?

   _____

3. November 2016, Surgery: Musculoskeletal System (page 9). Is code 27236, Open treatment of femoral fracture, proximal neck, internal fixation or prosthetic replacement the appropriate code to report the repair of a trochanteric fracture when the patient has an osteoporotic comminuted femoral neck fracture due to the fragility of the osteoporotic bone?

   _____

4. February 2016, Surgery: Nervous System (page 13). What is the appropriate code to report the placement of the Neuro-Stim System™ Electro-Auricular Device™ for pain management?

   _____

(Continued on next page)

Exercise 2.7   (Continued)

5. December 2016, Frequently Asked Questions (page 16). What CPT code is used to report a breast biopsy, when the only guidance used is tomographic guidance?

_____

6. February 2015, Surgery: Musculoskeletal System (page 10). Does code 23412 (Repair of ruptured musculotendinous cuff) include a partial acromioplasty or acromionectomy with or without coracoacromial ligament release?

_____

7. September 2015, Surgery: Digestive System (page 12). Which code is appropriate (45330 or 45378) when the physician is unable to advance the colonoscopy to the cecum?

_____

For the following questions, search the *CPT QuickRef* app by code number (enter the code number in the search box), click the code number and then click the green arrow for CPT Assistant.

8. Enter CPT code 11401 in the search box, click *CPT Assistant*, then choose Surgery: Integumentary System. What is the appropriate code to report for excision of epidermal or pilar cyst?

_____

9. Enter CPT code 12031 in the search box, *click CPT Assistant*, then choose the first entry for Surgery/Integumentary System. If the physician closed a laceration that extended into the subcutaneous tissue, would this be reported as simple or intermediate?

_____

10. Enter CPT code 20100 in the search box, click *CPT Assistant* and then choose the first entry for Surgery: Musculoskeletal System. Is removal of foreign body(s) included in the Wound Exploration codes?

_____

Exercise 2.8   *CPT® QuickRef App* Coding Vignettes

This exercise highlights a feature in the *CPT QuickRef* app called Vignettes. The vignettes provide clinical examples of a typical case that would be assigned to the selected code. All of the answers are provided in appendix C of this book. For each code below, provide a description of a clinical procedure that would be assigned according to the vignette. Search the CPT code number, then select the Vignettes tab on the app.

1. What vignette describes use of code 11400 (Excision, benign lesion)?

_____

2. What vignette describes use of code 10120 (incision and removal of foreign body, subcutaneous tissues; simple)?

_____

3. What vignette describes use of code 20550 (Injection, single tendon sheath, or ligament, aponeurosis?

_____

4. What vignette describes use of code 49084 (Peritoneal lavage, including imaging guidance, when performed)?

_____

5. What vignette describes use of code 64910 (Nerve repair, with synthetic conduit or vein allograft, each nerve)?

_____

Centers for Medicare and Medicaid Services (CMS)

The federal government provides some interpretative guidance on the use of CPT codes and modifiers as an element of HCPCS. The HCPCS guidelines are published in the form of transmittals, manuals, and other documents. For example, CMS publishes the National Correct Coding Initiative (NCCI) Policy Manual for Medicare Services, which includes coding and billing guidance. NCCI is introduced in chapter 3 of this textbook. Most of the Medicare and Medicaid manuals are available for downloading from the CMS website.

> Although CMS regulates Medicare and Medicaid, other payers often follow their lead on general policies.

American Hospital Association

The American Hospital Association publishes _Coding Clinic for HCPCS_, a subscription service that focuses on CPT coding and HCPCS Level II (National) codes. However, because this is not an official coding reference published by the AMA, the notations within the CPT code book do not highlight this publication.

Chapter 2 Review

Answers to odd-numbered questions can be found in appendix C of this book. The answers to even-numbered questions are located in the instructor materials and are available to approved instructors.

Answer the following questions in the spaces provided.

1. Which symbol indicates that a procedure code is new in CPT?

_____

2. The surgeon documents surgical removal of metatarsophalangeal joint. Translate the procedure description in order to assign the correct CPT code.

_____

(Continued on next page)

Chapter 2 Review   (Continued)

3. Which category of CPT codes is reserved for emerging technology?

_____

4. Refer to CPT codes 11730 and 11732. Assume that a physician performed a complete avulsion of the nail plate of the thumb and index finger. What would be the correct code assignment?

_____

5. Refer to CPT codes 40840 through 40844. Assume that a surgeon performed a unilateral, posterior vestibuloplasty. Which code should be assigned?

_____

6. Refer to CPT code 56630. What documentation in the operative report would be needed to support the use of this code?

_____

7. Refer to CPT code 43275. If the surgeon performed an ERCP and removed two stents for the pancreatic duct, would you list the code twice?

_____

8. Refer to CPT codes 25071 through 25076 (note that the CPT codes are out of sequence). Assume that a surgeon removed a 3.5 cm soft tissue mass from the forearm that extended into the deep fascia. Which code should be assigned?

_____

9. Refer to CPT codes for ERCP beginning with 43260. If the surgeon fully examined the hepatobiliary system without performing any other procedure, what would be the correct code assignment?

_____

10. Refer to CPT codes 15200 and 15201. If the surgeon performed a free skin graft of the back that totaled 45 sq cm, what would be the correct code assignment?

_____

11. Refer to the CPT code range of 21930–21933. If the surgeon excised a 6.0 cm benign soft tumor of the back that extended beyond the subcutaneous layer of skin and invaded the subfascia, what would be the correct code assignment? What would be the correct code assignment if the documentation stated that the tumor was cutaneous in nature (confined to layers of the skin)?

_____

12. The surgeon performed a laparoscopic reconstruction of the ureter. Refer to code 50700. Is this the correct code for the laparoscopic approach? If not, what is the correct coding action?

_____

13. Refer to CPT codes 42310 and 42320. Assume that a surgeon drained an external submaxillary abscess. Which code should be assigned?

_____

Modifiers

3

Learning Objectives

- Describe the uses of modifiers.
- Differentiate between hospital-only and physician-only modifiers.
- Distinguish between CPT and National modifiers.

- Explain the uses of NCCI edits.
- Demonstrate how to use the NCCI file to research codes.
- Given a scenario, correctly identify the applicable modifier that may be appended to a CPT code.

(Please note that for purposes of instruction and for ease in reading, this book uses a dash to separate each five-character Current Procedural Terminology (CPT) code from its two-character modifier. However, dashes are not used in actual code assignments and reimbursement claims, which report seven-character codes with no spaces between the characters when the assignment of modifiers is appropriate.)

Modifiers may be reported along with a CPT code to indicate that a particular event modified the service/procedure, but with no change to its basic definition. Modifiers may indicate any of the following situations:

- A service/procedure has both a professional component and a technical component.
- A service/procedure was performed by more than one physician or in more than one location.
- A service/procedure has been increased or reduced in scope.
- A service was performed only partially.
- An adjunctive service was performed.

- A bilateral procedure was performed.
- A service/procedure was performed more than once.
- An unusual event occurred during the service/procedure.

Example of Modifier:

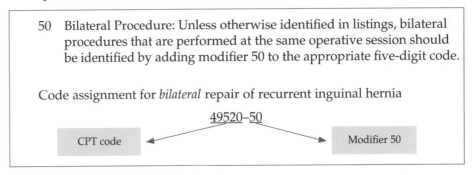

> 50   Bilateral Procedure: Unless otherwise identified in listings, bilateral procedures that are performed at the same operative session should be identified by adding modifier 50 to the appropriate five-digit code.
>
> Code assignment for *bilateral* repair of recurrent inguinal hernia
>
> 49520–50
>
> CPT code   ←   →   Modifier 50

There is a distinct advantage to conveying as much information as possible to the third-party payer to ensure appropriate payment when billing for professional physician services or services provided by an ambulatory surgery or service center. Use of a modifier, in selected cases, allows the healthcare provider to explain special circumstances that surround the charge for the service and may affect claim payment. Use of an appropriate modifier also can prevent a claim from being denied. When using modifiers, it is important to note that an individual third-party payer may have their own policies for reporting modifiers.

Appendix A of the CPT code book includes a complete list of currently accepted modifiers and their descriptions. Coding professionals should examine modifier descriptions carefully for conditions that may limit use of a modifier to a specific section of CPT. For example, modifier 25 is limited by definition to evaluation and management codes and would not be appended to a code from the surgery section. Modifier 78 (Return to Operating Room for a Related Procedure During the Postoperative Period) would only be appended to a CPT surgical code.

Use of Modifiers

Uses of modifiers are often determined by the payer.

The CPT and *Healthcare Common Procedure Coding System* (HCPCS) systems for describing and reporting medical procedures and services include the use of special supplementary codes called modifiers. Modifiers are two-character codes that can be appended to some of the CPT Level I codes and the HCPCS Level II codes to provide additional information.

Different sets of modifiers apply to different services and settings. For example, two-digit numerical modifiers can be appended to CPT codes for reporting additional information relevant to physician and outpatient hospital services. In addition, two-digit alphabetic or alphanumeric modifiers permit more concise reporting of services in Level II (National) HCPCS codes.

Several specific CPT modifiers are required for reporting hospital outpatient services and are designated for hospital use only.

Use of Modifiers for Physician Services

In most cases, modifiers applicable to the codes for physician services are simply appended to the appropriate CPT code, as in the following example:

Example:

> 35840–78   Exploration for postoperative hemorrhage, thrombosis or infection; abdomen
> Postoperatively, a patient is taken to the operative room for exploration of postoperative hemorrhage.

Some third-party payers have special reporting requirements that affect the assignment of modifiers. For example, they may ask that claims for surgical procedures performed bilaterally include the appropriate surgical code twice, with modifier 50 assigned only on the second listing of the code to indicate that the same procedure was performed twice. This practice does not follow the American Medical Association's (AMA) guidelines for reporting bilateral procedures, and the Centers for Medicare and Medicaid Services (CMS) requires a one-line method of reporting bilateral procedures for Medicare claims.

Example:

> 49500
> 49500–50   Required reporting by some payers
> 49500–50   AMA and CMS method of reporting

In addition to the CPT modifiers, HCPCS Level II National Codes include many modifiers for more concise reporting of procedures performed by physicians. A complete list of HCPCS Level II Modifiers can be located on the CMS website. Use the CMS website's search engine to locate HCPCS Release and Code Sets. These two-digit alphanumeric modifiers can be used to identify:

- The specific finger or toe involved (for example, F3 for left hand, fourth digit)
- A visit for a second or third opinion (for example, SM for second opinion)
- A service provided by someone other than a physician (for example, GN for outpatient speech language services)
- Right or left-side involvement (for example, RT for right side)

Modifiers Approved for Hospital Outpatient Use: CPT Level I Modifiers

The following CPT modifiers are available for use by hospitals for outpatient Medicare services. The modifiers should be reported as two digits appended to the appropriate CPT code in field location 44 of the CMS-1450 form (UB-04). (Refer back to figure 1.5).

25   Significant, separately identifiable evaluation and management service by the same physician (or other qualified healthcare professional) on the same day of a procedure or other service

27   Multiple outpatient hospital E/M encounters on the same date

33   Preventive services

50   Bilateral procedure

52   Reduced services

58   Staged or related procedure or service by the same physician during the postoperative period

59   Distinct procedural service

73   Discontinued outpatient procedure prior to the administration of anesthesia

74   Discontinued outpatient procedure after anesthesia administration

76   Repeat procedure or service by same physician or other qualified healthcare professional

77   Repeat procedure or service by another physician or other qualified healthcare professional

78   Unplanned return to operating/procedure room by the same physician or other qualified healthcare professional following initial procedure for a related procedure during the postoperative period

79   Unrelated procedure or service by the same physician during the postoperative period

91   Repeat clinical diagnostic laboratory test

Level II (HCPCS/National) Modifiers

In addition, the following Level II modifiers are acceptable for hospital use:

Anatomic Site Modifiers

LT   Left side (used to identify procedures performed on the left side of the body)

RT   Right side (used to identify procedures performed on the right side of the body)

E1   Upper left, eyelid

E2   Lower left, eyelid

E3   Upper right, eyelid

E4   Lower right, eyelid

FA   Left hand, thumb

F1   Left hand, second digit

F2   Left hand, third digit

F3   Left hand, fourth digit

F4   Left hand, fifth digit

F5   Right hand, thumb

F6   Right hand, second digit

F7   Right hand, third digit

F8   Right hand, fourth digit

F9   Right hand, fifth digit

TA   Left foot, great toe

T1   Left foot, second digit

T2   Left foot, third digit

T3   Left foot, fourth digit

T4   Left foot, fifth digit

T5   Right foot, great toe

T6   Right foot, second digit

T7   Right foot, third digit

T8   Right foot, fourth digit

T9	Right foot, fifth digit
LC	Left circumflex coronary artery
LD	Left anterior descending coronary artery
LM	Left main coronary artery
RC	Right coronary artery
RI	Ramus intermedius coronary artery

Other Modifiers

GG	Performance and payment of a screening mammogram and diagnostic mammogram on the same patient, same day
GH	Diagnostic mammogram converted from screening mammogram on same day
QM	Ambulance service provided under arrangement by a provider of services
QN	Ambulance service furnished directly by a provider of services

Example of use of Level II Modifier:

Surgical procedure: exploratory arthrotomy of left elbow
24000–LT   Arthrotomy, elbow, including exploration, drainage, or removal of foreign body
Level II modifier LT is appended to indicate the procedure was performed on the left

A complete list of CPT modifiers is located in beginning of appendix A in CPT 2019. Appendix A also includes CPT modifiers approved for Ambulatory Surgery Center (ASC) hospital outpatient use. After the hospital-approved CPT modifiers, there is a list of Level II (HCPCS/National) modifiers. A complete list of Level II (HCPCS/National) modifiers can be found on CMS's website. Most healthcare providers maintain an internal list of the most common modifiers used for their specialty. For example, note the following group of modifiers for Anesthesiology services:

HCPCS National Modifiers:

AA	Anesthesia Services Performed Personally by Anesthesiology
AD	Medical Supervision by a Physician: More than Four Concurrent Anesthesia Procedures
G8	Monitored Anesthesia Care (MAC) for Deep Complex, Complicated, or Markedly Invasive Procedure
G9	Monitored Anesthesia Care for Patient Who Has History of Severe Cardio-Pulmonary Condition
QK	Medical Direction of Two, Three, or Four Concurrent Anesthesia Procedures Involving Qualified Individuals
QS	Monitored Anesthesia Care Service
QX	CRNA Service: With Medical Direction by a Physician
QY	Medical Direction of One Certified Registered Nurse Anesthetist (CRNA) by an Anesthesiologist
QZ	CRNA Service: Without Medical Direction by a Physician

Application of modifiers for use with surgical codes is provided in figure 3.1.

Figure 3.1.   Modifiers for use with surgical codes

22   Increased Procedural Services

Modifier 22 is intended only for use by physicians. The modifier is assigned to indicate that the work required was substantially greater than typically required. Carriers may or may not increase the fee as a result. It may be necessary to submit supportive documentation to justify the use of this modifier.

Example:

Because of the patient's extreme obesity, a physician required an additional 30 minutes to perform a cholecystectomy. He should report 47600–22.

47   Anesthesia by Surgeon

Modifier 47, also for physician use only, may be reported to indicate that the surgeon provided regional or general (not local) anesthesia for a surgical procedure. This modifier should not be reported with the anesthesia codes (00100–01999).

Example:

Obstetrician performs emergency cesarean delivery for an out-of-town patient visiting relatives. He also administers a pudendal block (regional anesthesia). Moreover, he will provide postpartum care for the patient until she is able to return home. The physician should report 59515–47 (C-section) and 64430 (Injection of pudendal nerve block).

50   Bilateral Procedure

Modifier 50 may be reported by both physicians and hospitals to identify bilateral procedures that are performed during the same operative episode. However, if the code describes the procedure as bilateral, modifier 50 should not be reported.

Example:

Physician performs a complex anterior packing of both nares for a nosebleed. Both physicians and hospitals providing this service for Medicare patients should report 30903–50.

51   Multiple Procedures

Modifier 51 may be reported to identify that multiple procedures (other than E/M services, physical medicine or rehabilitation services, or provision of supplies) were performed at the same session by the same provider. The procedure listed first should identify the major or most resource-intensive -procedure, which usually is paid at 100 percent of the allowed reimbursement. Subsequent or secondary procedures should be appended by modifier 51, and payment may be reduced according to the terms of the health plan. Policies on payment of multiple procedures vary depending on the payer, so a complete understanding of the individual payer's policies is required to ensure appropriate reimbursement. It is not appropriate to

There is a lack of consistency among payers for use of modifiers. An example is modifier 51; some payers require its use on secondary procedure codes while others do not require the modifier.

Figure 3.1.   Modifiers for use with surgical codes (Continued)

append modifier 51 to CPT codes listed in appendix D of the book. This is a *physician-only* modifier and is not used in the hospital setting.

Example:

Physician performed an excision of a chalazion and a dacryolith from the lacrimal passage. She should report 68530 (Removal of dacryolith) and 67800–51 (Excision of chalazion)

Some procedures in the CPT code book are not intended to stand alone, so they are reported as add-on codes to describe a more extensive procedure. Modifier 51 should not be appended to these codes.

Example:

Percutaneous transluminal pulmonary artery balloon angioplasty is performed on two vessels. The physician should report 92997 and 92998. Modifier 51 should not be reported in this situation because code 92998 is considered an add-on code and thus must be reported with code 92997.

52   Reduced Services

Modifier 52 may be reported by physicians (or other qualified healthcare professional) and hospitals to indicate that a service or procedure is partially reduced in scope or eliminated at the discretion of the physician.

Although this modifier serves the purpose of identifying a reduction in the procedure or service, many physicians also use it to report a reduction in the charge for a particular procedure because the complete procedure was not performed. However, CMS directs hospitals to use modifier 73 instead of 52 when a procedure is partially reduced or eliminated at the physician's election before anesthesia is induced. This would apply when the patient has been prepared and taken to the room for surgery, but the surgery is not carried out due to specified circumstances. Modifier 73 was added to differentiate the definitions between physicians and hospitals for this situation.

Example:

Patient was taken to the operating room (OR) for excisional debridement of a decubitus ulcer (CPT code 11042). However, before anesthesia was administered, the physician was called for emergency surgery of a trauma patient, and the ulcer surgery was postponed until a later date. In this case, the hospital would report the appropriate code for the excisional debridement, along with modifier 73 to indicate that, at the discretion of the physician, the surgery was not performed. The physician would not report a procedure code because no professional services were rendered.

53   Discontinued Procedure

Modifier 53 is appropriate in circumstances where the physician (or other qualified healthcare professional) elects to terminate or discontinue

Note that modifier 51 is appended to the lower-paying CPT code because it will be paid at 50 percent. A physician payment look-up tool is discussed in chapter 12.

(Continued on next page)

Figure 3.1. Modifiers for use with surgical codes (Continued)

a surgical or diagnostic procedure, usually because of a risk to the patient's well-being. However, this modifier should not be used to report the elective cancellation of a procedure prior to the patient's surgical preparation or prior to the induction of anesthesia. Also, the appropriate ICD-10-CM code should be assigned to identify the reason for the procedure's termination or discontinuation. For hospital reporting, the CMS guidelines state that modifier 74, not 53, should be used when a procedure must be discontinued at the physician's election after the induction of anesthesia or after the procedure is underway. Elective cancellation of a procedure by the patient is not reported in this way.

Example:

Patient was admitted for a cystourethroscopy with bladder biopsy. Twenty minutes into the procedure, the patient developed some arrhythmia and the surgery was stopped. The physician should report 52204–53. The hospital should report 52204–74.

54 Surgical Care Only

Modifier 54 may be reported by physicians (or other qualified healthcare professionals) only to indicate that one physician performed the surgical procedure and another provided the preoperative and postoperative care.

Example:

Dr. Reynolds is asked to perform an extracapsular cataract extraction for his partner, Dr. Owens, who is detained out of town. Dr. Owens provided the preoperative care and will provide postoperative care for his patient. Dr. Reynolds should report 66940–54.

55 Postoperative Management Only (*for physician use only*)

Modifier 55 may be reported to identify that the physician (or other qualified healthcare professional) provided only postoperative care services for a particular procedure.

Example:

Patient sustains a fracture of the distal femur while skiing in Colorado. The physician in Colorado performed a closed treatment of the fracture with manipulation. However, the patient's postoperative care will be provided by his hometown physician, Dr. Rogers. Dr. Rogers should report 27510–55.

56 Preoperative Management Only

Modifier 56 may be reported by physicians (or other qualified healthcare professionals) to indicate that the physician provided only preoperative care services for particular procedure.

Example:

Dr. Smith provides preoperative care services for his patient, who will be transferred later the same day to another hospital to undergo a lower lobectomy of the right lung. The physician should report 32480–56.

Figure 3.1. Modifiers for use with surgical codes (Continued)

58 Staged or Related Procedure or Service by the Same Physician (or other qualified healthcare professional) During the Postoperative Period

Both hospitals and physicians (or other qualified healthcare professionals) may report modifier 58 to indicate that a staged or related procedure performed by the same physician is provided during the postoperative period. This procedure may have been planned (staged) prospectively at the time of the original procedure, it may be more extensive than the original procedure, or it may be for therapy following a diagnostic surgical procedure.

Example:

Physician performed the first stage of a hypospadias repair 1 month ago. The patient now returns for the second-stage repair, which includes a urethroplasty with a free skin graft obtained from a site other than genitalia. The physician should report the following for the second-stage procedure: 54316–58.

59 Distinct Procedural Service

Modifier 59 may be used by physicians and hospitals to identify that a procedure/service was distinct or independent from other services provided on the same day. Furthermore, modifier 59 is useful when circumstances require that certain procedures/services be reported together, even though they usually are not. Use of this modifier often signifies a different session or patient encounter, a different procedure or surgery, a different site or organ system, a separate incision/excision, or a separate lesion or injury not ordinarily encountered or performed on the same day by the same physician. Modifier 59 should not be reported if another modifier can more appropriately describe the circumstance. Coding professionals are encouraged to use applicable Level II (HCPCS National) Modifiers when appropriate (XE- Separate encounter, XS-Separate structure, XP-Separate practitioner, XU-Unusual non-overlapping services) for identification of subsets for modifier 59. Although CMS will continue to recognize modifier 59, it may selectively require the more specific modifier for billing certain codes at risk for incorrect billing.

> Because modifier 59 can bypass edits, it is often the focus of coding audits.

Example:

Procedures 23030 (Incision and drainage of shoulder area; deep abscess or hematoma) and 20103 (Exploration of penetrating wound; extremity) are performed on the same patient during the same operative session. Ordinarily, if these codes were reported together without a modifier, code 20103 would be denied as integral to code 23030. Because incision and drainage of the shoulder is the definitive procedure, any exploration of the area (code 20103) preceding this would be considered an inherent part of the more comprehensive service. If the exploration procedure were performed on the other limb, modifier 59 (or XS) explains that the codes are distinct from each other and both services are eligible for reimbursement from the health plan.

62 Two Surgeons

Physicians may report modifier 62 to identify that two surgeons were required to perform a particular procedure. Each surgeon should report

(Continued on next page)

Figure 3.1. Modifiers for use with surgical codes (Continued)

his or her distinct operative work by adding the modifier to the procedure code and any associated add-on code(s) for that procedure as long as both surgeons continue to work together as primary surgeons. If a co-surgeon acts as an assistant in the performance of additional procedure(s), other than those reported with the modifier 62, during the same surgical session, those services may be reported using separate procedure code(s) with modifier 80 or modifier 82 added. To expedite payment, the operative note dictated by each physician should be sent to the third-party payer.

63   Procedure Performed on Infants Less than 4 kg

Modifier 63 may be appended to codes in the 20000 through 69999 series when a procedure or service is performed on a neonate or infant with a body weight of up to 4 kg. Use of this modifier indicates that the procedure involved significantly increased complexity of physician work, which is commonly associated with these patients. Modifier 63 should only be assigned by physicians and should not be appended to any CPT code listed in the evaluation and management services, anesthesia, radiology, pathology and laboratory, or medicine sections.

66   Surgical Team

Modifier 66 may be reported by physicians only to identify a complex procedure performed by a team of physicians and other highly skilled personnel.

Example:

Patient is admitted for a liver transplant. All the physicians involved in performing this complex procedure should report 47135–66.

73   Discontinued Outpatient Procedure Prior to Anesthesia Administration

Modifier 73 is approved for hospital use only. If a surgical patient is taken to the operating room (or cystoscopy suite, gastrointestinal laboratory, and so on) and is prepared for surgery, but the surgery is cancelled before anesthesia is administered, the intended procedure code, along with modifier 73, is assigned. This modifier is not to be reported for an elective cancellation of a procedure. The medical record documentation should reflect the circumstances surrounding the cancellation.

Example:

Patient is scheduled for a knee arthroscopy for a lateral meniscus repair. The patient is taken to the OR and prepped, but it was noted that before anesthesia was administered, the patient was experiencing severe hypotension. The procedure was cancelled. The correct code assignment would be 29882–73.

74   Discontinued Outpatient Procedure After Anesthesia Administration

Modifier 74 is reported by hospitals only when a patient's surgery is cancelled after administration of anesthesia or after the procedure was begun (for example, after an incision was made or after an endoscope was inserted). The procedure in progress at the time of cancellation should be reported, not all intended procedures.

Figure 3.1. Modifiers for use with surgical codes (Continued)

Example:

Patient is scheduled for a knee arthroscopy for a lateral meniscus repair. The patient is taken to OR, prepared for surgery, and anesthesia is administered. Ten minutes into the procedure, the patient develops cardiac arrhythmia and the surgery is cancelled. The correct code assignment would be 29882–74.

76 Repeat Procedure or Service by Same Physician (or other qualified healthcare professional)

Modifier 76 may be reported by hospitals and physicians (or other qualified healthcare professionals) to identify a procedure or service that was repeated by the physician who performed the original procedure/service. Use of this modifier will help to clarify that the provider is not submitting a duplicate claim. Some third-party payers may require supportive documentation. Hospitals also may report this modifier.

Example:

Patient is admitted with significant pleural effusion and congestive heart failure, and the physician performs a thoracentesis. Later in the day, the lungs again fill up with fluid and the same physician performs a second thoracentesis. The physician or hospital should report the following: 32554 (first thoracentesis); 32554–76 (second thoracentesis identified as a repeat procedure with modifier 76).

77 Repeat Procedure by Another Physician (or other qualified healthcare professional)

Modifier 77 may be reported by hospitals and physicians to identify a procedure that was repeated by a physician other than the one who performed the original procedure. As with modifier 76, some third-party payers may require supportive documentation. Hospitals also may report this modifier as appropriate.

Example:

Dr. Reynolds performs a percutaneous transluminal balloon angioplasty of the renal artery. Later in the day, a diagnostic evaluation determines that the artery has occluded again. Because Dr. Reynolds cannot be reached, Dr. Smith repeats the earlier procedure. Dr. Reynolds should report 37246 to identify the first angioplasty performed, and Dr. Smith should report 37246–77 to identify the repeat angioplasty.

78 Unplanned Return to the Operating/Procedure Room by the Same Physician (or other qualified healthcare professional) Following Initial Procedure for a Related Procedure During the Postoperative Period (approved for physician and facility use)

This modifier reflects circumstances when it is necessary for a patient to return to the operating room (unplanned) during the postoperative period. The procedure performed for the subsequent surgery is related to the initial procedure. It is important to note that the modifier specifically states that the subsequent surgery is performed by the *same* physician.

(Continued on next page)

Figure 3.1.   Modifiers for use with surgical codes (Continued)

Example:

Dr. Bailey performs an excision of a hydrocele (CPT code 55040). Two days later, the patient develops a postoperative wound abscess. Dr. Bailey takes the patient to the operating room and performs an incision and drainage of the abscess (CPT code 10180). Modifier 78 would be reported with CPT code 10180.

79   Unrelated Procedure or Service by the Same Physician (or other qualified healthcare professional) During the Postoperative Period (approved for physician and facility use)
Modifier 79 is applicable to situations when a procedure is performed during the postoperative period that was unrelated to the original procedure (by the same physician).

Example:

Patient is seen for an excision of a 2.0-cm soft tissue tumor of the back (CPT code 21930). Three days later, the same general surgeon performs an emergency laparoscopic cholecystectomy (CPT code 47562). Modifier 79 would be appended to code 47562. The modifier conveys to the payer that the two procedures are not related and the cholecystectomy was not part of the global surgical period.

80   Assistant Surgeon
Modifier 80 may be reported by physicians only to indicate that the physician provided surgical assistant services for a particular procedure. The surgeon who assists another physician reports the code for the procedure that was performed along with modifier 80. The operating surgeon should not report modifier 80. (Assistant surgeons are usually assumed to have been present throughout the entire surgical procedure.)

Example:

Dr. Reynolds performs a total abdominal hysterectomy with removal of fallopian tubes and ovaries. Dr. Jones provides surgical assistance. Dr. Reynolds should report 58150, and Dr. Jones should report 58150–80

81   Minimum Assistant Surgeon
Modifier 81 may be reported by physicians only to indicate that a physician provided minimal surgical assistance when another surgeon's presence typically is not required throughout the entire procedure. The physician who provided minimal assistance reports the code for the procedure performed, along with modifier 81. As in the case of modifier 80, the operating surgeon should not report modifier 81.

82   Assistant Surgeon (when qualified resident surgeon not available)
Modifier 82 may be reported by physicians only when a physician provides surgical assistance to another surgeon and a resident surgeon is unavailable. This situation occurs primarily in teaching facilities where resident surgeons typically assume the role of assistant surgeon. When

Figure 3.1. Modifiers for use with surgical codes (Continued)

a qualified resident surgeon is unavailable, another physician may serve as an assistant surgeon and report the appropriate procedure code along with modifier 82. As in the case of modifiers 80 and 81, the operating surgeon should not report modifier 82.

95 **Synchronous Telemedicine Service Rendered via a Real-Time Interactive Audio and Video Telecommunications System**

96 **Habilitative Services**

97 **Rehabilitative Services**

99 **Multiple Modifiers**
Modifier 99 may be reported by physicians only to alert third-party payers that more than one modifier is being submitted on a claim. Many health plans have limitations on the number of modifiers recognized.

Other Uses of Modifiers

Modifier 33 (Preventive Service) is to be appended to a service when the primary purpose is the delivery of an evidence-based service in accordance with a US Preventive Services Task Force (USPSTF) A or B rating. The entire list of services is available on the website of the task force. The following is an excerpt from the list:

Topic	Description	Grade	Date in Effect
Syphilis screening: pregnant women	The USPSTF recommends that clinicians screen all pregnant women for a syphilis infection	A	May 2009

Category II Modifiers

Category II performance measurement modifiers indicate that a service specified in the measure(s) was considered but, due to either medical or patient circumstances(s), was not provided. The new modifiers are as follows:

1P Performance Measure Exclusion Modifier due to Medical Reasons
2P Performance Measure Exclusion Modifier due to Patient Reasons
3P Performance Measure Exclusion Modifier due to System Reasons
8P Performance Measure Reporting Modifier—Action Not Performed, Reason Not Otherwise Specified

Category II modifiers should only be reported with Category II codes and the circumstances must be documented in the medical record.

Use of Physical Status Modifiers

The Anesthesia section of CPT contains a list of six levels for ranking the physical status of patients. The codes are alphanumeric and appended to the appropriate Anesthesia CPT code. The following is a list of the physical status modifiers:

P1 A normal healthy patient
P2 A patient with mild systemic disease
P3 A patient with severe systemic disease

(Continued on next page)

Figure 3.1.   Modifiers for use with surgical codes (Continued)

P4   A patient with severe systemic disease that is a constant threat to life
P5   A moribund patient who is not expected to survive without the operation
P6   A declared brain-dead patient whose organs are being removed for donor purposes

These modifiers provide additional information about the condition of the patient and the complexity of the case.

Medicare Transmittals

Chapter 1, Part E of NCCI Policy Manual for Medicare Services is an excellent resource for coding professionals. Download and highlight the important information in that document pertaining to coding and use of modifiers.

Periodically, CMS issues its own guidelines or clarification memos pertaining to coding issues. Whenever CMS sees the need to alter or provide additional clarification on the correct usage of CPT codes or modifiers for Medicare reimbursement, it issues one of these memorandums. These guidelines are published as transmittals and an archive of these documents can be found on the CMS website by searching the key word Transmittals.

For example, Transmittal 1422, issued on August 14, 2014, defines four HCPCS modifiers that are subsets of Distinct Procedural Services (-59 modifier). The modifiers were defined as:

XE   Separate Encounter, A Service that is Distinct Because it Occurred During a Separate Encounter
XS   Separate Structure, A Service that is Distinct Because it was Performed on a Separate Organ/Structure
XP   Separate Practitioner, A Service that is Distinct Because it was Performed by a Different Practitioner
XU   Unusual Non-Overlapping Service, the Use of a Service that is Distinct because it does not Overlap Usual Components of the Main Service

National Correct Coding Initiative (NCCI) and Modifiers

Some software editing programs can help with NCCI edits.

The National Correct Coding Initiative (NCCI) was implemented to promote correct coding. The Excel-formatted tool includes modifier edits and procedure-to-procedure (PTP) code-pair edits to prevent improper billing for codes that should not be reported together. NCCI PTP edits list two columns that have CPT codes that normally would not be performed at the same patient encounter because the two procedures were mutually exclusive based on anatomic, temporal, or gender considerations (see figure 3.2). Occasionally modifiers are appended to CPT codes to bypass the NCCI edits and explain the circumstances. For example, if a surgeon excised a benign skin lesion from the patient's left arm (CPT code 11401) and another 1.0 cm benign skin lesion from the patient's right arm (CPT 11401), then listing 11401 and 11401–59 would be appropriate to explain the use of these two codes together. Otherwise it would appear as a duplicate code. It is important to note that modifier 59 is being monitored for misuse; therefore, documentation must support the assignment.

A manual editing spreadsheet tool is published by CMS that explains the appropriate use of modifiers by CPT code numbers (explained in chapter 4 of this textbook). The PTP edits include a modifier indicator of 0, 1, or 9. The modifier of "0" means that an edit can never be bypassed, even if a modifier is used. If the modifier column has a "1," it means that an edit may be bypassed with use of an appropriate modifier. The number "9" indicates that edits are not applicable. CMS publishes a booklet that describes how to use the NCCI tools.

Figure 3.2 is an excerpt from the publication on how to read the tables. Note the second entry for column 1, code 99215 for Office or other outpatient visit, should not be billed with G0102 (HCPCS code or prostate cancer screening; digital rectal examination). Column 6 reveals the modifier indicator of 0 (for code pairs 99215 and G0102). As noted in the key, the 0 means that a modifier (such as 59) is not allowed to bypass the edits. The last column provides a rationale for the edit. In this case, the standards of practice include rectal examinations in office visit codes.

Figure 3.2. NCCI tables

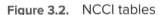

1	2	3	4	5	6	7

Column 1	Column 2	* = In existence prior to 1996	Effective Date	Deletion Date *=no data	Modifier 0=not allowed 1=allowed 9=not applicable	PTP Edit Rationale
99215	G0101		19980401	19980401	9	More extensive procedure *
99215	G0102		20000605	*	0	Standards of medical / surgical practice *
99215	G0104		19980401	19980401	9	More extensive procedure *
99215	G0105		19980401	19980401	9	More extensive procedure *
99215	G0106		19980401	19980401	9	More extensive procedure *
99215	G0107		19980401	19980401	9	More extensive procedure *
99215	G0117		20020101	*	0	Standards of medical / surgical practice *
99215	G0118		20020101	*	0	Standards of medical / surgical practice *
99215	G0120		19980401	19980401	9	More extensive procedure *
99215	G0245		20020701	*	0	Standards of medical / surgical practice *

Figure 2: Column 1/Column 2 table with 99215 in Column 1

1   Column 1 indicates the payable code.

2   Column 2 contains the code that is not payable with this particular Column 1 code, unless a modifier is permitted and submitted.

3   This third column indicates if the edit was in existence prior to 1996.

4   The fourth column indicates the effective date of the edit (year, month, date).

5   The fifth column indicates the deletion date of the edit (year, month, date).

6   The sixth column indicates if use of a modifier is permitted. This number is the modifier indicator for the edit. (The Modifier Indicator Table, shown on page 6 of this booklet, provides further explanation.)

7   The seventh column provides the underlying basis for each PTP edit.

Source: CMS.gov. "How to Use the Medicare National Correct Coding Initiative (NCCI) Tools." Centers for Medicare and Medicaid Services. January, 2018. Accessed October, 2018. https://www.cms.gov/Outreach-and-Education/Medicare-Learning-Network-MLN/MLNProducts/Downloads/How-To-Use-NCCI-Tools.pdf.

Chapter 3 Review

Answers to odd-numbered questions can be found in appendix C of this book. The answers to even-numbered questions are located in the instructor materials and are available to approved instructors.

Refer to appendix A of the CPT 2019 code book to identify the appropriate modifiers to be reported for the procedures.

1. The modifier that can be appended to a code to indicate that two surgeons were required to perform the procedure.

_____

2. April 1: Patient treated for a tibial fracture. May 15: Patient returns complaining of pain at the site of the external fixator. The surgeon immediately returns the patient to OR to remove the fixator. What physician modifier would be appended to the removal of the external fixator due to pain?

_____

3. The modifier that is to be used when a surgical procedure took a great deal of extra work and time due to the complexity of the case.

_____

4. The modifier that is to be appended to CPT code 90792 Psychiatric diagnostic evaluation, to indicate that the service was performed using synchronous telemedicine.

_____

5. The modifier that is to be used when a procedure was begun but had to be discontinued because of deterioration in the patient's condition (coding is for physician services, not hospital).

_____

6. A patient is seen in the dermatologist's office for follow-up after having a cancerous lesion removed last year. The physician performs a comprehensive history/examination with moderate-complexity decision-making. During the examination, a suspicious lesion is found on the patient's arm, which was biopsied using a shaving technique. In addition to the skin biopsy code (11102) the physician wishes to report the E/M code. What modifier would explain that the E/M services were significantly and separately identified from the services normally provided for just a biopsy?

_____

For items 7 through 17, assign the correct CPT code(s) and the appropriate modifiers (CPT and HCPCS National).

7. The patient underwent a percutaneous core needle biopsy of the right breast with the use of stereotactic guidance.

_____

(Continued on next page)

Chapter 3   Review   (Continued)

8. The physician performed a partial avulsion of the nail plate of the left thumb.

_____

9. A patient was taken to the outpatient surgery suite for an excisional debridement of the skin that extended into the muscle. The patient was prepared for surgery, but before anesthesia was administered, the physician was called for an emergency surgery of a trauma patient and the outpatient surgery was cancelled. (Assign code[s] to be reported by the hospital.)

_____

10. Chemodenervation of salivary glands (two glands injected).

_____

11. The surgeon performed a laparoscopic cholecystectomy. The procedure was complicated due to the fact that the patient had extensive adhesions that required over 2 hours to lysis. Assign the appropriate code with a modifier for the surgeon's service.

_____

12. A patient undergoes carpal tunnel releases on both the left and right wrists.

_____

13. The surgeon performed an open reduction with internal fixation for a right, fifth metatarsal fracture.

_____

14. The surgeon excised a chalazion of the left lower eyelid.

_____

15. According to _CPT Assistant_, October 2001, Cystourethroscopy Procedures, is it appropriate to append modifier 50 (bilateral procedure) to CPT code 52320 (Cystourethroscopy, with ureteroscopy and/or pyeloscopy; diagnostic?

_____

16. According to _CPT Assistant_, December 2012 (_Mobile APP Pathway under Island Pedicle Flaps, scrolling down to Frequently Asked Questions_), what modifier is recommended for reporting 15734 twice?

_____

17. According to _CPT Assistant_, July 2018, page 14 (Frequently Asked Questions), what modifier is used when an esophagogastroduodenoscopy (EGD) with biopsy (CPT code 43239) is performed with a dilation procedure (CPT code 43249) on the same date of service?

_____

(Continued on next page)

Chapter 3   Review   (Continued)

18. Locate the NCCI edits from the CMS website. Download the group that contains codes for the Digestive System. Complete the following table with the modifier indicator and PTP edit rationale. In the last column, use reasoning and knowledge of how procedures are performed to describe the intent of the edit.

Column 1 CPT Code	Column 2 CPT Code	Modifier 0 = not allowed 1 = allowed 9 = not applicable	PTP Edit Rationale	Explanation
43633 Gastrectomy, partial, distal; with Roux-en-Y reconstruction	44005 Enterolysis (freeing of intestinal adhesions) (separate procedure)			
45307 Proctosigmoidoscopy, rigid; with removal of foreign body	46601 Anoscopy; diagnostic			
45402 Laparoscopy, surgical; proctopexy	45540 Proctopexy; abdominal approach			

Surgery

4

Learning Objectives

- Identify the components of a surgical package.
- Distinguish between the CPT and CMS definitions of a surgical package.
- Define and cite examples of a separate procedure.
- Describe the purpose of NCCI edits.
- Given an operative statement or operative report, apply coding guidelines and abstract clinical information to assign correct codes.

To assign codes accurately from the surgery section, physicians and coding professionals must work together to ensure that the documentation in the health record supports the code(s) selected. In the hospital setting, as in the office setting, the operative or procedure report serves as the source document when identifying the type of procedure that has been performed.

Introduction to Surgery Section

The Surgery section provides codes for procedures performed by physicians of any specialty type (general surgeons, ophthalmologists, cardiovascular surgeons, neurosurgeons, and so on). It is further divided into subsections, such as Integumentary System, Musculoskeletal System, and Respiratory System.

This chapter reviews the guidelines and conventions for surgical coding and introduces specific subsections (links to various websites pertinent to the discussion in this chapter are located in the downloadable student resources for this book).

Surgical Packages

The term *surgical procedure* refers to any single, separate, systemic process upon or within the body that is complete in itself. Surgical procedures are performed for a number of purposes, including:

- To restore disunited or deficient parts
- To remove diseased or injured tissues
- To extract foreign matter from the body
- To assist in obstetrical delivery
- To provide diagnostic information

Each individual *surgical operation* includes one or more surgical procedures performed at one time for one patient via a common approach or for a common purpose. For example, consider a patient who has had an initial, incisional hernia repair with implantation of mesh. The surgical operation is the herniorrhaphy, which includes several surgical procedures such as incision, removal of hernia and implantation of the mesh, and closing of the wound. In this surgical case, the *Current Procedural Terminology* (CPT) code 49560 would be assigned for the repair of the hernia, and an additional code of 49568 is assigned for implantation of mesh. The incision, closure of the wound, and other minor intraoperative procedures are not assigned a code, because they are considered an integral part of the operation.

CPT Definition of Surgical Package

The term *surgical package* refers to a combination of individual *services* provided during one surgical operation. A surgical package is treated as one single service for purposes of reimbursement, and a single payment is issued for each package of related surgical services. The services covered in each surgical package include the following:

- The actual surgical procedure(s)
- Local infiltration, metacarpal/metatarsal/digital block, or topical anesthesia
- After the decision to perform surgery has been made, one related evaluation and management (E/M) encounter on the date of, or immediately prior to, the date of the procedure (including history and physical)
- Immediate postoperative care, including dictation of operative notes and talking with the family and other physicians

- Preparation of orders
- Evaluation of the patient in the postanesthesia recovery area
- Typical postoperative follow-up care

This reimbursement concept is sometimes referred to as global surgery payment. For example, if a physician performed a surgical operation and a few days later saw the patient in her office for standard follow-up care (for example, removal of sutures), the follow-up visit provided by the physician would not be reported separately. It would be included under the code(s) for the surgical procedure(s) performed during the first encounter, and both encounters would be submitted as a single reimbursement claim. In some cases, however, the code for the postoperative follow-up visit (99024) might also be reported for documentation purposes.

Example:

Four weeks ago, Dr. Smith repaired a closed tibial shaft fracture without manipulation. Today, the patient has returned to Dr. Smith's office to have his cast removed. Dr. Smith may bill only for the repair of the fracture, which includes the normal, uncomplicated follow-up care, including cast removal. Thus, only code 27750 is reported on his claim. The subsequent visit for removal of the cast is not billed separately; however, for tracking purposes only, code 99024 may be assigned for that encounter.

Services other than standard postoperative care, however, would not be included in the same surgical package. Follow-up visits for the treatment of complications resulting from the surgical procedure (for example, wound infection at operative site) would be reported with codes for the appropriate E/M level of service, along with the appropriate ICD-10-CM code, to describe the complication.

Example:

Two weeks ago, Dr. Smith performed a cholecystectomy. Today, the patient returns with complaints of redness, inflammation, and oozing from the wound site. Dr. Smith determines that the patient has developed an infection at the operative wound site and treats it appropriately. For the second office visit, Dr. Smith should report the appropriate E/M level of service code and assign an ICD-10-CM code (such as T81.4XXA for Infection following a procedure, initial encounter) that describes the reason for this visit.

Medicare guidelines for reimbursement for services involving complications are slightly different from CPT. These guidelines can be referenced in the manuals published by the Centers for Medicare and Medicaid Services (CMS). A complete list of manuals, including the Medicare Claims Processing Manual, can be located on the CMS website.

The surgical package or global surgery concept does not apply in the hospital outpatient setting. Hospitals may report postoperative visits that occur on subsequent days by using standard billing procedures, such as assigning the appropriate ICD-10-CM diagnosis code to describe the reason for the visit.

Example:

> Patient returns to the outpatient clinic of Central Hospital for a change of surgical dressing. The hospital assigns ICD-10-CM code Z48.01 (Encounter for change or removal of surgical wound dressing) to identify the reason for the visit. The E/M code appropriate to the circumstance (new or established) reflects the service rendered.

Medicare Definition of a Surgical Package

The services included in a surgical package may vary depending on individual third-party payer requirements. Unlike CPT, the postoperative period for Medicare claims is not open-ended. Medicare assigns postoperative global periods of 90 days for major surgeries and 0 to 10 days for minor surgeries and endoscopies. The Medicare global surgery definition for major surgeries includes the following types of services:

- The actual surgical procedure
- Preoperative services after the decision is made to operate beginning with the day before the day of surgery for major procedures and the day of surgery for minor procedures
- Follow-up visits during the postoperative period of the surgery that are related to recovery from the surgery
- Complications following surgery: All additional medical or surgical services required of the surgeon during the postoperative period of the surgery because of complications that do not require additional trips to the operating room
- Postsurgical pain management provided by the surgeon
- Insignificant surgical procedures not performed in the operating room, including dressing changes, removal of operative packs, and care of the operative incision site; removal of sutures, staples, wires, lines, tubes, drains, casts, and splints; insertion, irrigation, and removal of urinary catheters; routine peripheral intravenous lines; removal of nasogastric tubes and rectal tubes; care of tracheostomy tubes

Follow-up Care for Diagnostic and Therapeutic Procedures

Follow-up care for diagnostic or therapeutic procedures includes only that care related to recovery from the diagnostic procedure itself or care that is usually part of the surgical service. When follow-up care involves the initiation of treatment for the condition that has been diagnosed or for a complication, the treatment should be coded and reported separately. Complication, exacerbation, or recurrence, or the presence of other diseases or injuries requiring additional services should be reported with the appropriate code for that procedure.

Separate Procedures

The CPT code book defines a separate procedure as one that, when performed in conjunction with another service, is considered an integral part of the major service; therefore, it should not be coded separately. In normal circumstances, it is fraudulent to report the codes separately and charge separate fees for each procedure.

However, the separate procedure may be coded when it is performed independently and not in conjunction with the so-called larger or major procedure. A modifier, such as modifier 59 (Distinct Services), may be added to explain special circumstances where the separate procedure was not performed integral to the larger procedure. For example, assume that the following procedures were performed on a patient:

Example:

> 58720 Salpingo-oophorectomy, complete or partial, unilateral or bilateral (separate procedure)
>
> 58150 Total abdominal hysterectomy (corpus and cervix), with or without removal of tube(s), with or without removal of ovary(s)

Assignment of code 58720 would be appropriate in circumstances where *only* a salpingo-oophorectomy was performed. If the salpingo-oophorectomy was done as part of a larger procedure, as described in code 58150, an additional code of 58720 is inappropriate and would be considered unbundling of services. Unbundling is the practice of using multiple codes that describe individual components of a procedure rather than an appropriate single code that describes all steps in the procedure performed.

In another example, assume the physician performed a flexible bronchoscopy with cell washings (CPT code 31622) and a transbronchial lung biopsy (CPT code 31628). In this example, only CPT code 31628 is reported. CPT code 31622 is a separate procedure code and would not be assigned with 31628.

National Correct Coding Initiative (NCCI)

A list of coding edits has been developed by CMS in an effort to promote correct coding nationwide and to prevent the inappropriate unbundling of related services. The National Correct Coding Initiative (NCCI) (also known as CCI) edits help CMS to detect inappropriate codes submitted on claims and are based on CPT coding guidelines, current standards of medical/surgical coding practice, and advice from specialty societies. There are two major types of coding edits: the comprehensive/component edit and the mutually exclusive edit. Both of these files are consolidated into the Column One/Column Two Correct Coding edit file available on the CMS website.

Procedure-to-Procedure (PTP) Code Pair Edits

The PTP code pair edits pertains to *Healthcare Common Procedure Coding System* (HCPCS) codes that should not be used together by the same physician for the same patient on the same day. The prepayment edits prevent improper payment when certain codes are submitted together for Part-B covered services. Note the following table as an example of a NCCI listing. Under the NCCI, if bills contain a procedure in both the comprehensive code column and the component code column for the same patient on the same date of service, only the code in the comprehensive code column is covered (provided that code is on the list as an approved procedure for reimbursement). For example:

Column 1	Column 2
43260	31525

In the preceding example, Column 1 is the CPT code 43260 describing an endoscopic retrograde cholangiopancreatography (ERCP) and Column 2 is the CPT code 31525 that describes a laryngoscopy. It is not anatomically logical for these two procedures to be reported together.

Mutually Exclusive Edit

The mutually exclusive edit applies to improbable or impossible combinations of codes. For example, code 69601, Revision mastoidectomy; resulting in complete mastoidectomy, would never be performed with code 69604, Revision mastoidectomy; resulting in tympanoplasty. These edits are incorporated into the Column 1 and Column 2 format for editing.

Many coding/billing software programs contain these edits and warn coders about assigning inappropriate coding pairs. The software vendors are responsible for maintaining up-to-date edits to support the coding/billing function. More information about NCCI edits can be found on the CMS website.

Medical Unlikely Edits

For Part B claims, CMS has developed medical unlikely edits to reduce error rates for items on the claim form that reference units of service. For each HCPCS/CPT code, the edits list the maximum units of service that a provider would report under most circumstances for a single beneficiary on a single date of service.

Figure 4.1 is a screenshot from the CMS website that outlines the links to the necessary editing documents.

Figure 4.1. CMS website links to coding edits

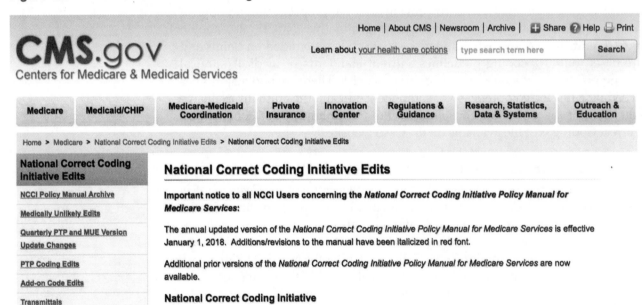

Source: CMS.gov. "National Correct Coding Initiatives Edits." Digital Images. Centers for Medicare and Medicaid Services. June, 2018. Accessed October, 2018. https://www.cms.gov/medicare/coding/nationalcorrectcodinited/ncci-coding-edits.html.

Policy Manual

CMS publishes a manual called National Correct Coding Initiative Coding Policy Manual for Medicare Services (Coding Policy Manual) that is referenced by carriers and fiscal intermediaries (FI) to explain the rationale for the NCCI edits. For an example, if a surgeon attempts a laparoscopic appendectomy but must convert the procedure to open, CMS directs coding professionals to only code the open procedure.

Integumentary System

Learning Objectives

- Differentiate between fine needle aspiration biopsy and core needle biopsy.
- Differentiate between the techniques for skin biopsy procedures.
- Apply coding guidelines for multiple skin biopsy techniques during the same encounter.
- Describe the decision pathways for determining coding for debridement.
- Differentiate between coding benign and malignant lesions.
- Define *excisional diameter* for measuring skin lesions.
- Distinguish between destruction and excision of lesions.
- Identify the difference between simple, intermediate, and complex wound repairs.
- Differentiate between the types of skin grafts.
- Describe the procedures for breast biopsies and mastectomy procedures.

The integumentary system subsection includes codes for procedures performed on the following body parts:

- Skin and subcutaneous structures, including excision of skin lesions, wound closure, skin grafting, burn treatment, Mohs' chemosurgery, incision and drainage, and debridement
- Nails, including debridement, excision, and reconstruction of nail bed
- Breast, including needle, incisional, and excisional biopsies, and all types of mastectomies

Figure 4.2 shows the skin and its components. For surgical coding, knowledge of anatomy is vital.

The integumentary system subsection includes many definitions that are located at various levels within the subsection. A careful review of each definition is necessary before codes are assigned.

Fine Needle Aspiration (FNA) Biopsy

A fine needle aspiration (FNA) biopsy uses a thin, hollow needle to extract cells or fluid from body tissue for examination under the microscope. The CPT codes, beginning with 10021, can be differentiated by the use of imaging and whether or not more than one biopsy was performed. Note that the code description states "first lesion" or "each additional lesion." The term *lesion* identifies an organ or tissue that has undergone abnormal change due to injury or disease. Typically, fine needle aspiration biopsies extract fluid or cells from cysts, nodules, masses, infected sites, and so on.

Figure 4.2. Anatomy of the skin

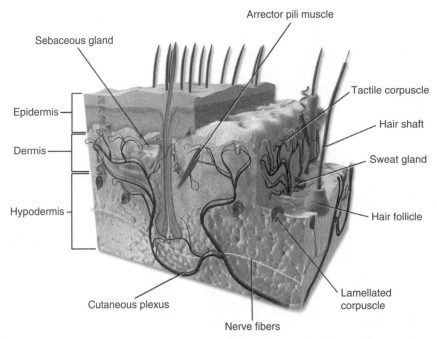

Source: Blaus, Bruce. "Skin Anatomy." Digital Image. Wikimedia Commons. January 2014. Accessed September, 2018. https://commons.wikimedia.org/wiki/File:Blausen_0810_SkinAnatomy_01.png.

Example:

Under ultrasound guidance, a fine needle aspiration biopsy of the kidney was performed. The correct code would be 10005.

FNA versus Core Needle Biopsy

Due to the nature of the tissue, the surgeon may elect to use a larger hollow needle to remove suspicious tissue. An important note appears below code 10012; it guides coding professionals to cite specific codes for core needle biopsy procedures.

Example:

Under ultrasound guidance, a core needle biopsy of the kidney was performed. The correct coding assignment is as follows:
50200 Renal biopsy; percutaneous, by trocar or needle
76942 Ultrasonic guidance for needle placement (e.g., biopsy, aspiration, injection, localization device), imaging supervision and interpretation)

Note that in the first example for FNA of kidney, the ultrasound guidance was bundled into the description of the code. In the core needle example, a CPT note under 50200 prompted the coding professional to report a radiological supervision and interpretation code (see 76942, 77002, 77012, 77021) because 50200 was not bundled with guidance.

Biopsy

A biopsy is taking a sample of tissue to be analyzed in a laboratory. In procedures such as excision of lesion, it is expected that the specimen will be sent to the pathology department for analysis; therefore, the CPT code for biopsy would not be reported separately. The skin biopsy codes (11102–11107) are only used when the procedure is *solely* for taking tissue for pathological examination and is unrelated or distinct from the other procedures performed. The skin biopsy codes can be differentiated by technique (such as punch or shaving), and in the case of FNA biopsy, the use of imaging is captured. Table 4.1 provides a quick reference for identifying skin biopsies by technique.

Table 4.1. Skin biopsy techniques

Type of Biopsy	Technique	Documentation for Coding
Tangential biopsy	Shaving, curette, scoop, saucerize	• Scraping (or shaving) tissue that needs to be examined
Punch biopsy	A circular tool removes a small section of skin (see figure 4.3).	• One lesion or more
Incisional biopsy	A piece of tissue is cut out using a blade. Also includes wedge biopsy.	• A portion of the tissue is taken (not the entire lesion/mass) • One lesion or more

CPT coding guidance is provided for multiple biopsies and multiple techniques. When multiple techniques are performed during the same encounter, only one primary lesion biopsy code is reported along with corresponding add-on codes. For example, if one punch biopsy were performed for a skin lesion of the arm, and two more tangential biopsies were performed for lesions on the leg, the coding assignment would be as follows:

11104   Punch biopsy of skin; single lesion
11103   each separate/additional tangential biopsy
11103   each separate/additional tangential biopsy

Figure 4.3 depicts a punch biopsy for laboratory analysis.

Debridement

CPT provides a variety of codes to reflect the treatment of damaged or infected tissue. A good coding practice is to review a selection of codes and identify the unique characteristics. For example, scan the codes in the following list and differentiate each.

- 11000: This code reflects the treatment via debridement for infected skin and eczema. The wound size is dependent on the percent of body surface.
- 11004–11006: Code 11004 starts a family of codes used to identify a more serious type of infection (necrotic soft tissue infection) that can extend to the depth of bone. Site includes external genitalia, perineum, and abdominal wall.
- 11008: This code involves removal of prosthetic material associated with an abdominal wall infection. A plus sign (+) in front of this code indicates that it is an add-on code and should not be reported separately.

Review the reference of biopsy codes (listed before code 11102) that are coded from other sections, such as biopsy of ear (69100).

A punch biopsy of one lesion would be reported with CPT code 11104.

Figure 4.3. Skin punch biopsy

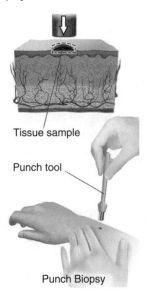

Source: Blaus, Bruce. "Punch Biopsy." Digital Image. Wikimedia Commons. July, 2017. Accessed September, 2018. https://commons.wikimedia.org/wiki/File:Skin_Punch_Biopsy.png.

- 11010–11012: This family of codes is reserved for debridement associated with open fractures. The hierarchy of codes is related to the depth (11011 extends to the muscle, while 11012 extends to the bone).
- Note the series of entries under code 11012 that refers a coder to different sections of CPT if the debridement is associated with burns (16020–16030) or active wound care management codes (97597–97602) located in the Medicine chapter.

Wound debridement (11042–11047) is a surgical method in which a patient's dead, damaged, or infected tissue is removed to assist the healing process. The coding selection is differentiated by depth (subcutaneous, bone, muscle) and size. CPT provides the following guidelines to support an accurate code assignment:

- For a single wound, report the depth using the deepest level of tissue removed.
- For multiple wounds, sum the surface areas that are at the *same depth* (do not combine sums from different depths).

Example 1:

The physician debrided a 3.0-sq cm wound of the buttocks (in the muscle) and another 4.0-sq cm wound (in the muscle) of the heel.

Coding rationale: Both wounds were at the same depth (*in the muscle*), so a sum of the wounds would be reported (3.0 sq cm + 4.0 sq cm = 7.0 sq cm). Code 11043

Example 2:

The physician debrided a 3.0-sq cm wound of the buttocks (*in the muscle*) and another 4.0-sq cm wound (*in the bone*) of the heel.

Coding rationale: The wounds are *not* at the same depth. The wound of the buttocks was debrided in the muscle, but the wound of the heel extended down to the bone. The correct coding assignment would be 11043 (wound of buttocks) and 11044 (wound of heel).

Note: The sequencing of these codes, for reporting on a claim form, would require knowledge of reimbursement amounts and payer guidelines offered by current software programs. Typically, the more resource-intensive code (in this case 11044) is sequenced first on the claim form.

Exercise 4.1 Integumentary System—Debridement

Answers to odd-numbered questions can be found in appendix C of this book. The answers to even-numbered questions are located in the instructor materials and are available to approved instructors.

Assign appropriate CPT code(s) to the following debridement procedures. Assign only CPT surgical codes (no E/M codes) and append any applicable modifiers.

1. Patient has a Grade III ulcer of the left heel. The physician debrided the 4 cm × 2 cm × 0.5 cm ulcer to the subcutaneous tissue. The #15 blade removed the fibrinous tissue.

   Code(s): _____

2. The patient had a mesh inserted during an inguinal hernia repair a couple of years ago. The patient presents for removal of the infected mesh and debridement of the necrotic tissue. The physician performed a debridement of the wound, including the fascia, and removed the mesh.

   Code(s): _____

3. Patient was involved in a motorcycle accident and sustained a fractured fibula. The wound was debrided down through the subcutaneous tissue into the muscle for removal of debris (gravel and glass). (*Only assign CPT code for the debridement in this case.*)

   Code(s): _____

4. The surgeon performs debridement down to and including the fascia of the abdominal wall due to necrotizing fasciitis

   Code(s): _____

5. The patient is seen for treatment of a diabetic foot ulcer (4.0 cm × 3 cm). The surgeon performed a surgical debridement of the skin, subcutaneous tissue, and extensor digitorum brevis muscle.

   Code(s): _____

Lesions

A lesion is tissue that has suffered damage through injury or disease. Skin lesions can include moles, cysts, keloids, warts, or skin tags. Most are benign; however, they are sometimes removed if they are painful, unsightly, or restrictive of movement. Surgical removal is the most common treatment for most skin lesions. Warts are also removed by the use of liquid gas to freeze them off, or they may be treated with chemical paint. If the lesion is suspected of being malignant, a biopsy is taken and analyzed in a laboratory for any signs of cancerous cells.

Removal of Skin Lesions

There are a variety of methods used to remove skin lesions. The physician may elect to remove the lesion by any of the following techniques: shaving, paring, excising, or with the use of laser. Coding professionals should read the documentation to determine the method used to remove the lesion. Depending on the method of removal and the CPT code description, other documentation is also necessary. Table 4.2 displays the supportive documentation required for different methods of removing different types of skin lesions.

Table 4.2. Necessary documentation for removal of skin lesions

Method of Removal	Necessary Documentation	CPT Code Range
Paring of lesions	• Diagnosis of benign hyperkeratotic lesion • Number of lesions removed	11055–11057
Removal of skin tags	• Diagnosis of skin tag(s) • Number of skin tags removed	11200–11201
Shaving of epidermal or dermal lesions	• Diagnosis of epidermal or dermal lesion • Diameter of lesion • Location of lesion	11300–11313
Excision of benign lesion(s)	• Diagnosis of benign skin lesion • Excised diameter • Location of lesions	11400–11471
Excision of malignant lesion(s)	• Diagnosis of malignant skin lesion • Excised diameter • Location of lesions	11600–11646
Destruction of benign or premalignant lesions	• Diagnosis of benign or premalignant skin lesion • Lesion removed by methods such as electrosurgery, cryosurgery, laser, or chemical treatment • Number of lesions removed	17000–17004 17110–17250
Destruction of malignant lesions	• Diagnosis of malignant skin lesion • Lesion removed by destruction • Diameter of lesion • Location of lesion	17260–17286

Excision of Lesions

Two separate code ranges can be found in this subsection to describe the excised site of benign (11400–11471) and malignant (11600–11646) lesions. Both series of codes are further subdivided, first by body part and then by lesion size. To accurately code excision of lesions, the coding professional must be able to answer the following questions:

- *Is the lesion malignant or benign?* Careful review of the operative report and, more important, the pathology report is required to determine the lesion type. Coding from superbills or encounter forms, which do not reveal pathology results, often leads to inappropriate code assignment.

- *What site or body part is involved with the lesion?* The operative report should be reviewed for this information.

- *How large is the excised area (in centimeters, including margins, if applicable)?* During surgery, physicians may take some normal-looking skin around the growth. Removal of the normal-looking skin is known as taking margins. This is done to be sure no cancer cells are left behind. The total size of the excised area, including margins, is needed for accurate coding (see figure 4.4). Usually, this information is provided in the operative report. It is very important that surgeons be educated and trained to provide accurate lesion size information. The pathology report typically provides the specimen size rather than the lesion or excised size. Because the specimen tends to shrink, this is not an accurate measurement according to the intent of the code assignment. Inches should be converted to centimeters, when necessary.

> If the lesion is irregular, the maximum width is used to measure the lesion. For example, excision of a 1.0 cm × 2.0 cm lesion of the hand would be assigned 11422.

1 mm = 0.1 cm
10 mm = 1.0 cm
1 inch = approximately 2.54 cm
1 cm = 0.4 inch

Figure 4.4. Melanoma excision

> If the documentation stated that the melanoma (skin lesion) was 1.0 cm and required wide excision of 0.3 cm margins on each side, the code assignment would be 11602 (1.0 cm + 0.3 cm + 0.3 cm = excised diameter of 1.6 cm of arm).

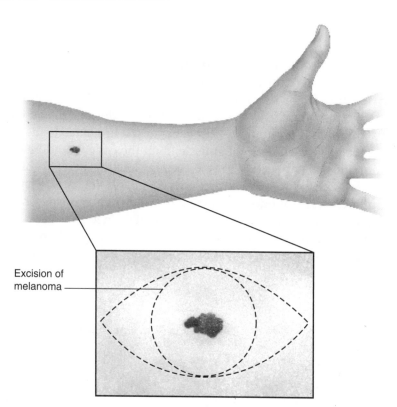

Excision of melanoma

Source: ©AHIMA.

- *What type of wound closure was performed?* Both series of codes (11400–11471 and 11600–11646) include simple closure. Separate codes should be reported when the excision requires more than simple closure, such as an intermediate repair.

When more than one dimension for an excised area is provided, the size is equal to the largest dimension of the excision, including margins.

Excised Diameter Example:

The physician excised a malignant melanoma of the back that was reported as 3.0 cm × 2.0 cm. Documentation in the operative report states that 0.5 cm margins were excised around the lesion. For coding purposes, the size of the excision was 3.0 cm + 0.5 cm + 0.5 cm = 4.0 cm in total. The correct code assignment would be 11604.

Excision of Lesion Followed by Adjacent Tissue Transfer

> Excision of a 2.0 cm malignant lesion of the arm followed by an adjacent tissue skin graft would be assigned only 14020.

When excision of a malignant or benign lesion involves repair by adjacent tissue transfer—such as Z-plasty, W-plasty, V-Y plasty, rotation, advancement, or double pedicle flap—codes 14000–14350 should be reported. It should be noted that these codes include both the excision and the tissue transfer or rearrangement. A separate code should not be reported for the lesion excision. A more detailed discussion of adjacent tissue transfer techniques follows in the section on skin grafts later in this chapter.

Every excised lesion should be reported individually with the correct CPT code. Multiple lesion excisions are not treated as a single excision.

Excision of Lipomas

> Lipomas may be coded to Integumentary or Musculoskeletal Systems depending on the depth. Soft tissue involvement codes are located in the Musculoskeletal chapter.

Lipomas are usually benign fatty tumors commonly found in superficial tissue, although they can also be present in subfascial and submuscular locations. Whether the lipoma is confined to the skin or extends into the deeper tissues will be the deciding factor for accurate code assignment. For example, if the patient has a lipoma of the back that extends into the dermis, then a code for excision of skin lesion is appropriate. However, if the lipoma extends into the soft tissue of the back, including the muscle, then the code would be selected from the musculoskeletal section. For example, looking at code 21930 for Excision, tumor, soft tissue of back or flank, *soft tissue* refers to tissues that connect, support, or surround other structures and organs of the body. Soft tissue includes muscles, tendons (bands of fiber that connect muscles to bones), fibrous tissues, fat, blood vessels, nerves, and synovial tissues (tissues around joints). In addition, codes for removal of soft-tissue tumors are differentiated by site and size.

Example:

21555	Excision, tumor, soft tissue of neck or anterior thorax, subcutaneous; less than 3 cm
#21552	3 cm or greater

Note that the symbol (#) indicates that the codes are out of numerical sequence.

Exercise 4.2   Integumentary System—Lesions and Skin Biopsies

Answers to odd-numbered questions can be found in appendix C of this book. The answers to even-numbered questions are located in the instructor materials and are available to approved instructors.

Assign appropriate CPT code(s) to the following procedures. Assign only CPT surgical codes (no E/M codes) and append any applicable modifiers.

1. Physician excises three benign skin lesions. The excised areas are 2.0 cm from arm, 0.8 cm of hand, and 1.0 cm from neck.

   Code(s): _____

2. Physician excised a 1.0-cm squamous cell carcinoma from the forehead. The excision required margins of 1.0 cm around the lesion.

   Code(s): _____

3. Physician excises a lesion from the chin. The excised dimension is 1.5 cm. Pathology report reveals malignant melanoma.

   Code(s): _____

4. In the physician's office, the patient had a punch biopsy of a 1.0 cm skin lesion of the neck.

   Code(s): _____

5. Physician excised an area 3.0 cm × 2.0 cm × 1.5 cm from the patient's back. The pathology report shows a lipoma in the subcutaneous layer of skin.

   Code(s): _____

6. Laser removal of sixteen benign skin lesions from the back.

   Code(s): _____

7. Excision of malignant melanoma of the forehead (1.0 cm) and nose (0.5 cm).

   Code(s): _____

8. Paring of three hyperkeratotic lesions from the patient's foot.

   Code(s): _____

9. The raised suspicious skin lesion of the arm was biopsied using a curette to shave the top of the lesion for pathological evaluation.

   Code(s): _____

10. A wedge of tissue was biopsied from a mass on the patient's back. The sample was sent to pathology for analysis. In addition, another lesion of the arm was shaved with a scalpel for biopsy.

    Code(s): _____

Exercise 4.3   Integumentary System—Operative Reports

Answers to odd-numbered questions can be found in appendix C of this book. The answers to even-numbered questions are located in the instructor materials and are available to approved instructors.

Operative Report #1

Operative Report

Preoperative Diagnosis:	Sebaceous cyst, left face
Postoperative Diagnosis:	Same
Procedure:	Excision of left-face sebaceous cyst
Anesthesia:	Local with IV sedation

The patient is a 69-year-old woman who has a sebaceous cyst, which has started to grow larger, on the left side of her face. She presents now for excision of the cyst.

The patient was brought to the OR and placed on the operating table in the supine position. She was given 50 mg of Demerol and 1 mg of Versed IV. The left face was prepped and draped in the usual sterile fashion. The area overlying the cyst was anesthetized with 1% lidocaine with epinephrine. An elliptical incision was made of the cyst in the direction of the facial wrinkles. The cyst itself was 1 cm in diameter. The underlying cyst was dissected away from the surrounding tissues, taking care to remove the entire cyst, with an excised area of 2.0 cm × 0.5 cm. Hemostasis was obtained using electrocautery. The wound was then closed with 3-0 Vicryl. It was then dressed with Masticel and Steri-Strips. The patient tolerated the procedure well and was taken to the recovery room in stable condition.

Pathology Report

Clinical Diagnosis:	Cyst of the face
Specimen:	Ellipse of skin measuring 2.0 × 0.5 × 0.2 cm
Pathological Diagnosis:	Epidermal inclusion cyst with rupture, marked acute and chronic inflammation
	Assign only CPT surgical codes (no E/M codes) and append any applicable modifiers.

Code(s): _____

Operative Report #2

Operative Report

Preoperative Diagnosis: Epidermoid nevus of scalp

Postoperative Diagnosis: Same

Procedure: Shave excision of 4.0-cm benign scalp lesion

This patient is on chronic anticoagulation. A subgaleal lipoma has previously been removed. At that time, he was not interested in having his seborrheic keratosis removed from his scalp, although the offer was made to do so. He has had a very nice result from his original surgery and is now willing and wishing to undergo removal of what I believe is a seborrheic keratosis. Although, according to the history, it has been there as long as he can remember, it may be an epidermal nevus. A small portion is sent for biopsy to create the definitive diagnosis. The patient understands the risks of bleeding.

The patient was brought to the operating room and made comfortable in a supine position on the table. The area to be worked up was infiltrated with 1% lidocaine with 1:100,000 parts epinephrine. The area was then prepared and draped in the usual sterile fashion. A #15 blade was used to remove a small portion of the lesion, which was carefully labeled and sent to pathology for examination. The rest was then shaved off at the level of the dermis, where there was punctate bleeding. Hemostasis was achieved with cautery. A dressing of Gelfoam soaked in thrombin was placed over this, and the patient was allowed to return to the recovery room with stable vital signs. The estimated blood loss was less than 15 cc, which was replaced with crystalloid solution only. Sponge, needle, and instrument counts were reported as correct.

Assign only CPT surgical codes (no E/M codes) and append any applicable modifiers.

Code(s): _____

Wound Repair/Closure

The CPT code book describes three types of wound repair/closure: simple, intermediate, and complex.

Simple Wound Repair

A simple repair is a superficial repair that primarily involves the epidermis, dermis, or subcutaneous tissues without involvement of deeper structures. This repair usually requires simple suturing of only one layer of skin.

Intermediate Wound Repair

An intermediate repair, like a simple wound repair, is considered a superficial repair, requiring that one or more of the deeper layers of the subcutaneous tissue and superficial (nonmuscle) fascia, as well as the skin (epidermal and dermal), be closed in layers. In other words, wounds that require closure of subcutaneous tissue or more than one layer of tissue beneath the dermis should be coded as intermediate, unless the criteria for a complex closure are met. Wounds that are closed with only one layer, but which are so heavily contaminated that they require extensive cleaning or removal of foreign material, such as gravel or glass, also may be classified as an intermediate repair.

Example:

Surgeon documents the defect is to the epidermis, dermis, and subcutaneous tissue. Procedure description includes that the absorbable sutures were placed within the subcutaneous tissue and deep dermis. In order to close the defect, epidermal sutures were placed in interrupted or running fashion (intermediate closure).

Complex Wound Repair

A complex repair of a wound goes beyond a layer closure and may include documentation of scar revision, debridement, extensive undermining, stents, or retention sutures. Wounds described as angular, jagged, irregular, or stellate may require complex repair. Layered closure is part of this wound repair.

Example:

Wound edges were undermined extensively. Buried absorbable sutures were used to close the subcutaneous and dermal components of the defect. Simple interrupted sutures were used to approximate the epidermal edges.

Coding of Wound Repairs/Closures

Coding professionals can add the sum of the wound closures if they are the same category (simple, intermediate, or complex) and the same anatomical grouping.

To accurately code wound closures, the following questions must be answered:

- *What type of repair is being performed: simple, intermediate, or complex?*
- *What site or body part is involved, and what is the extent of the wound?* The operative report should be reviewed for mention of blood vessel, tendon, or nerve involvement. The wound repair codes include simple ligation of blood vessels and simple exploration of the nerves, vessels, or tendons, so they should not be reported separately. However, a separate code is warranted if the extent of the laceration requires repair of the nerves, vessels, or tendons.
- *What is the length of the repair (in centimeters)?*

When multiple wounds are repaired, the coding professional should add together the lengths of those in the same classification and from all anatomic sites that are grouped together into the same code descriptor. For example, add together the lengths of intermediate repairs to the trunk and extremities. Do not add lengths of repairs from different groupings of anatomic sites (for example, face and extremities). Also, do not add together the lengths of different classifications (for example, intermediate and complex repairs).

Example 1:

Simple wound repair of two lacerations of the arm measuring 2.5 cm and 1.5 cm. The sum of the two lacerations is 4.0 cm, and the code reported is 12002.

Example 2:

Emergency department physician documents a simple repair of the following lacerations: 2.0 cm of arm, 3.0 cm of leg, and 1.5 cm of cheek. In addition, the physician documented the following layered wound closures: 2.0 cm of foot, 1.5 cm of leg, and 3.0 cm of knee. Note the correct code assignment:

Simple Repairs	Intermediate Repairs
2.0 cm arm 3.0 cm leg 1.5 cm cheek	2.0 cm foot 1.5 cm leg 3.0 cm knee
Add 2.0 cm of arm and 3.0 of leg and assign CPT code 12002 (5.0-cm repair). *An additional code, 12011, would be assigned for the repair of the cheek.*	*Add 1.5 cm of leg and 3.0 cm of knee to assign CPT code 12032 (4.5-cm repair).* *An additional code, 12041, would be assigned for the 2.0-cm repair of the foot.*

When more than one classification of wounds is repaired, the most complicated repair is listed first, followed by the less complicated repairs. Modifier 51 (for physician billing) also should be reported to identify the performance of more than one procedure. It is important to note that the payers determine use of modifier 51. Debridement may be reported separately only when gross contamination requires prolonged cleansing, considerable amounts of devitalized or contaminated tissue are removed, or debridement is carried out separately without immediate primary closure.

A note under the wound repair subheading refers the coding professional to codes 20100 through 20103 if the wound required any of the following:

- Enlargement
- Extension of dissection
- Debridement
- Removal of one or more foreign bodies
- Ligation or coagulation of minor subcutaneous and/or muscular blood vessel(s)

Superficial wound repairs requiring only Steri-Strips or bandages are reported with the appropriate E/M services code. Surgical codes are inappropriate because no surgical repair was performed. Repairs with tissue adhesive, such as 2-cyanoacrylate (Dermabond), are reported using the appropriate code from the repair category.

Tissue Adhesives

It is important to note that Medicare requires a Level II HCPCS code to identify a wound closed with tissue adhesives. Instead of assigning the CPT code for wound repair, the following code should be assigned: G0168, Wound closure utilizing tissue adhesive(s) only (HCPCS Level II codes are discussed further in chapter 10).

Exercise 4.4   Integumentary System—Wound Repairs

Answers to odd-numbered questions can be found in appendix C of this book. The answers to even-numbered questions are located in the instructor materials and are available to approved instructors.

Assign appropriate CPT code(s) for the following procedures. Assign only CPT surgical codes (no E/M codes) and append any applicable modifiers.

1. The patient is treated in the emergency department for a deep 7.0-cm wound of the back. A routine cleansing and deep nonmuscle layer closure was required.

   Code(s):_____

2. A child is seen in the physician's office for a superficial laceration of the right knee. The physician repairs the 2.5-cm laceration with simple suturing.

   Code(s):_____

3. A patient is treated for multiple wounds of the right forearm, hand, and knee. The physician sutured the following: simple repair, 2.5 cm forearm; intermediate repair, 1.5 cm hand; 2.0 cm simple repair, knee.

   Code(s):_____

Exercise 4.5   Integumentary System—ED/ Operative Reports

Answers to odd-numbered questions can be found in appendix C of this book. The answers to even-numbered questions are located in the instructor materials and are available to approved instructors.

ED Report #1

Emergency Department Record

Chief Complaint:	Laceration, left hand
History of Present Illness:	Patient is a 67-year-old woman who tripped over a brick. As she tried to break her fall, she somehow cut her left hand. She has a laceration at the base of her fifth finger on the palm side, but no other injuries.

Past Medical History:	Unremarkable
Medications:	None
Allergies:	None
Physical Examination:	
General:	Alert female in no acute distress
Extremities:	Left upper extremity examination reveals a 2.5-cm full-skin-thickness laceration on the palm side of the left hand just at the base of the finger over the volar metacarpal phalangeal joints. She has full active and passive range of motion.
Procedure:	Anesthesia local injection 2 cc 1% lidocaine plain; prepped and routine exploration revealed no foreign body. No neurovascular tendon injury noted. Repaired with six 5-0 nylon sutures. Polysporin ointment and dressing placed on the wound.
Diagnosis:	2.5-cm simple laceration, left hand
Disposition and Plan:	Wound care instructions given and advised to have sutures taken out in 10 to 12 days

Assign only CPT surgical codes (no E/M codes) and append any applicable modifiers.

Code(s): _____

ED Report #2

Emergency Department Record

Chief Complaint:	Right arm laceration
History of Present Illness:	This 24-year-old man presents here after attempting to punch out a window in his garage door with his elbow in an attempt to enter his own house.
Medications:	None
Allergies:	Keflex
Last Known Tetanus:	Unknown
Review of Systems:	No shoulder pain, no wrist pain. Complains of multiple lacerations of the forearm.
Extremities:	Right elbow and right forearm reveal multiple lacerations in various lengths from proximal and working distally. Over the area of the olecranon, there is noted to be a 3-cm superficial laceration. There is also noted to be several simple lacerations distally: approximately four measuring 1 cm and three others measuring 2 cm each. There is noted to be a 5-cm laceration involving deeper layers of skin.
Procedure:	After adequate anesthesia was obtained with local infiltration of all lacerations with 1% lidocaine with

(Continued on next page)

Exercise 4.5 (Continued)

epinephrine, the wounds were explored. No foreign bodies were appreciated. Each wound was vigorously irrigated and draped individually in a sterile fashion. Initially, the 3-cm laceration along the area of the olecranon was closed with two interrupted sutures of 4-0 Ethilon. The remaining smaller wounds were closed with simple sutures. The 5-cm laceration required closing with 3-0 Vicryl for the subcutaneous layer and 4-0 Vicryl to close the skin. Wound edges were painted with Benzoin and Steri-Strips applied. The patient tolerated the procedure well.

Assign only CPT surgical codes (no E/M codes) and append any applicable modifiers.

Code(s): _____

ED Report #3

Emergency Department Operative Note

Chief Complaint: Head laceration

History of Present Illness: This 85-year-old man was found in his basement with a bleeding head laceration. Examination revealed a scalp laceration, which is at the superior occiput. The laceration was approximately 8 cm and required a complex repair. The wound was irrigated as well as possible with normal saline. Subsequently, using 4-0 Vicryl suturing, some of the deeper structures were reapproximated with some hemostasis. Approximately three Vicryl sutures were placed deep in these structures. Multiple 4-0 nylon interrupted sutures were placed, with eventual control of the hemostasis. Several other staples were placed as well for further cosmetic closure of the skin. The procedure did provide complete resolution of the symptoms. There was a very complex and deep wound with active hemorrhage. Subsequent to this, it was cleansed and Neosporin was placed. Please note that multiple areas of hair were trimmed with scissors prior to this procedure.

Assign only CPT surgical codes (no E/M codes) and append any applicable modifiers.

Code(s): _____

Operative Report #4

Operative Report

Preoperative Diagnosis: Pigmented nevus, arm

Postoperative Diagnosis: Melanoma

Operation: Excision 1.5-cm nevus of arm

The patient was brought into the surgery center and prepped and draped in the usual manner. Local anesthesia was injected under the lesion. The lesion with 0.5-cm margins was excised taking full-thickness skin, transversely oblique. Hemostasis was obtained with cautery. The skin was closed in layers of 3-0 Vicryl in fascia, 5-0 Vicryl subcuticular, and 6-0 nylon in the skin. Dressing was applied.

Assign only CPT surgical codes (no E/M codes) and append any applicable modifiers.

Code(s): _____

Skin Grafting

Skin grafting is a method of treating damaged or lost skin in which a piece of skin is taken from another area of the body and transplanted to the area of the damaged or missing section. There are several code ranges to identify skin graft procedures.

Adjacent Skin Grafts

The first series of codes (14000–14350) identify grafts that maintain their own blood supply. If a lesion is removed and it results in an adjacent skin graft to cover the defect, the excision of the lesion is included in the skin graft procedure. Examples of tissue transfer or rearrangement (also known as local skin flaps) are: Z-plasty, W-plasty, V-Y plasty, rotation, advancement, or double pedicle flap. These codes are categorized first by body part involved and then by size of defect in square centimeters.

An additional code may be reported to describe any skin grafting required to close the secondary defect.

The following definitions are helpful when coding adjacent tissue transfer or arrangement procedures:

- *Advancement:* The sliding of a pedicle graft into its new position.
- *Pedicle graft:* Grafted tissue that remains connected to its vascular bed.
- *Z-plasty:* A tissue transfer that surgically releases tension in the skin caused by a laceration, contracted scar, or a wound along the flexion crease of a joint. It is characterized by a Z-shaped incision that is above, through, and below the scar or defect. This type of technique is used to reposition a scar so that it more closely conforms to the natural lines and creases of the skin, where it will be less noticeable.
- *W-plasty:* A tissue transfer performed to release tension along a straight scar. A W-shaped incision creates a series of triangular flaps of skin. The triangle flaps on both sides of the scar are removed, and the remaining skin triangles are moved together and sutured into place.
- *V-Y plasty:* A tissue transfer that begins with a V-shaped skin incision and with advancement and stretching of the skin and tissue. The defect is covered and forms a Y when sutured together.

- *Rotational flap:* These flaps are curved or semicircular and include the skin and subcutaneous tissues. A base is left, and the remaining portion of the flap is freed and rotated to cover the defect and then sutured into place.

Skin Replacement Surgery

The next range of skin graft codes are categorized into two groupings: Autograft (or tissue cultured autograft) and Skin Substitute Grafts. The subsection begins with surgical preparation codes (15002–15005).

Surgical Preparation

Codes 15002–15005 include surgical preparation of a site by excision of open wounds, eschar, or scar, including subcutaneous tissue. The code selection also includes incisional/excisional release of scar contracture. Code differentiation is made by the site and size of the area. A percentage of body surface for adults (and children age 10 years and older) is measured in increments of 100 square centimeters. The measure of infants and children (younger than 10 years) is in percentages of body surface area.

Autograft (or Tissue Cultured Autograft) Grafts

The next series of codes describes autograft skin grafts. Skin transplanted from one location to another on the same individual is termed an autograft (see figure 4.5 for an illustration of a skin graft).

> If the operative note stated that this was a 2.5 cm split-thickness graft taken from the thigh to replace the skin on the finger (figure 4.5), the code assignment would be 15120.

Figure 4.5. Skin graft harvest

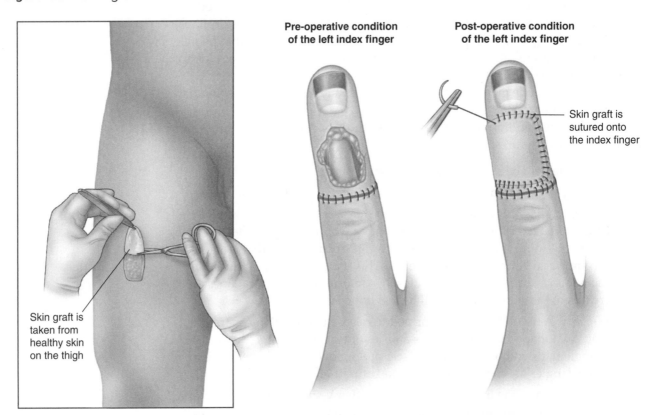

Pre-operative condition of the left index finger

Post-operative condition of the left index finger

Skin graft is sutured onto the index finger

Skin graft is taken from healthy skin on the thigh

Source: ©AHIMA.

These codes are categorized by type of graft (for example, pinch graft, split-thickness graft, or full-thickness graft), body part involved, and size of defect in square centimeters (except for pinch grafts, which are measured in centimeters). If the donor site requires skin grafting or local flaps, an additional code should be reported. CPT code 15040 is to be assigned for harvesting of skin for tissue-cultured skin autograft.

The following definitions are helpful when coding skin grafts:

- *Pinch graft:* This is a piece of skin graft about 0.25 inch in diameter that is obtained by elevating the skin with a needle and slicing it off with a knife.

- *Split-thickness graft:* This graft consists of only the superficial layers of the dermis.

- *Full-thickness graft:* This graft is composed of skin and subcutaneous tissues (see figure 4.6 for an illustration of depth of split-thickness and full-thickness grafts).

- *Allograft:* This graft is obtained from a genetically dissimilar individual of the same species (one individual to another). It is also known as allogenic graft and homograft.

- *Autograft:* A graft transferred from one part of the patient's body to another part.

- *Dermal autograft:* An autograph from which epidermis and subcutaneous fat has been removed; can be used in place of fascia.

- *Epidermal autograft:* An autograft consisting primarily of epidermal tissue including keratinocytes cells but with little dermal tissue.

- *Skin substitute:* Biomaterial engineered tissue or a combination of material and cells or tissues that can be substituted for skin autograft or allograft in a clinical procedure

- *Tissue-cultured*: Skin cells are removed from the patient and used to grow new skin for replacement.

Figure 4.6. Depth of split-thickness and full-thickness grafts

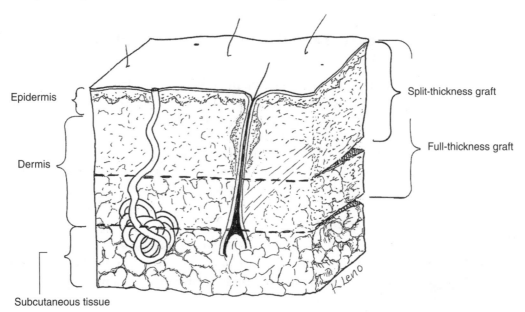

Source: ©AHIMA.

- *Xenograft:* This graft is obtained from a species different from the recipient (for example, animal to human). It is also called xenogenic graft, heterograft, and heterotransplant. Currently, pig skin is the most popular xenograft.

Tissue-Cultured Autograft

CPT codes 15150–15157 are assigned for tissue-cultured autograft procedures. For this technique, living, healthy skin cells are removed from a patient and used to grow thin sheets of new cells in a laboratory. The harvested cells are then placed in a cultured medium and cocultured with mouse cells, where the tissue is nutritionally supported and grown to the size of a playing card. This method is often used to treat deep dermal or full-thickness burns comprising a total body surface area of greater than or equal to 30 percent. Studies have supported the fact that these grafts are not rejected by the patient's immune system because they are recognized by the immune system as being part of the person's own body. Codes are differentiated by the size and location of the recipient site.

Epicel® is an example of a tissue-cultured autograft process.

Skin Substitute Grafts

Codes 15271–15278 are used to identify application of skin substitute grafts that are not autologous. The product may be from natural cells (such as human cadavers or pig skin) or a synthetic substitute. Common skin substitute grafts include:

- Biobrane®—consists of a nylon mesh, which acts as a dermis, and a silicon membrane, which acts as an epidermis
- Integra®—a silicone membrane is used as an epidermal layer
- Alloderm®—a skin substitute derived from a cadaveric dermis

Free Skin Grafts

Included in the Autograft subsection is a range of codes to identify full-thickness free skin grafts (15200–15261). If the dermis is included in its entirety, the appropriate term is full-thickness skin graft. Mirroring the other skin graft codes, the coding selection is based on site and size.

Removal of Skin Lesion with Skin Replacement/Substitute Graft

When an excision of a lesion requires a skin replacement/substitute graft (such as a split-thickness skin graft) for repair of the defect, the coding professional is directed to also assign a code to identify the excision of the lesion using a code from the range 11400 through 11471 or 11600 through 11646. This coding guidance differs from the guidance for an excision of a lesion with an adjacent skin graft. Review the note before code 14000, which indicates that the excision of a lesion is included in adjacent skin graft codes.

Flaps (Skin and/or Deep Tissues)

This series of codes (15570–15738) includes procedures describing pedicle flaps, muscle, myocutaneous or fasciocutaneous flaps, and delayed flap transfers. The codes are categorized first by type of flap (for example, pedicle) and then by recipient body part.

To differentiate between a flap and a graft: the blood source is intact with flaps but not for grafts.

Codes 15600 through 15630, which describe delayed transfer, identify the donor site, not the recipient site. An additional code should be reported when repair of the donor site requires skin grafting or local flaps.

The following definitions are helpful when coding flaps:

- *Pedicle flap:* This flap consists of detached skin and subcutaneous tissue in which the attached end or base contains an adequate blood supply. It is partially transferred to the recipient site with the base still attached to the donor site. After the recipient site has established a good blood supply, the base or pedicle is cut off and the graft completed.

- *Myocutaneous flap:* This flap involves the transfer of intact muscle, subcutaneous tissue, and skin as a single unit rotated on a relatively narrow blood supply of the muscle.

Free flap codes (15756–15758) describe procedures in which the tissue is completely removed from the site (free) but the vascular network comes along with the skin/muscle.

Other Flaps and Grafts

The last range of codes for skin grafts (15740–15776) identifies specialty procedures such as punch graft for hair transplants and neurovascular pedicle procedures. Add-on code 15777 is used for implantation of biologic implant. For example, use of acellular dermal matrix for breast reconstruction would include both the reconstruction code and 15777.

Exercise 4.6   Integumentary System—Skin Grafts

Answers to odd-numbered questions can be found in appendix C of this book. The answers to even-numbered questions are located in the instructor materials and are available to approved instructors.

Assign appropriate CPT code(s) for the following procedures. Assign only CPT surgical codes (no E/M codes) and append any applicable modifiers.

1. A 35-year-old patient sustained third-degree burns three weeks ago. A small skin graft was harvested at the time and submitted for tissue culturing. The patient is now admitted for grafting of the cultured tissue. A total of 20 sq cm is grafted onto the patient's arm during this encounter.

   Code(s): _____

2. Physician performs a wide resection of a 3.0-cm malignant skin lesion of the left leg. The defect required an adjacent tissue transfer measuring 15 sq cm.

   Code(s): _____

3. Surgeon performs a full-thickness skin graft, harvesting skin from the buttocks to the chest covering the 2 cm × 4 cm defect.

   Code(s): _____

4. The surgeon performed a tubed pedicle flap from the forehead to cover the defect on the nose.

   Code(s): _____

Exercise 4.7 Integumentary System-Operative Reports

Answers to odd-numbered questions can be found in appendix C of this book. The answers to even-numbered questions are located in the instructor materials and are available to approved instructors.

Operative Report #1

Operative Report

Preoperative Diagnosis: Basal cell carcinoma of the forehead

Postoperative Diagnosis: Same

Procedure: Excision of basal cell carcinoma with split-thickness skin graft

The patient was given a local IV sedation and taken to the OR suite. The face and left thigh were prepped with Phisohex soap. The cancer was outlined for excision and measured 5 × 4 cm. The forehead was infiltrated with 1% Xylocaine with 1:100,000 epinephrine.

The cancer was excised and carried down to the frontalis muscle. A suture was placed at the 12 o'clock position. The specimen was sent to pathology for frozen section.

Attention was then turned to the skin graft. A pattern of the defect was transferred to the left anterior thigh using a new needle. A local infiltration was performed on the thigh. Using a freehand knife, a split-thickness skin graft was harvested. The thigh was treated with Tegaderm and a wraparound Kerliz and Ace wrap. The skin graft was applied and sutured to the forehead defect with running 5-0 plain catgut.

Xeroform with cotton soaked in glycerin was sutured with 4-0 silk. A sterile dressing was applied. The patient tolerated the procedure well, with no complications or blood loss.

Assign only CPT surgical codes (no E/M codes) and append any applicable modifiers.

Code(s): _____

Operative Report #2

Operative Report

Preoperative Diagnosis: Open wound, left thigh, status post fasciotomy

Postoperative Diagnosis: Same

Procedure: Split-thickness skin graft, left thigh, donor site from left thigh. Graft was approximately 12 × 5 cm.

The patient is status post trauma. A tree fell on him and he sustained a significant injury to his thigh.

He had compartment syndrome of his thigh, requiring a fasciotomy. He presents today for a skin graft to the fasciotomy site.

The patient was brought to the operating room and placed supine on the operating table. Following the adequate induction of general anesthesia, his left thigh and fasciotomy site were prepped and draped in the standard surgical fashion. Attention was first directed to the patient's anterior thigh. The Betadine prep was gently removed with normal saline. We then applied mineral oil to the anterior thigh. We then used a dermatome to harvest an approximately 12 × 5-cm split-thickness skin graft in the depth of 0.015. Following removal of our donor site, an epinephrine-soaked sponge was applied to the donor site. We then went in to the back table and meshed our graft 1:1. Following this, we prepared our graft bed for graft placement. The excellent granulation tissue bed was roughed up using a gauze sponge, and the skin graft was applied and secured in place using surgical staples. The edge of the skin was then trimmed accordingly. Following adequate placement and securing our graft, we then fashioned the dressing. A Bacitracin-coated Adaptic was then applied over the graft and Reston foam was applied over that. Fine mesh gauze was then used to secure it in place, and the Reston and mesh gauze were secured also using surgical staples. There was an excellent compression against the graft. Following this, we turned our attention to the donor site. Epinephrine-soaked gauze was removed, and Calgiswab dressing was applied. There was excellent hemostasis from the donor site. Following this, a Kerlix roll was placed around the left thigh and secured with paper tape. The patient tolerated the procedure without complications. The patient was then taken to the PACU for recovery.

Assign only CPT surgical codes (no E/M codes) and append any applicable modifiers.

Code(s): _____

Mohs Micrographic Surgery

Mohs surgery (17311–17315) is a specialized treatment for skin cancer cases that usually involves several stages with histologic examination of 100 percent of the surgical margins. The selective removal of skin cancer allows for preservation of as much of the surrounding normal tissue as possible. After the removal of the visible portion of the tumor, the surgeon excises a thin layer of tissue that is processed and examined under the microscope. This process includes dividing the tumor specimen into pieces, and each individual piece is embedded into an individual tissue block that is histopathologically examined. If any tumor is seen during the microscopic examination, its location is established, and a thin layer of additional tissue is excised from the involved area. The microscopic examination is then repeated. The entire process is repeated until no tumor is found. The Mohs surgery codes are differentiated by the stage of the procedure, site, and number of tissue blocks.

Surgical Procedures of the Breast

Codes 19000 through 19499 describe procedures performed on the breast, such as biopsy, mastectomy, and reconstruction. These codes are categorized first by general type of procedure (incision, excision, reconstruction/repair) and then by specific procedure.

The codes describing breast procedures refer to unilateral procedures, and modifiers LT or RT should be appended. If a bilateral procedure is performed, modifier 50 should be reported.

Breast Biopsy

In coding breast biopsies, the coding professional must determine the type of biopsy performed: percutaneous, excisional, or incisional:

- *Percutaneous biopsy:* A biopsy that involves the insertion of a hollow needle to remove a biopsy specimen of breast tissue. This procedure is reported with code 19100. See figure 4.7.

- *Excisional biopsy:* The operative phrase excisional biopsy can be confusing. The documentation usually means that the entire lesion was removed, in contrast to an incisional biopsy in which only a sample of tissue is cut out. To make this determination, the coding professional should review both the operative report and the pathology report. The operative report should indicate that the lesion was removed completely. In the case of malignant lesions, the pathology report may indicate that the margins of the specimen are negative for malignancy or free of tumor. CPT code 19120 is reported when the entire breast lesion is removed.

- *Breast Biopsy with Localization Devices:* Surgeons may elect to identify the precise location of abnormal breast tissue with a localization device (such as clip or wire) before a breast biopsy procedure. For example, if a suspicious area was identified on a mammogram, a marker will confirm the location for the surgeon. Bundled codes have been created to describe breast biopsy procedures that include imaging guidance as well as placement of one or more localization devices. The range of codes (19081–19086) includes the biopsy procedure, placement of the device, and imaging. The codes can be distinguished by the type of imaging guidance and the number of lesions marked with the device. A separate range of codes (19281–19288) is provided to report just the placement of the device (without performing a biopsy).

- *Incisional biopsy:* A biopsy of the breast (19101) that typically involves removal of only a portion of the lesion for pathologic examination.

Figure 4.7. Needle breast biopsy

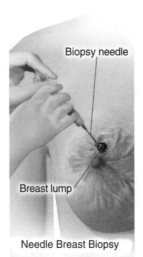

Source: Blaus Bruce. "Needle Breast Biopsy." Digital Image. Wikimedia Commons. February, 2016. Accessed October, 2018. https://commons.wikimedia.org/wiki/File:Needle_Breast_Biopsy.png.

> If the operative report stated that the core needle biopsy procedure was performed without guidance (figure 4.7), the correct code assignment would be 19100-RT.

Mastectomy

Codes 19300 through 19307 describe the various types of mastectomy:

- Code 19301, Partial mastectomy, refers to the partial removal of part of the breast tissue, leaving the breast almost intact. This also may be referred to as a lobectomy or lumpectomy. If an axillary lymphectomy is also performed, the correct coding assignment would be 19302.

- Code 19303, Simple, complete mastectomy, is assigned for the excision of all the breast tissue, with the lymph nodes and muscle left intact.

- Code 19304, Subcutaneous mastectomy, is used for excision of breast tissue with the skin and nipple intact. This is often referred to as a skin-sparing procedure.

- Code 19305, Radical mastectomy, refers to the excision of breast tissue including the pectoral muscles and the axillary lymph nodes.

- Code 19306, Radical mastectomy, is assigned for the excision of breast tissue including the pectoral muscles and axillary lymph nodes (see code 19305 above), and also includes the internal mammary lymph nodes.

- Code 19307, Modified radical mastectomy, is used for the excision of breast tissue including the axillary lymph nodes. The pectoralis minor muscles may or may not be removed, but the pectoralis major muscles are left intact. Figure 4.8 illustrates a modified radical mastectomy with removal of axillary lymph nodes.

Insertion of breast prosthesis may be reported as an additional code when performed at the same time as the mastectomy (19340) or when performed at a later date (19342).

Breast Reconstruction

A series of codes beginning with 19316 focuses on reconstruction of the breast, such as with muscle flaps. For example, code 19361 captures a latissimus dorsi flap where the surgeon uses a flap of skin, muscle, or blood vessels from the back, which is rotated to reconstruct the breast. Another type of flap, called a transverse rectum abdominis myocutaneous flap (TRAM), is depicted in figure 4.9.

Modified radical mastectomy with regional lymph nodes (figure 4.8) would be a combination code, 19307-RT.

Figure 4.8. Modified radical mastectomy

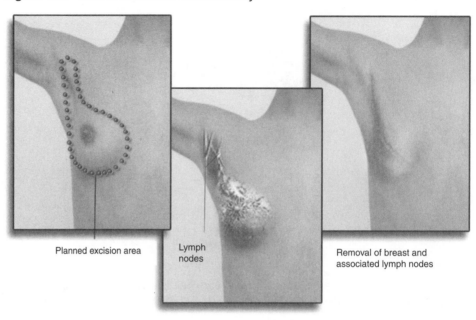

Planned excision area

Lymph nodes

Removal of breast and associated lymph nodes

Source: ©AHIMA.

Note that this TRAM procedure (figure 4.9) is a single pedicle. If the documentation stated that the blood vessels were also anastomosed to the reconstructed breast, the code would be 19368.

Figure 4.9. Transverse rectus abdominis myocutaneous flap (TRAM) for breast reconstruction

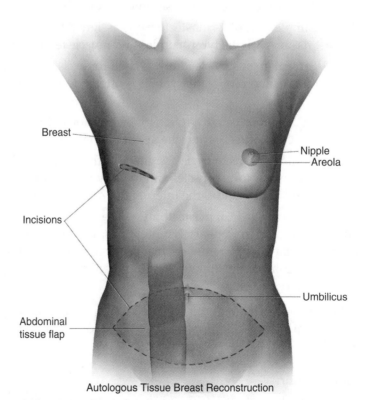

Breast

Nipple
Areola

Incisions

Umbilicus

Abdominal tissue flap

Autologous Tissue Breast Reconstruction

Source: Blaus Bruce. "Breast Reconstruction TRAM. Digital Image. Wikimedia Commons. January 2014. Accessed September, 2018. https://commons.wikimedia.org/wiki/File:Blausen_0140_BreastReconstruction_ TRAM.png.

Exercise 4.8   Integumentary System—Operative Reports

Answers to odd-numbered questions can be found in appendix C of this book. The answers to even-numbered questions are located in the instructor materials and are available to approved instructors.

Operative Report #1

Physician Office Operative Note

This patient has come to see me for follow-up for a cyst present in the left breast area. I did a needle aspiration biopsy, and fluid was sent out for cytology. If the biopsy is negative, I can see her back in the office in four months, or earlier if there are any problems.

The right breast feels benign. There is no axillary adenopathy. No cervical adenopathy.

Hospital pathology of a sample from a left breast aspiration revealed only a few benign lipocytes.

Assign only CPT surgical codes (no E/M codes) and append any applicable modifiers.

Code(s): _____

Operative Report #2

Operative Report

Preoperative Diagnosis: Abnormal mammogram, left breast

Postoperative Diagnosis: Same

The patient is a 61-year-old G3, P3 female with a family history of positive carcinoma of the breast. She underwent a screening mammogram in the spring of this year that demonstrated a localized density in the subareolar tissue of the left breast. Physical examination demonstrated no palpable abnormality in the area.

The patient was brought to the OR after undergoing placement of a hook wire localizing needle in the mammography suite by the radiologist. She was placed on the OR table in a supine position. After ensuring an adequate level of conscious sedation, her left breast and chest wall were prepped and draped in a sterile fashion. A needle/wire complex was protruding from the left breast approximately 2 centimeters above the nipple. The skin surrounding the needle in the breast tissue in the subareolar area was infiltrated with 1% Xylocaine to achieve local anesthesia. A 5-cm incision was made around the localizing wire. Small superior and inferior skin flaps were elevated, exposing the underlying

(Continued on next page)

Exercise 4.8   (Continued)

subcutaneous fat. Dissection with electrocautery was begun into the breast about the wire. The needle wire complex was grasped using Allis clamps and drawn into the operative wound. The breast tissue and subcutaneous fat surrounding the needle were excised in this fashion until all the tissue surrounding the needle/wire complex was excised. The specimen was then forwarded to the radiology suite for specimen mammography.

As the specimen mammogram was being obtained, the wound was examined for hemostasis, which was thought to be complete. The deeper breast tissues were closed using interrupted 3-0 Vicryl figure-of-8 sutures. Subcutaneous tissues were approximated in a similar fashion. The wound was irrigated and again examined for hemostasis, which was thought to be complete. The skin was closed using a running 5-0 Maxon subcuticular suture. The wound was washed and dried and sterile dressings applied. The operative field was not disturbed until a call was received from the radiology suite indicating that the specimen contained the area of interest identified on the patient's original mammogram. At this point, the patient was transferred to the recovery area in stable condition.

Assign only CPT surgical codes (no E/M codes) and append any applicable modifiers.

Code(s): _____

Operative Report #3

Operative Report

Preoperative Diagnosis: Probable carcinoma of the right breast

Postoperative Diagnosis: Carcinoma of the right breast

Operation: Excisional biopsy

The patient was brought to the OR. Under satisfactory general endotracheal anesthesia, the right breast was prepped and draped in the usual manner. Through an elliptical incision in the upper outer quadrant, a small nodule was excised. Bleeders were electrocoagulated. The deep layer was closed with interrupted 3-0 Vicryl. The skin was closed with clips. A dry sterile dressing was applied, and the patient returned to the recovery room in good condition.

Pathology Report

Clinical Diagnosis: Right breast mass

Specimen: Mass, right breast, frozen section

Pathological Diagnosis: Breast mass, right: infiltrating ductal carcinoma, Grade 2/3, 0.7 cm; resected margins negative for carcinoma

Assign only CPT surgical codes (no E/M codes) and append any applicable modifiers.

Code(s): _____

Exercise 4.9   Integumentary System Review

Answers to odd-numbered questions can be found in appendix C of this book. The answers to even-numbered questions are located in the instructor materials and are available to approved instructors.

Assign appropriate CPT code(s) for the following procedures. Assign only CPT surgical codes (no E/M codes) and append any applicable modifiers.

1. Debridement and dressing of first-degree (partial-thickness) burn of the index finger

   Code(s): _____

2. Debridement of below-knee amputation stump. The necrotic wounds were sharply excised down to and including the fascia with a 10-blade scalpel (15 sq cm).

   Code(s): _____

3. Intermediate, layered closure of 2.0-cm laceration of right forearm and intermediate closure of 2.5-cm laceration of left elbow

   Code(s): _____

4. Fine needle aspiration biopsy of mass in chest, under fluoroscopic guidance

   Code(s): _____

5. Excision of malignant melanoma of left arm (3.0 cm × 1.5 cm, with 1.0-cm margins surrounding the lesion)

   Code(s): _____

6. Bilateral total mastectomy with reconstruction using double-pedicle TRAM

   Code(s): _____

(Continued on next page)

Exercise 4.9   (Continued)

7. Complete excision of nail and matrix, right great toe

Code(s): _____

8. With the use of ultrasound guidance, the surgeon placed a metallic clip to identify the suspicious tissue in the left breast. A percutaneous core needle biopsy was performed.

Code(s): _____

9. Electrosurgical fulguration was used to remove a 2.0-cm squamous cell carcinoma of the hand

Code(s): _____

10. Wide excision of a malignant lesion of back (5.0 cm × 3.0 cm) with adjacent skin graft

Code(s): _____

Musculoskeletal System

Learning Objectives

- Describe criteria for coding lipomas of the skin versus the musculoskeletal system.
- Identify documentation to support coding fractures and dislocations.
- Define *manipulation*.
- Distinguish between open fracture and open reduction.
- Identify when it is appropriate to assign a casting/strapping code.
- Differentiate between an open procedure and endoscopic technique (such as arthroscopy).
- Explain the organization of codes for arthrodesis of the spine.

For each new section, take a few minutes to flip through the code book pages and discover the organization of codes.

The musculoskeletal subsection is categorized first by body part and then by general type of procedure, with the individual codes describing the specific procedure performed. The first series of codes describes general musculoskeletal procedures such as bone biopsy, application of fixation device, bone graft, replantation of body part, wound exploration, and arthrocentesis. A lengthy note at the beginning of this subsection defines terms related to the treatment of fractures.

The codes listed in this subsection include the application and removal of the first cast and/or traction device. Subsequent replacement of the cast and/or traction device may be reported with codes 29000 through 29799 and codes located at the beginning of the general subsection.

Integumentary vs. Musculoskeletal Codes

In the integumentary system section, it was noted that procedure codes associated with skin abscesses/cysts (tumors) may be found in the Musculoskeletal system section. Fascia is a layer of fibrous connective tissue that surrounds muscles. Soft tissue tumors may extend beyond the skin into the subcutaneous fascia (located beneath the dermis) or in the subfascia (below [deep] fascia but not involving the bone). Coding professionals must read the documentation to determine the location and size of the soft tissue tumors. If the physician documents an incision of an abscess that extends beyond the skin into the soft tissues (muscle, fascia, or tendon), then the musculoskeletal code would be appropriate. Note the following examples:

Example 1:

Patient is seen in the physician's office for an infected epidermal inclusion cyst of the arm that requires an incision and drainage. (Integumentary code 10060)

Example 2:

Physician removes a 1.5-cm lipoma located in the subcutaneous layer of the scalp. (Musculoskeletal code 21011)

Example 3:

Physician excises a 1.5-cm lipoma located in the subfascial tissue of the scalp. (Musculoskeletal code 21013)

Fractures and Dislocations

To report the diagnosis and treatment of fractures and dislocations accurately, coding professionals must answer the following questions:

- *What body site is involved?* The operative report and/or any diagnostic tests performed, such as x-rays or computed tomography (CT) scans, should be reviewed.

- *Was the fracture/dislocation treatment open or closed or with percutaneous skeletal fixation?* This part of the coding decision-making refers to the fracture treatment not the physician's diagnosis. The diagnosis of a closed fracture is when the bone breaks but there is no puncture or open wound in the skin. An open fracture is one in which the bone breaks through the skin. Although the diagnosis determines the treatment options, the coding selection is based on the procedure performed.

  Treatment: There are several methods of reduction for fractures. **Closed treatment** refers to treatment of the fracture/dislocation without a surgical incision into the site. The physician manipulates the bone fragments without surgical exposure. **Open treatment** refers to the treatment of a fracture or dislocation that includes exposing the site via a surgical incision or when a fractured bone is opened remote from the fracture site in order to insert an intramedullary (through the marrow) nail across the fracture site (fracture site is not opened and visualized). **Percutaneous skeletal fixation** involves treatment of a fracture by

> Be careful with the description of the fracture and operative technique. It is common practice for the surgeon to perform an open reduction on a closed fracture.

placing fixation devices such as pins across the fracture site, usually under x-ray imaging.

- *Was the fracture/dislocation manipulated?* Many CPT codes include the choice of coding with or without manipulation (see example below). Manipulation refers to repositioning the bone back to its original position. Surgeons often refer to this procedure as a fracture reduction. If a fracture is nondisplaced it means that the pieces of the fractured bone are still aligned; therefore, manipulation is not needed. Treatment of a nondisplaced fracture may include rotational alignment, splinting, and taping or internal fixation.

Example:

28490	Closed treatment of fracture great toe, phalanx or phalanges; *without* manipulation
28495	*with* manipulation

- *Did the procedure include internal or external fixation?* Many of the code selections provide a reference to orthopedic devices. Note the examples below:

Example:

27253	Open treatment of hip dislocation, traumatic, *without internal fixation*
27254	Open treatment of hip dislocation, traumatic, with acetabular wall and femoral head fracture, *with or without internal or external fixation*

Application of Casts and Strapping

The series of codes (29000–29750) describing the application of casts and strapping can be reported in the following scenarios:

- To identify replacement of a cast or strapping during or after the period of normal follow-up care (global postoperative period)
- To identify an initial service performed without any restorative treatment or stabilization of the fracture, injury, or dislocation and/or to afford pain relief to the patient
- To identify an initial cast or strapping when the same physician does not perform, or is not expected to perform, any other treatment or procedure
- To identify an initial cast or strapping when another physician provided or will provide restorative treatment

CPT guidelines for hospital outpatient reporting of casting/strapping/splinting can be found in *CPT Assistant* (Vol. 12, Issue 4, April 2002).

Exercise 4.10 Musculoskeletal System—Fractures

Answers to odd-numbered questions can be found in appendix C of this book. The answers to even-numbered questions are located in the instructor materials and are available to approved instructors.

Assign appropriate CPT code(s) for the following procedures. Assign only CPT surgical codes (no E/M codes) and append any applicable modifiers.

1. Diagnosis: Closed fracture of ulnar shaft, left Procedure: Open reduction of ulnar shaft fracture

   Code(s): _____

2. Open reduction with internal fixation (screws), for a fracture of the left humeral shaft

   Code(s): _____

3. Closed reduction of proximal humerus fracture, right

   Code(s): _____

4. The orthopedic surgeon reduces a fracture of the left proximal fibula. After closed treatment and skeletal traction, the physician applies a short leg cast.

   Code(s): _____

5. The patient was diagnosed with a dislocated right patella. The surgeon performed a closed reduction with the patient under anesthesia.

   Code(s): _____

6. Open treatment with internal fixation of three rib fractures

   Code(s): _____

7. Patient is diagnosed with right humeral shaft fracture. The orthopedic surgeon performs an open treatment of the fracture using an intramedullary implant and locking screws.

   Code(s): _____

8. The surgeon performed open reduction with internal fixation of medial condylar fracture of the humerus.

   Code(s): _____

9. Open reduction with internal fixation (ORIF) of the proximal left tibia, unicondylar

   Code(s): _____

10. Open reduction with internal fixation (ORIF) of intertrochanteric fractured femur using Gamma nail.

    Code(s): _____

Exercise 4.11 Musculoskeletal System—ED/ Operative Reports

Answers to odd-numbered questions can be found in appendix C of this book. The answers to even-numbered questions are located in the instructor materials and are available to approved instructors.

ED Report #1

Emergency Department Record

Chief Complaint: Right ankle injury

History of Present Illness: The patient is a 39-year-old woman who injured her right ankle yesterday. While stepping around some puppies to avoid hitting them, she suffered an inversion injury to her ankle. She complains of lateral ankle and foot pain, and has pain on weight bearing.

Past Medical History: Status post hysterectomy

Medications: None

Allergies: Codeine, which causes nausea

Physical Examination: Alert female in no acute distress. Right lower extremity: proximal mid tibia-fibula are nontender. Ankle shows moderate diffuse swelling over the lateral ankle extending onto the dorsolateral foot with ecchymoses. Good distal neurovascular status. Decreased range of motion secondary to pain and swelling.

Emergency Department X-ray of right foot and ankle shows an avulsion fragment off the distal fibula.

Course: Otherwise soft tissue swelling.

Diagnosis: Acute right ankle sprain with avulsion fracture

Disposition and Plan: Short leg splint applied. Crutches. No weight bearing. Ice and elevate. Vicodin #30 1–2 q 4–6 h. She tolerates it well. Orthopedic referral.

Assign only CPT surgical codes (no E/M codes) and append any applicable modifiers.

Code(s): _____

Operative Report #2

Operative Report

Preoperative Diagnosis: Fracture of distal fibula, left

Postoperative Diagnosis: Same

Procedure: Closed reduction of fibular fracture

This 14-year-old gymnast feels pain in her left leg after vaulting at practice. She is unable to bear any weight on her foot.

Physical examination showed foot and ankle to be normal. The neurovascular status of the foot was normal. The ankle was nontender and not swollen. Findings were confined to the distal fibula, 2 inches proximal to the lateral malleolus. There was point tenderness in this area. An x-ray of the tibia and fibula shows a displaced fracture of the distal fibula.

The fracture was reduced and the patient placed in a short leg splint with extensive padding over the fracture site. She was given Tylenol #3 for pain and instructed to follow up with her physician in 10 days.

Assign only CPT surgical codes (no E/M codes) and append any applicable modifiers.

Code(s): _____

Arthroscopy

Procedures describing both diagnostic and therapeutic arthroscopy are reported with codes 29800 through 29909. These codes are categorized first by body part involved and then by type—surgical or diagnostic. The surgical arthroscopic codes are further divided to identify the specific procedure performed, such as synovectomy or debridement. A surgical arthroscopy always includes a diagnostic component that should not be reported separately.

All of the arthroscopic codes for musculoskeletal procedures are in the back of the code book chapter. This format is not followed in other sections of CPT.

Exercise 4.12   Musculoskeletal System— Arthroscopy

Answers to odd-numbered questions can be found in appendix C of this book. The answers to even-numbered questions are located in the instructor materials and are available to approved instructors.

Assign appropriate CPT code(s) for the following procedures. Assign only CPT surgical codes (no E/M codes) and append any applicable modifiers.

1. Arthroscopy of left shoulder with rotator cuff repair

   Code(s): _____

2. Arthroscopic synovectomy of the medial and lateral tibiofemoral compartments and the patellofemoral compartment of the left knee

   Code(s): _____

(Continued on next page)

Exercise 4.12 (Continued)

3. Arthroscopy of the right elbow with complete synovectomy

   Code(s): _____

4. Arthroscopy of the left wrist with repair of triangular fibrocartilage and joint debridement

   Code(s): _____

Exercise 4.13 Musculoskeletal System—Operative Report

Answers to odd-numbered questions can be found in appendix C of this book. The answers to even-numbered questions are located in the instructor materials and are available to approved instructors.

Operative Report #1

Operative Report

Preoperative Diagnosis: Tear of the right medial meniscus

Postoperative Diagnosis: Same

Operation: Meniscus repair

The patient was brought to the OR and anesthetized. An inflatable tourniquet was placed about the proximal thigh, and the operative area was prepared and draped in a sterile fashion with the leg placed in the instrument maker leg holder. Following this, incisions were made for insertion of the arthroscope inflow cannula and probe. Video arthroscopy was then carried out. He was found to have a tear of the posterior horn of the medial meniscus, and this was repaired. The anterior cruciate ligament was examined and found to be intact. The lateral meniscus also appeared to be intact. The patellofemoral joint was within normal limits. While the patient was asleep, the knee was examined and stressed. There was no opening of the medial collateral ligament region and no instability in that area. After completion of the arthroscopy, the instruments were withdrawn from the wound and the incisions closed. The incisions were injected marginally with local anesthetic for postoperative analgesia. After closure of the incisions, Betadine ointment and dressings were placed over the knee, and the patient was returned to the recovery room in stable condition.

Assign only CPT surgical codes (no E/M codes) and append any applicable modifiers.

Code(s): _____

Spine Surgery

The musculoskeletal chapter contains codes for reporting spinal fusion, beginning with code 22532. Spinal fusion is often performed to join together two or more vertebrae into a single immobile structure. It is typically performed to stop pain caused by movement. CPT organizes this section based on approach (for example, anterior or posterior), location (such as cervical or lumbar), and number of vertebral segments. A *vertebral segment* consists of two vertebral bones with a space between, called interspace. Figure 4.10 provides an anterior and posterior view of vertebrae stacked with two bones (bodies) separated by an intervertebral disc. For example, the surgeon may document that the fusion occurred at L4-L5—that is, two vertebrae separated by one interspace (disc), or one segment.

> Coding spinal procedures is considered an advanced skill that requires thorough knowledge of both anatomy and how the procedures are performed.

Note the code description for code 22554:

22554   Arthrodesis, anterior interbody technique, including minimal discectomy to prepare interspace (other than for decompression); cervical below C2

In plain language, code 22554 explains that the patient had vertebral bones fused in the cervical column below the level C2 (front side of the neck). The surgeon took the disc out and replaced this interbody structure with a bone graft. It is important to note that spinal fusion must include some sort of bone graft or a composite of body graft material for the fusion to work. A device may be used to hold the graft material, but the device alone does not create fusion; the bone graft creates the fusion. If additional segments of the same site were also fused, it would be reported with an add-on code, 22585.

> If the operative report stated that the patient had a posterior spinal fusion at L2-L3 using an interbody technique, the correct code would be 22630.

Coding spinal procedures often requires additional codes for obtaining a bone graft or using spinal instrumentation. This advanced coding concept is illustrated in the following case study.

Figure 4.10.   Vertebra

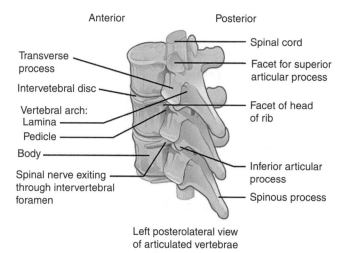

Left posterolateral view
of articulated vertebrae

Source: BodyParts3D/Anatomography. "Left posterolateral view of articulated vertebra." Digital Image. Wikimedia Commons. July, 2014. Accessed October, 2018. https://commons.wikimedia.org/wiki /File:Vertebra_Posterolateral.jpg.

Case Study ··

The patient had an anterior cervical fusion at C4-C5 for decompression. A discectomy was performed and replaced with a polyetheretherketone (PEEK) intervertebral device packed with morselized allograft bone.

CPT Code Assignment

22551 Arthrodesis, anterior interbody, including disc space preparation, discectomy, osteophytectomy and decompression of spinal cord and/or nerve roots; cervical below C2

22853 Insertion of interbody biomechanical device(s) (e.g., synthetic cage, mesh) with integral anterior instrumentation for device anchoring (e.g., screws, flanges), when performed, to intervertebral disc space in conjunction with interbody arthrodesis, each interspace (List separately in addition to code for primary procedure)

20930 Allograft, morselized, or placement of osteopromotive material, for spine surgery only (List separately in addition to code for primary procedure)

Exercise 4.14   Musculoskeletal System Review

Answers to odd-numbered questions can be found in appendix C of this book. The answers to even-numbered questions are located in the instructor materials and are available to approved instructors.

Assign appropriate CPT code(s) for the following procedures. Assign only CPT surgical codes (no E/M codes) and append any applicable modifiers.

1. Closed reduction of two metatarsal fractures of left foot

    Code(s): _____

2. Repair of hammertoe, second digit of right foot

    Code(s): _____

3. Open reduction of fracture of right posterior malleolus with internal fixation

    Code(s): _____

4. Removal of splinter embedded deep in the left knee

    Code(s): _____

5. Incision and drainage of hematoma of the thigh

    Code(s): _____

6. Arthroscopy of the right wrist with complete synovectomy

    Code(s): _____

7. Metatarsophalangeal arthrodesis, great toe

   Code(s): _____

8. Repair of medial collateral ligament of right elbow using local tissue

   Code(s): _____

9. Excision of bone cyst, toe (third digit of left foot)

   Code(s): _____

10. Surgical exploration of stab wound of chest with included coagulation of blood vessels and enlargement of the wound.

    Code(s): _____

11. Anterior lumbar interbody fusion (ALIF) with PEEK cage device packed with morselized bone allograft.

    Code(s): _____

Respiratory System

Learning Objectives

- Describe general guidelines for coding nasal endoscopy procedures.
- Differentiate between direct, indirect, and flexible laryngoscopy procedures.
- Define *bronchoscopy*.
- Describe an EBUS procedure.
- Differentiate between a pneumonectomy, lobectomy, wedge resection, and segmental resection.
- Distinguish between diagnostic and therapeutic procedures.
- Differentiate between thoracotomy procedures and VATS.

The respiratory subsection includes surgical procedures involving the nose and sinuses, larynx, trachea and bronchi, and lungs and pleura. Figures 4.11 and 4.12 illustrate the respiratory system.

Nasal Sinus Endoscopy

Beginning with 31231, the codes describe nasal sinus endoscopic procedures. These procedures allow the physician to visualize the interior of the nasal cavity, the middle and superior meatus, the turbinates, and the sphenoethmoid recess. The purpose of the procedures may be either diagnostic or surgical in nature. A surgical endoscopy may be performed to control a nosebleed or to perform a maxillary antrostomy or sphenoidotomy. The coding professional should always review the documentation carefully to clarify the extent of the procedure. A surgical endoscopy includes the diagnostic component. The diagnostic

Figure 4.11.   The upper respiratory system

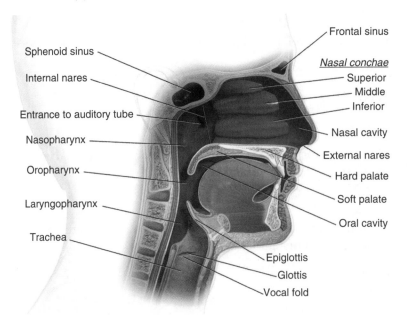

Source: Blaus, Bruce. "The Upper Respiratory System." Digital Image. Wikimedia Commons. August, 2013. Accessed September, 2018. https://commons.wikimedia.org/wiki/File:Blausen_0872 _UpperRespiratorySystem.png.

Figure 4.12.   The lower respiratory system

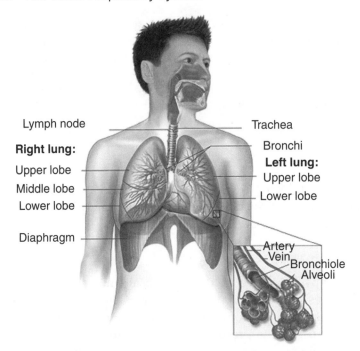

Source: ©AHIMA.

endoscopy should not be reported separately when performed during the same operative episode. Also, if performed, a sinusotomy is considered part of the endoscopic procedure and not reported separately.

Unless otherwise stated, the codes in this section are assumed to be unilateral. When the documentation indicates that a bilateral procedure was performed

and the specific code does not state *bilateral,* modifier 50 may be assigned. Key
points to remember include:

- Separate codes should not be assigned to identify a diagnostic nasal/
  sinus endoscopy when it is performed in conjunction with a surgical
  nasal/sinus endoscopy.
- A surgical endoscopy includes a sinusotomy. Only the code for the
  surgical endoscopy should be assigned when both are performed during
  the same operative episode.
- Modifier 50 should be assigned to identify a bilateral procedure only if
  the code does not specify bilateral.

Exercise 4.15   Respiratory System—Endoscopy

**Answers to odd-numbered questions can be found in appendix C of this
book. The answers to even-numbered questions are located in the instructor
materials and are available to approved instructors.**

Assign appropriate CPT code(s) for the following procedures. Assign only CPT
surgical codes (no E/M codes) and append any applicable modifiers.

1. Bilateral nasal endoscopy with total ethmoidectomy

   Code(s): _____

2. Left nasal endoscopy for control of epistaxis

   Code(s): _____

3. Diagnostic maxillary sinusoscopy, bilateral

   Code(s): _____

4. Endoscopic anterior and posterior ethmoidectomy with sphenoidotomy
   and frontal sinus exploration

   Code(s): _____

Exercise 4.16   Respiratory System

**Answers to odd-numbered questions can be found in appendix C of this
book. The answers to even-numbered questions are located in the instructor
materials and are available to approved instructors.**

Operative Report #1

Operative Report

Preoperative Diagnosis: Deviated nasal septum, chronic maxillary sinusitis,
turbinate hypertrophy, nasal obstruction

Postoperative Diagnosis: Same

(Continued on next page)

Exercise 4.16 (Continued)

Procedure Performed:

1. Septoplasty

2. Nasal endoscopy, with bilateral maxillary antroscopy, removal of maxillary polyp

3. Submucous resection of the inferior turbinates, bilaterally

This 26-year-old woman was seen by ENT service for complaints of chronic sinusitis and difficulty breathing through the nose. She was noted to have a severely deviated septum toward the right with turbinate hypertrophy, nasal obstruction (CT scans confirmed this), as well as obstruction of the ostiomeatal complexes with mucosal thickening. A decision for the above-stated procedure was then made after she had failed conservative care.

The patient was brought to the operative suite, given general anesthetic, and properly prepped and draped. 5% cocaine pledgets were placed in each nasal chamber. 1% lidocaine with 1:100,000 epinephrine was injected into the caudal columnar region into the septum, as well as the middle uncinate middle turbinate region. Then, with the #1 scalpel blade, an incision was made along the left caudal columnar region in the septum, down to the mucoperichondrium. The mucoperichondrium was carefully elevated off the nasal septum cartilage, exposing a portion of the deviation. The contralateral portion was also freed up. With a Seiler knife, a portion of the deviation was removed. A large septal spur, touching the lateral wall, was carefully freed up and removed.

After the patient exhibited a much improved nasal septum, a piece of cartilage was morcellized and inserted between the septal mucosa layers, and the submucosa was closed with 4-0 plain suture in interrupted form. Attention was then brought to the middle turbinates, which were found to be lateralized. A decision to medialize them was made by placing 4-0 Vicryl to the left middle turbinate, sent through the right middle turbinate, back to the septum, and tied off on the left side.

Next, with the scope, the left nasal chamber was examined. The natural os was located. With the frontal probe, it was further enlarged with microbiter straight shot and back-biters. There was a moderate amount of mucosal thickening around this opening, just on the inside. After it was widely patent and cleaned out, attention was brought to the right side. The right os was located in a similar fashion and widely enlarged with the microbiter straight shot and back-biters. Again, a moderate amount of mucosal thickening was noted around this opening. When this was completed, attention was brought to the inferior turbinates.

The inferior turbinates were infractured and clamped with a Carmel clamp for five minutes, then submucosal resection was performed in the usual fashion. The rods of the turbinates were then cauterized with suction cautery. This was repeated in a similar fashion bilaterally. Silastic splints were sewn into place along the septum with 3-0 Ethilon, and tampons coated in Bactroban were inserted into both nasal chambers. The oral cavity was suctioned of all serosanguineous debris, and the patient exhibited good hemostasis. She recovered from the anesthetic and was transferred to the recovery room in stable condition.

Assign only CPT surgical codes (no E/M codes) and append any applicable modifiers.

Code(s) to be submitted for the hospital services: _____

Laryngoscopy

A laryngoscopy is an endoscopic procedure that allows the physician to visualize the larynx, or voice box. This examination may be diagnostic only or may be performed for surgical purposes such as for a biopsy or removal of a lesion. Codes 31505–31579 describe these diagnostic and surgical endoscopic procedures.

Indirect Laryngoscopy

Codes 31505 through 31513 refer to an indirect laryngoscopy. An indirect laryngoscopy is the simplest way to examine the larynx. One technique involves the use of a small mirror placed in the back of the throat. With the aid of a light source, the image of the larynx can be visualized in the mirror. The physician may view the image of the oropharynx, posterior third of the tongue, lateral laryngeal walls, posterior pharyngeal wall, epiglottis, valleculae, and piriform sinuses. He or she also may be able to view the aryepiglottic folds, posterior epiglottis, and vocal cords. Although an indirect laryngoscopy is the simplest and least expensive way to examine the larynx, it does require a great deal of skill on the part of the physician. Moreover, this technique may be impossible to perform on a patient who has a strong gag reflex, and it cannot be used on small children.

Direct Laryngoscopy

Codes 31515 through 31571 are used to identify a direct laryngoscopy. This range of codes identifies the performance of procedures such as biopsy, removal of a lesion, arytenoidectomy, and removal of a foreign body. Laryngoscopes that are commonly used include Kleinsasser, Jako, Dedo, Jackson, Lindholm, Nagashima, Holinger, and Benjamin. During this complex procedure, the physician looks directly at the larynx. The patient is usually placed under general anesthesia to avoid the difficulties associated with the gag reflex. A microscope also may be used during the procedure to magnify the image of the larynx. Because the code assignment will be affected, the coding professional should review the operative report carefully for any mention of a microscope or for terms such as microlaryngoscopy. It is inappropriate to use code 69990, Use of operating microscope, in addition to any laryngoscopy code identified as being done with an operating microscope.

Flexible Laryngoscopy

Codes 31575 through 31578 are used for a laryngoscopy performed with flexible equipment. After administration of a topical anesthesia and vasoconstrictor, the instrument is passed through the nasal cavity. This type of laryngoscope provides a more comfortable approach to visualizing the larynx, the pharynx, and the nasal cavity.

Code 31579 identifies a laryngoscopy with stroboscopy. A strobe light provides a very bright light in short flashes. Because of the flashing produced by the stroboscopy, the physician is better able to examine moving vocal cords.

The following questions should be answered before assigning codes for laryngoscopies:

- *What was the purpose of the laryngoscopy?*
- *Which type of laryngoscope was used: direct, indirect, or flexible?*
- *Was stroboscopy used?*

In cases during which an operating microscope was used, the combination code should be assigned and not code 69990.

Exercise 4.17   Respiratory System—Laryngoscopy

Answers to odd-numbered questions can be found in appendix C of this book. The answers to even-numbered questions are located in the instructor materials and are available to approved instructors.

Assign appropriate CPT code(s) for the following procedures. Assign only CPT surgical codes (no E/M codes) and append any applicable modifiers.

1. Direct laryngoscopy with stripping of vocal cords

Code(s): _____

2. Flexible laryngoscopy performed for removal of a dime lodged in the patient's larynx

Code(s): _____

3. Using an operating microscope, the surgeon performs a laryngoscopy with excision of a polyp

Code(s): _____

4. Flexible laryngoscopy with laser destruction of lesion, vocal cord

Code(s): _____

5. Flexible laryngoscopy with removal of lesion using microdebrider

Code(s): _____

Exercise 4.18   Respiratory System—Operative Report

Answers to odd-numbered questions can be found in appendix C of this book. The answers to even-numbered questions are located in the instructor materials and are available to approved instructors.

Operative Report #1

Operative Report

Preoperative Diagnosis: Laryngeal lesion

Postoperative Diagnosis: Same

Operation: Direct laryngoscopy and biopsy of vocal cord lesion using an operating microscope

The patient was placed on the OR table in the supine position, induced under general anesthesia, and intubated. The Dedo laryngoscope was introduced into the oral cavity, slipped under the tip of the epiglottis, and suspended from the Lewy suspension apparatus. The lesion involved the entire left vocal cord and extended through the ventricle to the false vocal cord and into the anterior commissure area. It also slightly involved the anterior portion of the right vocal cord. In addition, some subglottic extension was present. A biopsy was taken and sent out for frozen section. The laryngoscope was then removed and the procedure terminated. The patient tolerated the procedure well and left the room in good condition.

Assign only CPT surgical codes (no E/M codes) and append any applicable modifiers.

Code(s): _____

Bronchoscopy

A bronchoscope is an instrument that can be inserted into either the nose or the mouth and passed through the trachea, past the larynx, and into the bronchial tubes. Indications for this procedure include hemoptysis, a persistent cough that is unresponsive to medication, shortness of breath, an acute upper airway obstruction, or an abnormal chest x-ray or infection.

A physician may elect to use a flexible or rigid bronchoscope. The rigid scope, also referred to as an open-tube bronchoscope, is inserted through the mouth and most often is used to remove foreign objects or to secure a larger-than-normal biopsy sample. The more commonly performed flexible bronchoscopy consists of a flexible tube with many small glass fibers that allow the transmission of light. Codes in the 31622 through 31651 range are used to identify a variety of procedures using either type of bronchoscope.

The note at the beginning of this section advises coding professionals that a surgical bronchoscopy includes a diagnostic bronchoscopy. It is important to note that codes 31622–31646 include fluoroscopic guidance, if performed. Fluoroscopic equipment serves as an image intensifier and is frequently used during bronchoscopies. It is incorrect to use an additional code to identify fluoroscopy.

Frequently, the purpose of the bronchoscopy is to obtain tissue to allow the physician to make an accurate diagnosis. Specimens may be collected in several ways. Cell washings may be obtained by introducing saline solution into the airways, which then is removed and sent to the laboratory for cytological examination. Code 31622 identifies a bronchoscopy *with* or *without* cell washings.

Brushings of tissue is another method of specimen collection. One advantage to this method is that brushings allow the diagnosis to be made on the basis of tissue that could not be obtained normally with biopsy forceps. Either a fixed brush or a protected specimen brush (PSB) may be introduced through the bronchoscope. A PSB is a brush contained in a double catheter. A wax plug at the top prevents contamination of the specimen by upper airway flora. Code 31623 is assigned when a bronchoscopy is performed to collect specimen(s) with either a fixed brush or a PSB.

Code 31624 identifies a bronchoscopy with bronchial alveolar lavage (BAL). This procedure is performed to collect cells from peripheral lung tissue. During a BAL, sterile saline is instilled into the airway in aliquots of 20 mL up to 50 mL. The saline is suctioned out and sent for cytological examination.

CPT provides two codes for placement of fiducial markers during a bronchoscopic procedure. Code 31626 describes a stand-alone code for placement of fiducial markers, which help mark the position of a tumor, especially providing guidance to locate lesions in the distal regions of the lung. Code 31627 (computer assisted image-guided navigation) is an add-on code for the fiducial marker placement.

Code 32997 is assigned for total lung lavage (unilateral).

When a lesion can be visualized with the bronchoscope, the physician may elect to use forceps to obtain a sample of tissue. This procedure allows a more precise sample of tissue to be obtained for pathological diagnosis. Code 31625 is used to identify a bronchoscopy with bronchial or endobronchial biopsy, single or multiple sites.

When the diagnosis of a lung disease requires a sample of lung tissue, a transbronchial lung biopsy may be performed. During the bronchoscopy, forceps are used to puncture the bronchus and take samples of the lung tissue. This procedure is less invasive than an open-lung biopsy and thus carries less risk of morbidity. Code 31628 is assigned to identify a bronchoscopy with a transbronchial lung biopsy of a single lobe. To report transbronchial lung biopsies performed in additional lobes, assign add-on code 31632.

The following questions should be answered before assigning a code for a bronchoscopy:

- *Why was the bronchoscopy performed?*
- *Was a diagnostic bronchoscopy performed in conjunction with a surgical bronchoscopy?* If so, only the code for the surgical procedure should be assigned.
- *Was the procedure one of the bronchoscopies described by a code from the series 31622 through 31651?* If so, a separate code to identify fluoroscopy should not be assigned because fluoroscopic guidance is considered part of the procedures identified by that series of codes.

Endobronchial Ultrasound (EBUS)

CPT codes 31652–31654 are used to identify a procedure used in the diagnosis of lung cancer, lung infections, and other diseases that cause enlarged lymph nodes in the chest. Endobronchial ultrasound (EBUS) is a minimally invasive procedure that allows physicians to sample lung masses and lymph nodes with the use of ultrasound guidance. The technique begins with a bronchoscope inserted into the mouth. A specialized endoscope is fitted with an ultrasound processor and a fine-gauge aspiration needle for performing the biopsy. The real-time imaging allows physicians to view the hard to reach areas. The two codes can be differentiated by the number of samplings.

An add-on code (31654) was included to identify when EBUS is used for diagnostic or therapeutic intervention for peripheral lesion(s). The imaging combined with bronchoscopy video helps to access the peripheral airways.

Lung Procedures

The codes associated with removal of the lung or a portion of the lung (32440–32540) refer to surgical procedures such as resection of segment, pneumonectomy, or wedge resection. Note the following definitions that differentiate between the procedures:

- Pneumonectomy—removal of entire lung
- Lobectomy—removal of one lobe of the lung; removal of two lobes is called bilobectomy
- Wedge resection—removal of small, wedge-shaped portion of the lung
- Segmental resection—removal of a large portion of the lung lobe (larger than a wedge resection)

Diagnostic vs. Therapeutic Procedures

Many procedures, within the coding section for lung procedures, differentiate between diagnostic and therapeutic. CPT provides guidance in the form of a Note before code 32035. As an example, a *diagnostic* biopsy of a lung nodule using a wedge technique requires only a tissue sample, in contrast to a *therapeutic*

Figure 4.13. Lung procedures

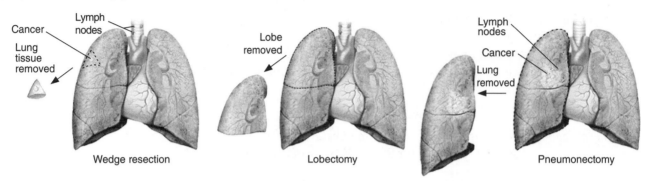

Wedge resection   Lobectomy   Pneumonectomy

Source: ©AHIMA.

Assuming the three lung procedures shown in figure 4.13 were performed via open approach, the coding assignment would be as follows:

   Wedge resection (therapeutic) 32505

   Lobectomy 32480

   Pneumonectomy 32440

wedge resection that includes attention to margins and a complete resection of the area. For example, if a surgeon uses a wedge resection to remove cancerous tissue, then a therapeutic CPT code would be assigned. Careful analysis of the documentation will support the coding decisions for diagnostic vs. therapeutic.

Figure 4.13 illustrates the following lung procedures: therapeutic wedge resection, lobectomy, and pneumonectomy.

Thoracoscopy (Video-Assisted Thoracic Surgery [VATS])

A special coding selection (32601–32674) is provided to identify video-assisted thoracic surgery (VATS). During this surgery, a tiny camera (thoracoscope) and surgical instruments are inserted in the chest through small incisions. The thoracoscope transmits images of the inside of the chest onto a video monitor, guiding the surgeon in performing the procedure. VATS can be used for many purposes, including biopsies to removal of tumors or lobes of the lungs. Note the following comparison between CPT codes for therapeutic wedge resection performed via the traditional incision (thoracotomy) method versus the VATS procedure:

Thoracotomy	VATS
32505 Thoracotomy with therapeutic wedge resection (e.g., mass, nodule), initial	32666 Thoracoscopy, with therapeutic wedge resection (e.g., mass, nodule), initial unilateral

Exercise 4.19   Respiratory System—Bronchoscopy

Answers to odd-numbered questions can be found in appendix C of this book. The answers to even-numbered questions are located in the instructor materials and are available to approved instructors.

Assign appropriate CPT code(s) for the following procedures. Assign only CPT surgical codes (no E/M codes) and append any applicable modifiers.

1. Bronchoscopy with excision of lesion

   Code(s): _____

2. Bronchoscopy with transbronchial biopsy of lung

   Code(s): _____

3. Flexible bronchoscopy with cell washings, brushings, and biopsy

Code(s): _____

4. Bronchoscopy with EBUS-guided transbronchial sampling of two mediastinal lymph nodes

Code(s): _____

Exercise 4.20   Respiratory System—Operative Report

Answers to odd-numbered questions can be found in appendix C of this book. The answers to even-numbered questions are located in the instructor materials and are available to approved instructors.

Operative Report #1

Operative Report

Preoperative Diagnosis: Persistent cough, dyspnea

Postoperative Diagnosis: Probable bronchitis

Procedure: Bronchoscopy

Medications: Versed 13 mg given just prior to and during the procedure; topical aerosolized lidocaine and atropine 0.4 mg IM and aerosolized albuterol 2.5 mg

The left nares was cannulated. The posterior nasopharynx was normal. The vocal cords, although with exogenous tissue consistent with obesity, were normal and normally apposed. The main carina was normal as was the trachea itself. The left lower lobe anatomy was a variant of normal with two main subsegments, each having three sub-subsegments in the left upper lobe. Very slight erythema is seen in the medial aspect of the left upper lobe subsegment. Brushings were obtained from this area.

The right inside anatomy was entirely normal. No endobronchial lesions were seen throughout.

Pathology Report

Gross Description: Received are two prepared slides

Microscopic Description: The bronchial brushing slides demonstrate benign bronchial epithelial cells and macrophages. The background contains mucus with minimal inflammation. There is no atypia or malignancy.

(Continued on next page)

Exercise 4.20   (Continued)

Diagnosis: Lung, left upper lobe, bronchial brushings. Negative for malignant cells.

Assign only CPT surgical codes (no E/M codes) and append any applicable modifiers.

Code(s): _____

Operative Report #2

Operative Report

Preoperative Diagnosis: Left upper lobe lung mass

Postoperative Diagnosis: Left upper lobe lung mass

Operations: Flexible bronchoscopy with transbronchial biopsy and bronchial washings and brushings.

Indications for Procedure: The patient recently was diagnosed with a left upper lobe lung mass. The PET scan was negative in his mediastinum.

The patient was brought to the operating room and placed in supine position on the operating room table. After general endotracheal anesthesia was performed, the Olympus bronchoscope was placed in the ET tube down and into the patient's trachea. The carina was observed. The right lobe appeared free of lesions. The bronchoscope was then removed and placed in left main bronchus. The main stem and lower lobe was inspected and found to have no irregularities. The left upper lobe was then examined. Bronchial washings were obtained and sent for cytology. Using fluoroscopic guidance to ensure that we were in the appropriate segment, the tip of the bronchoscope was placed into the posterior segment of the left upper lobe of the bronchus and bronchial brushings were obtained. After this, the transbronchial biopsy forceps were used to biopsy this area. Three samples were obtained for frozen section and three samples were obtained for permanent section. After removing the last specimen, the bronchoscope was removed. The patient was extubated in good condition and sent to recovery.

Code(s): _____

Exercise 4.21   Respiratory System Review

Answers to odd-numbered questions can be found in appendix C of this book. The answers to even-numbered questions are located in the instructor materials and are available to approved instructors.

Assign appropriate CPT code(s) for the following procedures. Assign only CPT surgical codes (no E/M codes) and append any applicable modifiers.

1. Thoracoscopy [VATS] with resection of upper left lobe of the lung

    Code(s): _____

2. Percutaneous drainage of pleural cavity via indwelling catheter, with imaging

    Code(s): _____

3. Partial excision of inferior turbinate

    Code(s): _____

4. Flexible bronchoscopy with bronchial brushings and cell washings

    Code(s): _____

5. Nasal endoscopy total ethmoidectomy and sphenoidotomy

    Code(s): _____

6. Patient treated in the emergency department for severe epistaxis (first visit for this condition); physician performs posterior packing, bilateral

    Code(s): _____

7. Flexible laryngoscopy with biopsy of tissue

    Code(s): _____

8. Bronchoscopy for removal of tumor using argon plasma coagulation

    Code(s): _____

9. Removal of pebble from child's nasal passage, performed in the physician's office

    Code(s): _____

10. The patient has a history of persistent hoarseness. The surgeon performs a flexible laryngoscopy to evaluate the larynx.

    Code(s): _____

Cardiovascular System

Learning Objectives

- Describe the components of a pacemaker system.
- Identify the documentation necessary to accurately code pacemaker procedures.
- Describe a CABG procedure and explain CPT guidelines for the coding assignment.
- Explain endocatheter procedure techniques.

- State the components of interventional radiology.
- Differentiate between selective and nonselective catheterization.
- Differentiate between AV fistulas and AV grafts.
- Describe the documentation requirements for coding central venous device procedures.

To become familiar with cardiovascular procedures, students may want to search the internet for professional videos.

The cardiovascular subsection includes surgical procedures involving the heart and pericardium, arteries, and veins. The codes are categorized first by body part involved and then by procedure performed, such as insertion of pacemaker, coronary artery bypass, embolectomy, and venipuncture. Assignment of codes for many of the cardiac procedures requires advanced knowledge and skill. The reference section of this book provides a list of recommended resources for coding cardiac procedures.

Pacemaker or Implantable Defibrillator

Cardiac pacemakers are devices that send a small current through a lead (wire) to stimulate the heartbeat. There are two components to a pacemaker: generator (battery) and, attached to the generator, one or two leads. A pacemaker is usually implanted under local anesthesia and sedation. A small incision is made under the collarbone, and the generator is placed under the skin and subcutaneous tissue in a pocket created above the muscle. The lead or leads are passed to the heart via a vein and placed in the right atrium and/or right ventricle. Pacemakers may be either single chamber (either atrium or ventricle) or dual chamber (both atrium and ventricle).

An implantable defibrillator is a device that monitors heart rhythms and delivers shocks if dangerous rhythms are detected.

The CPT coding process involves reviewing documentation (that is, operative reports, physician notes, pathology reports, radiology reports) and applying it to the CPT code selection(s). Coding professionals need to determine the intent of the procedure (insertion, removal, replacement, upgrade) and components of the system that was implanted. In this subsection, some of the key documentation elements, or questions, include:

- *Was the electrode(s) inserted into the atrium, ventricle, or both?*
- *Was a single lead inserted? Dual leads? Multiple leads? (or electrodes)*
- *Did the procedure involve inserting, replacing, or repositioning the device(s)?*
- *Did the surgeon use the epicardial or transvenous approach?*

Pacemakers, pacing cardioverters, and defibrillator systems are classified with codes from the series 33202 through 33273. Guidelines in this section should be reviewed for descriptions of what comprises the various kinds of pacemaker and defibrillator systems.

Figure 4.14 illustrates an implanted pacemaker with the generator in the chest wall and electrodes in the right atrium and right ventricle.

Figure 4.14. Implanted pacemaker

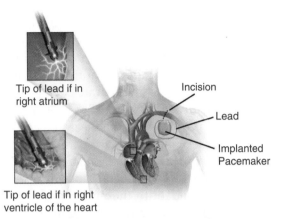

Tip of lead if in right atrium

Incision

Lead

Implanted Pacemaker

Tip of lead if in right ventricle of the heart

Source: Blaus, Bruce. "Implanted Pacemaker." Digital Image. Wikimedia Commons. May, 2014. Accessed September, 2018. https://commons.wikimedia.org/wiki/File:Blausen_0696_PacemakerPlacement.png.

If the operative report supports the insertion of a new permanent pacemaker with leads placed in the right atrium and left ventricle (figure 4.14), the correct code assignment would be 33208.

Cardiac Valves

Procedures performed on cardiac valves have traditionally been performed as an open procedure. A selection of CPT codes for transcatheter aortic valve replacement (TAVR) identify placement of a collapsible aortic heart valve via a catheter that is inserted through a small incision such as in the leg (femoral artery approach). An extensive set of Notes for reporting is printed before code 33361. Figure 4.15 illustrates a transcatheter mitral valve repair (TMVR).

Figure 4.15. Transcatheter mitral valve repair (TMVR)

The code assignment for a TMVR (figure 4.15) would be 33418.

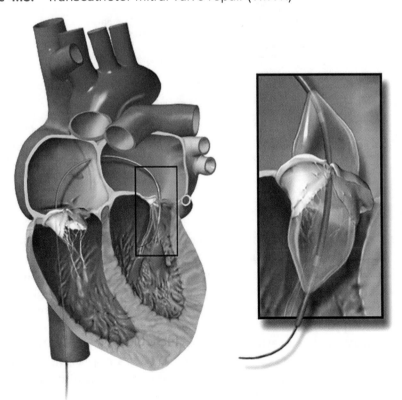

Source: Blaus, Bruce. "Mitral Valvuloplasty." Digital Image. Wikimedia Commons. 2013. Accessed September, 2018. https://commons.wikimedia.org/wiki/File:Blausen_0889_MitralValvuloplasty.png.

Coronary Artery Bypass Grafting (CABG)

Codes 33510 through 33548 describe procedures related to coronary artery bypass grafting (CABG). The first series of codes (33510–33516) is reported when the CABG uses <u>only</u> venous grafts, such as those obtained from the saphenous vein. These codes are not to be reported when the bypass requires both arterial and venous grafts. In addition, harvesting of the saphenous vein is included in the bypass procedure and not reported as a separate code. Combined arterial and venous grafts are reported with 33517 through 33523. As previously mentioned, the saphenous vein usually provides the venous grafts and the arterial graft is usually created from the internal mammary artery. To fully code arterial-venous bypass grafting, two codes must be assigned: one from the 33517 through 33523 series to identify the number of venous grafts performed, and one from the 33533 through 33536 series to identify the number of arterial grafts. Careful review of the operative report is required to determine the type and number of grafts performed.

Figure 4.16 illustrates a double coronary artery bypass graft (CABG) procedure. For this procedure, the left internal mammary artery is used as an arterial graft to bypass the coronary artery blockage. The saphenous vein is harvested from the leg to create the second bypass. For the double bypass, code 33533 is reported for the single arterial graft and code 33517 is also reported to capture the combine arterial-venous grafting with use of a single vein graft.

Figure 4.16.   Coronary artery bypass graft (CABG) procedure

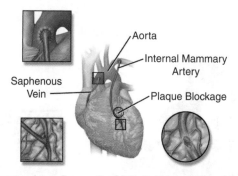

Source: Blaus, Bruce. "Coronary Artery Bypass Graft." Digital Image. Wikimedia Commons. December, 2013. Accessed October, 2018. https://commons.wikimedia.org/wiki/File:Blausen_0151_CABG_02.png.

Endovascular Surgery

Endovascular surgery describes a minimally invasive surgical technique designed to access many regions of the body via major blood vessels. The term "endovascular" means "inside blood vessels." Typically, the procedure begins with an introduction of a catheter inserted percutaneously into a large blood vessel. During surgical interventions, surgeons may insert stents, coils and other vascular prostheses. For example, an endovascular stent graft is used to reinforce a weak spot in an artery called an aneurysm. See figure 4.17 that shows an example of a graft that is inserted within the aorta to prevent an aneurysm from bursting. CPT provides several ranges of codes to identify endovascular surgery procedures. Guidance for use of the codes is documented before each family of codes.

Figure 4.17. Endovascular repair of aneurysm

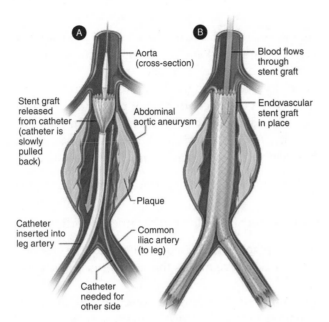

Source: National Institutes of Health. "Endovascular Repair." Digital Image. Wikimedia Commons. January, 2011. Accessed September 2018. https://commons.wikimedia.org/wiki/File:Aneurysm_endovascular.jpg.

Extracorporeal Membrane Oxygenation (ECMO) or Extracorporeal Life Support Services (ECLS) (33946–33989)

This series of codes identify extracorporeal membrane oxygenation (ECMO) and extracorporeal life support services (ECLS) procedures for cardiac or respiratory support to patients whose heart and lungs are so severely damaged that they can no longer serve their function. The codes can be differentiated by the age of the patient, service provided (insertion, removal, or reposition), and type of cannulation (such as peripheral or central).

Interventional Radiology Procedures for Cardiovascular Conditions

Coding interventional radiology procedures for cardiovascular conditions requires a thorough understanding of coding guidelines and anatomy. Coding professionals often refer to anatomic diagrams of the vascular families to assist with accurate coding assignment. Appendix L of the CPT book provides a reference list for the vascular families. The Society of Interventional Radiology publishes a book titled *The Interventional Radiology Coding Users' Guide*, and AHIMA has offered several audio seminars that concentrate on CPT coding in this area. The purpose of this lesson is to provide an overview of coding guidelines. In order to be proficient at interventional radiology coding, more advanced study and practice are necessary.

Interventional Radiology is a specialty section of CPT that requires advanced study.

Angiography

Most interventional angiography procedures have two components: a surgical component (involving, for example, injection of contrast solutions, implantation of devices, and removal of strictures with angioplasty balloons), and an imaging (radiology) component, which includes supervision and interpretation (S&I) of images.

Coding guidelines state that codes must be assigned for both the catheter placement (surgical component) and the imaging procedure (S&I component), unless the procedures are bundled into one code.

CPT coding decisions for angiography are based on whether the physician performed a selective or nonselective catheter placement. Nonselective catheter placement is one in which the vascular catheter is left in the vessel it punctured and not advanced any further; or it is advanced into the aorta and not beyond. Examples of nonselective catheter placement CPT codes are as follows:

- 36140 Introduction of needle or intracatheter, upper or lower extremity artery
- 36160 Introduction of needle or intracatheter, aortic, translumbar

Selective catheter placement is moved beyond the vessel punctured or beyond the aorta. Nonselective means the catheter is not advanced beyond the access site.

Review of the coding descriptions for selective catheter placement (36215–36248) reveals a reference to order, such as first order, second order, and so on. Appendix L provides guidance for the classification of vascular families. It is important to emphasize the need to review anatomic diagrams/definitions and reference materials before attempting to code interventional radiology cases.

The vascular family is divided into two parts:

- *Arterial vascular family:* A group of arteries fed by a primary branch of the aorta or a primary branch of the vessel punctured (that is, left common iliac artery, innominate artery, right renal artery)
- *Venous vascular family:* A group of veins that flows into a primary branch of the vena cava or a primary branch of the vessel punctured (that is, left iliac vein, right renal vein, left brachiocephalic vein)

Coding guidelines instruct coding professionals to assign a code to the highest-order catheter placement within a vascular family. Each vascular family that is catheterized is coded separately. A code for nonselective catheter placement should not be assigned in addition to a selective catheter placement code unless there are multiple accesses (punctures).

Example:

A catheter is inserted in the femoral artery and passed into the aorta, into the brachiocephalic artery, and then further into the right common carotid artery.

The brachiocephalic is a first-order vessel and the right common carotid artery is a second-order vessel within the same vascular family. A code (36216) would be assigned for the second order only.

S&I codes are used to describe the imaging component of the procedure. S&I codes are assigned based on the vessels that are imaged, not the vessels that are catheterized. Some CPT codes are bundled with the S&I codes, while others require an additional code. CPT provides guidance in the form of Notes throughout the code book.

Arteriovenous (AV) Fistulas and Grafts

Creating an arteriovenous (AV) fistula is the most desirable method for hemodialysis access because AV fistulas are less likely to clot or become infected than other methods, and they last longer. See illustration in figure 4.18. This procedure requires the surgeon to connect the artery to the vein. This abnormal connection between these two vessels causes more blood to flow from the artery directly to the vein under high arterial pressure. Eventually, the vein grows stronger and becomes thick-walled. This thick-walled vein becomes an ideal target to place the dialysis needles.

Figure 4.19 depicts an AV graft in which a synthetic tube connects the artery to the vein.

The connection between an artery and vein for an AV fistula does not use a device. An AV graft (or shunt) uses a man-made tube to make the connection.

Figure 4.18. Arteriovenous (AV) fistula

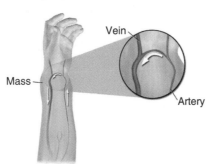

Source: Blaus, Bruce. "Arteriovenous Fistula." Digital Image. Wikimedia Commons. February 2014,. Accessed September, 2018. https://commons.wikimedia.org/wiki/File:Blausen_0049_ArteriovenousFistula.png.

If the operative report described a radiocephalic AV fistula (cephalic vein and radial artery at the wrist), the correct code would be 36821.

The CPT coding decision is based on whether the fistula was created by vein transposition or direct anastomosis. Codes for vein transposition are assigned according to the vein used:

- 36818 Upper arm (cephalic or brachiocephalic)
- 36819 Upper arm basilic vein
- 36820 Forearm vein (proximal radial artery and median antecubital vein)
- 36821 Direct, any site (e.g., Cimino type). Includes radiocephalic at the wrist.

The direct anastomosis method (36821) involves attaching an artery and a vein directly.

If an AV fistula is not possible because the patient's veins are too small or too far apart or there is not enough time to perform the procedure, the surgeon may elect to perform an AV graft (36825–36830) that connects the artery to the vein using a conduit. An AV graft is typically made of synthetic material, although some surgeons use a vessel from a human or cadaver to form the connection. AV fistulas require weeks or months to mature, but AV grafts require less time. A major disadvantage of AV grafts is that they often produce blood clots or become infected. CPT codes for AV grafts are 36825–36830. Figure 4.19 illustrates an AV graft.

If documentation supports that the graft is made of synthetic material (figure 4.19), the correct code assignment is 36830.

Figure 4.19. Arteriovenous (AV) graft

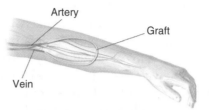

Source: Blaus, Bruce. "Arteriovenous Graft." Digital Image. Wikimedia Commons. February, 2014. Accessed September, 2018. https://commons.wikimedia.org/wiki/File:Blausen_0050_ArteriovenousGraft.png.

Complications of AV Fistulas and Grafts

Common complications of AV fistulas and grafts include clotting, obstruction, and narrowing of the access. Several CPT codes are provided for the procedures necessary to correct these complications.

There are several methods of treatment for stenosis, including angioplasty, stent placement, and thrombectomy. Thrombectomies can be performed with or without a revision of the graft, and CPT provides several codes to describe the various procedures:

- 36831 Thrombectomy, open, without revision
- 36832 Revision, open, without thrombectomy
- 36833 Revision, open, with thrombectomy

Percutaneous thrombectomy of a graft is coded with 36904, which includes all the work required to restore flow to the access. For this procedure, the thrombus may be removed pharmaceutically (that is, urokinase) or mechanically (AngioJet, small Fogarty-type balloons).

CPT has a category called Dialysis Circuit which includes codes that capture diagnostic and interventions associated with the peripheral or central dialysis circuit. The anatomical markers for distinguishing between peripheral and central segments are outlined in the note before code 36901. The interventions (such as thrombectomy of AV graft) are performed percutaneously.

Examples:

- Surgeon performs an open thrombectomy for an AV graft (connecting brachial artery with basilic vein) used for dialysis. Correct code is 36831.
- Surgeon performs a percutaneous transluminal thrombectomy for the same graft described in the case above. Correct CPT code is 36904.

Note that all of the associated procedures such as imaging and fluoroscopic guidance are bundled with the code and not separately reported.

Central Venous Access Procedures

Many therapies can be administered via various types of catheters and ports. CPT coding for catheterization procedures depends on the type and use of the catheter. In general, CPT codes are assigned only to catheters inserted by physicians and not to catheters inserted by nursing personnel.

Central venous access devices (CVADs) are small, flexible tubes placed in large veins for patients who require frequent access to their bloodstream. CVADs are commonly used for the following purposes:

- Administration of medications (for example, antibiotics, chemotherapy)
- Administration of fluids and nutritional compounds (for example, hyperalimentation)
- Transfusion of blood products
- Multiple blood draws for diagnostic testing

Before assigning codes in this section, coding professionals should read the note that precedes code 36555. First, CPT classifies venous access procedures into five distinct categories:

- Insertion
- Repair
- Partial replacement
- Complete replacement
- Removal

The definitions for each of these categories are provided in CPT. Additional information must be abstracted from the health record to determine the correct code. As an example, refer to the decision tree in figure 4.20 for insertion of a central venous access device. From this decision tree, documentation is needed to determine the following:

- Catheter inserted centrally or peripherally
- Tunneled or nontunneled
- Pump or port
- Age of patient

A centrally inserted catheter is placed in the jugular, subclavian, or femoral vein, or inferior vena cava. The peripherally inserted catheters are typically placed in the arm and advanced forward into the larger subclavian vein. The documentation may state that the catheter was inserted into the basilic or cephalic vein. For the centrally inserted catheter, the coding professional must check the documentation to determine whether the catheter was tunneled. Tunneled catheters have an entrance site at a distance from where they enter the vascular system. These are tunneled through the skin and subcutaneous tissue to a great vein. Typically, these catheters are for long-term use. The code descriptions also differentiate between the use of subcutaneous ports or pumps. Implanted ports are placed below the skin, and blood is drawn or medication is delivered by placing a tiny needle through the overlying skin into the port or reservoir. A coding decision table can be found in the professional edition of CPT code book.

Figure 4.20 illustrates an example of insertion of a central venous catheter with port.

Unlike centrally inserted central catheters, peripherally inserted central catheter (PICC) lines are not inserted into the central vein but rather into a peripheral vein, such as basilic or cephalic veins.

CPT provides codes for the removal of CVADs (36589–36590) but instructs the coding professional not to assign the codes for nontunneled central venous catheters. Removal of some catheters does not warrant a separate code when no surgical procedure is required and the catheter is simply pulled out.

Figure 4.20. Port-a-cath

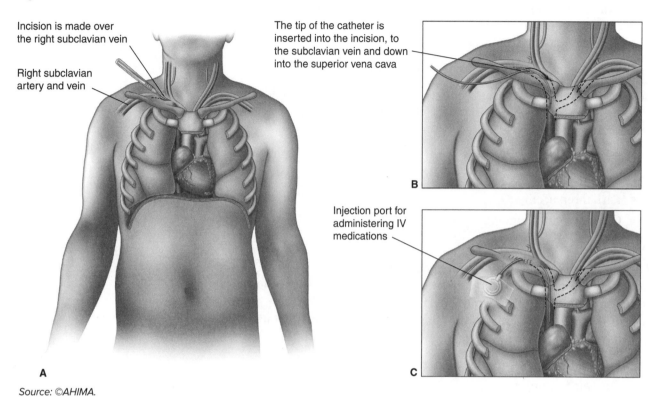

Incision is made over
the right subclavian vein

Right subclavian
artery and vein

The tip of the catheter is
inserted into the incision, to
the subclavian vein and down
into the superior vena cava

Injection port for
administering IV
medications

A

B

C

Source: ©AHIMA.

Endovascular Revascularization (Open or Percutaneous, Transcatheter)

Peripheral artery disease (PAD) occurs when plaque builds up in the arteries and reduces the blood flow to the patient's limbs. With the advent of catheter-based interventional therapies, endovascular physicians have become able to improve arterial perfusion in lower extremities through the use of balloon angioplasty and stenting. A series of CPT codes (37220–37235) identify these procedures and are differentiated by site (for example, iliac, femoral/popliteal, or tibial/peroneal vascular territory) and by additional procedures performed during the revascularization procedure (stent placement, atherectomy).

Coding professionals should carefully read the Notes section preceding code 37220 that provides guidance for selection of the appropriate code. General guidelines include:

* Only one code from the family should be reported for each lower extremity vessel.
* When coding for treatment of multiple territories in the same leg, one primary lower extremity code is used for each territory treated.
* Use add-on codes for additional vessels treated within the territory.
* If a lesion extends across the margins of one vessel vascular territory to another but can be opened with a single therapy, the single code should be reported.

Figure 4.21 illustrates a transluminal atherectomy.

Figure 4.21. Transluminal atherectomy

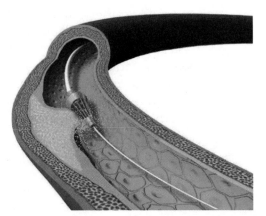

Source: Blaus, Bruce. "Atherectomy Transluminal." Digital Image. Wikimedia Commons. February, 2016. Accessed September, 2018. https://commons.wikimedia.org/wiki/File%3AAtherectomy_Transluminal.png.

If the operative report stated that the endovascular balloon angioplasty and atherectomy was performed on the femoral popliteal artery (figure 4.21), the code 37225 would be assigned.

Ligation, Division, and Stripping of Saphenous Veins

Varicose veins are gnarled, enlarged veins. Any vein may become varicose, but the veins most commonly affected are those in the saphenous veins of the leg. Surgical treatment includes ligation, division, and stripping of the affected veins (37718–37735). In ligation and division, the surgeon ties off all tributaries and then ties off the saphenous vein below the tributaries and divides it between the ligatures. Stripping involves completely removing the vein from the leg. Removing the veins does not affect the circulation of blood in the leg. Veins deeper in the leg take care of the larger volumes of blood.

Code 37700 is used for ligation and division of the long saphenous vein without stripping.

Exercise 4.22   Cardiovascular System—Operative Reports

Answers to odd-numbered questions can be found in appendix C of this book. The answers to even-numbered questions are located in the instructor materials and are available to approved instructors.

Operative Report #1

Operative Report

Preoperative Diagnosis: Heart block

Postoperative Diagnosis: Same

Procedure: Insertion of permanent pacemaker

The patient was premedicated before arriving at the OR. The patient was prepared and draped in the usual manner. A pocket was created for the pacemaker. The bipolar electrode was introduced, taken to the

(Continued on next page)

Exercise 4.22 (Continued)

pulmonary artery, and brought out slowly to the apex of the right ventricle. Measurements were taken, and the position was excellent. The electrode was anchored to the fascia over the sleeve and connected to the pacemaker battery. The wound was closed. Patient tolerated the procedure well and returned to the outpatient recovery area.

Assign only CPT surgical codes (no E/M codes) and append any applicable modifiers.

Code(s): _____

Operative Report #2

Operative Report

Preoperative Diagnosis: Breast carcinoma

Postoperative Diagnosis: Same

Operation: Removal of venous access port

The patient is a 44-year-old woman who had a left, modified radical mastectomy in 2010. In August she had a Port-a-cath placed in the right side. However, it has caused an extreme amount of discomfort, so she has requested that it be removed.

The patient was taken to the OR and placed in a supine position on the table. She was then prepared and draped in the usual sterile fashion. The area was anesthetized with 1% Carbocaine. An incision was made over the venous access device and carried down to the place of the device. After freeing it up and cutting the retention sutures, the venous access device was removed. Hemostasis was obtained with cautery and pressure. The wound was then closed in layers and a dressing applied. The patient tolerated the procedure well and was returned to the surgicenter in stable condition.

Assign only CPT surgical codes (no E/M codes) and append any applicable modifiers.

Code(s): _____

Operative Report #3

Operative Report

Preoperative Diagnosis: Renal failure

Postoperative Diagnosis: Same

Operation: Insertion of subclavian venous catheter

With this elderly patient in the head-down position, the entire left upper chest was prepared with Beta-dine scrub and draped in the usual sterile fashion.

Then, 1% lidocaine was used for local anesthetic. A percutaneously subclavian venous catheter was inserted without difficulty and secured at the skin level with 3-0 nylon, and a sterile dressing was applied. The catheter also was irrigated with heparin solution. Patient tolerated the procedure well. Will follow with a chest x-ray.

Assign only CPT surgical codes (no E/M codes) and append any applicable modifiers.

Code(s): _____

Exercise 4.23 Cardiovascular System Review

Answers to odd-numbered questions can be found in appendix C of this book. The answers to even-numbered questions are located in the instructor materials and are available to approved instructors.

Assign appropriate CPT code(s) for the following procedures. Assign only CPT surgical codes (no E/M codes) and append any applicable modifiers.

1. Relocation of pacemaker pocket

   Code(s): _____

2. Percutaneous thrombectomy of forearm AV graft that was inserted for dialysis treatment

   Code(s): _____

3. Repair of patent ductus arteriosus by division (18-year-old patient)

   Code(s): _____

4. A patient is seen for surgical treatment of an occlusion of the femoral artery, left. Percutaneously under guidance, the surgeon inserts a catheter to perform an atherectomy (lower extremity revascularization).

   Code(s): _____

5. Complete replacement of tunneled centrally inserted central venous catheter with subcutaneous port; replacement performed through original access site (45-year-old patient)

   Code(s): _____

6. Open revision of AV fistula with thrombectomy, patient receiving hemodialysis

   Code(s): _____

7. Catheter placement into the brachiocephalic artery (first-order)

   Code(s): _____

(Continued on next page)

Exercise 4.22   (Continued)

8. The patient has been diagnosed with severe aortic stenosis. Through a percutaneous incision in the leg (transfemoral), the surgeon performs a transcatheter aortic valve replacement (TAVR).

Code(s): _____

9. Removal of existing pacemaker pulse generator and insertion of new dual lead generator. The existing leads were attached to the new generator.

Code(s): _____

10. A coronary artery bypass graft (CABG) procedure was performed. The surgeon bypassed three coronary artery sites by grafting the left internal mammary artery (LIMA) and one site was treated by grafting the greater saphenous venous graft to the obtuse marginal from the aorta.

Code(s): _____

11. Patient is 34 year-old that had an insertion of PICC (peripherally inserted central venous catheter) line with no imaging.

Code(s): _____

12. Procedure; Excision of pseudoaneurysm of temporal artery. Operative note states that the artery was divided and aneurysm removed. Artery was ligated with fine Vicryl suture.

Code(s): _____

Digestive System

Learning Objectives

- Differentiate between EGD and ERCP procedures.
- Describe methods for removal of tumors and polyps.
- Explain coding guidelines for incomplete colonoscopy procedures.

- Differentiate between the surgical procedure codes for treatment of hemorrhoids.
- Identify documentation requirements for hernia repair procedures.

> Be careful in this section to distinguish between small and large intestine. For example, 44120 is reported for removal of a section of small intestine and 44140 is for large intestine.

The digestive subsection includes surgical procedures involving the lips, mouth and tongue, palate and uvula, salivary glands and ducts, pharynx, adenoids and tonsils, esophagus, stomach, intestines, appendix, rectum, biliary tract, abdomen, peritoneum, and omentum. The codes are categorized first by body part involved and then by procedure, such as herniorrhaphy, esophagotomy, ileostomy, cholecystectomy, and hemorrhoidectomy. Figure 4.22 shows the digestive system.

Figure 4.22. The digestive system

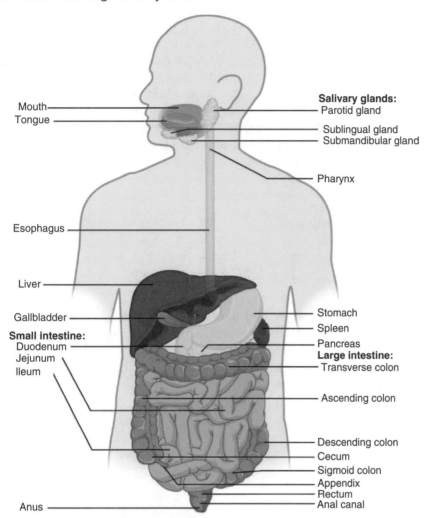

Source: OpenStax College. "Components of the Digestive System." Digital Image. Wikimedia Commons. June, 2013. Accessed September,, 2018. https://commons.wikimedia.org/wiki/File:2401_Components _of_the_Digestive_System.jpg.

Endoscopies

In general, gastrointestinal endoscopies are categorized by body part involved, type or purpose of endoscopy (diagnostic or surgical), and specific procedure performed, such as biopsy, ablation of tumor or polyp, and removal of foreign body. The endoscopy should always be coded as far as the scope was passed.

An esophagoscopy allows the physician to visualize the esophagus. Codes in the range 43180 through 43233 are used to report esophagoscopy procedures. The code ranges differentiate between rigid and flexible esophagoscopy procedures and approach (transoral, transnasal). Rigid esophagoscopy is performed by inserting a rigid endoscope through the mouth and down the throat into the esophagus. Flexible esophagoscopy is performed by inserting a thin, flexible endoscope either through the mouth (transoral) or through the nose (transnasal). If the scope goes beyond the esophagus, it would be considered an EGD.

Esophagogastroduodenoscopy (EGD)

An upper gastrointestinal endoscopy, also known as an esophagogastroduodenoscopy (EGD), or upper endoscopy, involves the visual examination of the esophagus, stomach and upper duodenum, or jejunum. Indications for these procedures include gastrointestinal (GI) bleeding, ulceration, or inflammation; abdominal pain; narrowing of the esophagus; and suspected tumors or polyps. EGDs are reported with codes in the range 43235 through 43270. In the CPT format for upper GI endoscopic procedures, the diagnostic procedure is listed first, followed by a list of descriptions for surgical treatment. According to CPT endoscopy guidelines, it is appropriate to list multiple codes if the documentation supports the coding selection.

Example:

During the EGD, the surgeon performs a snare removal of a polyp and removal of a foreign body.

Correct coding assignment: 43251 Snare removal

                                        43247 Removal of foreign body

> If the surgeon describes an EGD with removal of a piece of suspicious tissue from the first part of the duodenum (figure 4.23), the correct code would be 43239.

Note: For physician services, and according to payer policies, Modifier 51 (multiple procedures) may need to be appended to the second code to indicate that multiple procedures were performed by the same physician at the same session.

The code ranges can be located in the alphabetic index under Endoscopy, Gastrointestinal, Upper. There is no alphabetic entry for the abbreviation EGD. See figure 4.23 for illustration of upper GI endoscopy.

Figure 4.23.   Upper GI endoscopy

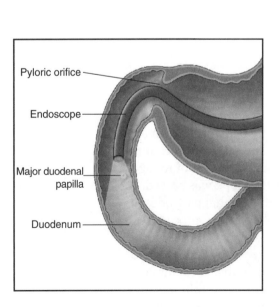
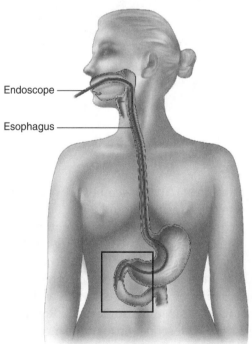

Pyloric orifice

Endoscope

Major duodenal papilla

Duodenum

Endoscope

Esophagus

Source: ©AHIMA.

Esophageal Dilation

CPT provides for two methods for esophageal dilation:

- *Endoscopic:* Through the endoscopy the physician selects a dilating balloon (43220) or plastic dilators over the guiding wire to stretch the esophagus (43226).

- *Manipulation (not with scope):* Surgeon sprays the throat with local anesthesia to pass a tapered dilating instrument through the mouth and guide it into the esophagus (43450–43460). Hurst and Maloney are common types of bougies used for esophageal dilation (43450).

Endoscopic Retrograde Cholangiopancreatography (ERCP)

Endoscopic retrograde cholangiopancreatography (ERCP) is a procedure that is used to diagnose conditions in the liver, gallbladder, bile ducts, and pancreas. The liver is a large organ that, among other things, makes a liquid called bile that helps with digestion. The gallbladder is a small, pear-shaped organ that stores bile until it is needed for digestion. The bile ducts are tubes that carry bile from the liver to the gallbladder and small intestine. These ducts are sometimes called the biliary tree. The pancreas is a large gland that produces chemicals that help with digestion, and hormones such as insulin.

ERCP combines the use of x-rays and an endoscope. Through the endoscope, the physician can see the inside of the stomach and duodenum and inject dyes into the ducts in the biliary tree and pancreas so they can be seen on x-rays. The CPT code range for these procedures is 43260–43278. Note the reference to alert the coding professional to the radiological supervision and interpretation codes.

Lower Gastrointestinal System Endoscopies

Lower GI endoscopies can be classified by the area of the intestine examined and if the procedure was performed through a stoma or not. The procedures performed through the natural orifice are as follows:

- *Proctosigmoidoscopy:* An examination limited to the rectum and may include a portion of the sigmoid colon (45300–45327).

- *Sigmoidoscopy:* An examination of the entire rectum, sigmoid colon and may also include a portion of the descending colon (45330–45350) (the depth visualization is typically 35 or 60 cm, depending on the instrument used).

- *Colonoscopy:* An examination of the entire colon, from the rectum to the cecum, that may include the terminal ileum or small intestine proximal to an anastomosis (45378–45398). Typically, a colonoscopy examines the entire colon, from the rectum to the cecum. Figure 4.24 illustrates the anatomy of the colon.

> If the operative report described removal of a polyp in the ascending colon by hot biopsy forceps, the correct coding assignment would be 45384.

Indications for performing lower GI procedures include an abnormal barium enema, lower GI bleeding, iron deficiency anemia of unknown etiology, and diarrhea. They may also be performed for follow-up examination after removal of a neoplastic growth.

When coding a colonoscopy, the coding professional must review the operative report to determine the approach and if it was performed for diagnostic or therapeutic reasons.

Figure 4.24. Anatomy of the colon

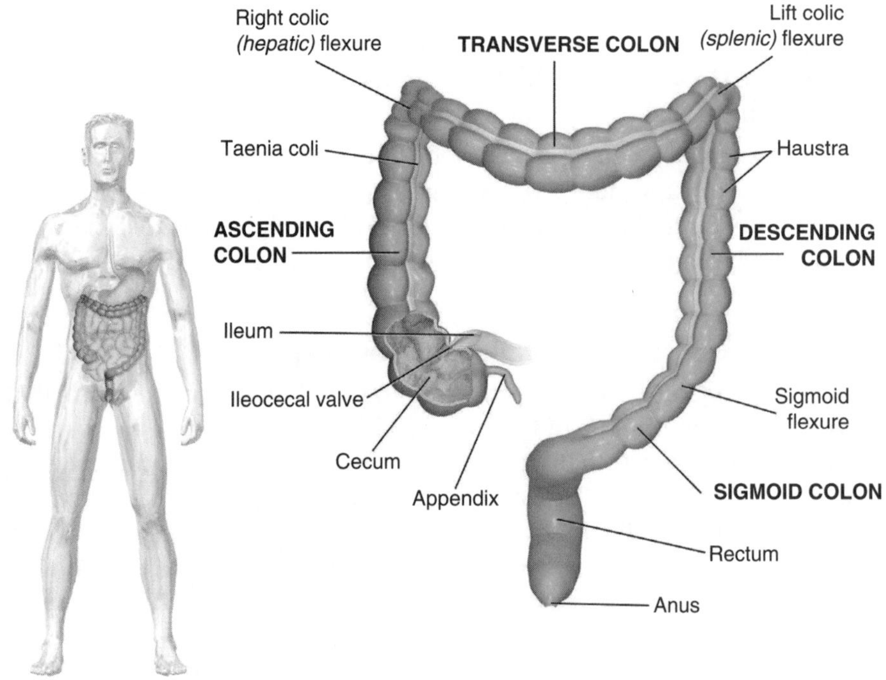

Source: Blaus, Bruce. "Large Intestine." Digital Image. Wikimedia Commons. October, 2013. Accessed September, 2018. https://commons.wikimedia.org/wiki/File:Blausen_0604_LargeIntestine2.png.

The following questions should be answered before a code is assigned for an endoscopy:

- *Was the diagnostic endoscopy performed as part of a surgical endoscopy?* If so, only the surgical endoscopy should be coded.
- *What was the purpose of the endoscopy?*
- *What approach was used to insert the endoscope?*

Removal of Tumors or Polyps

Because the endoscopic removal of a tumor or polyp can be accomplished with several techniques, the coding professional should review the documentation carefully before selecting a code. It is also possible for a physician to use different techniques to remove polyps during the same operative episode. In this case, an appropriate CPT code would be assigned to identify each technique.

One technique uses hot biopsy forceps or bipolar cautery. Hot biopsy forceps resemble tweezers connected to an electrosurgical unit. Grasping the polyp, the physician pulls the growth away from the wall of the structure. A portion of the neoplasm may be removed for pathological analysis. The remaining portion is destroyed with the electrocoagulation current. Bipolar cautery also uses electrical current to remove the polyp.

The snare technique uses a wire loop that is slipped over the polyp or tumor. The stalk is then cauterized and the growth removed.

Finally, the physician may elect to use a neodymium yttrium aluminum garnet (Nd:YAG) laser to remove the lesion. When a laser is used during the endoscopy, the coding professional should assign the code for the endoscopy that states with ablation of tumor(s), polyp(s), or other lesion(s) not amenable to removal by hot biopsy forceps, bipolar cautery, or snare technique.

Incomplete Colonoscopies

Causes of incomplete colonoscopies include poor bowel preparation, obstructing disease, or patient's inability to tolerate the procedure. There are several guidelines for coding discontinued procedures for physicians and hospitals (see chapter 3 of this book and appendix A of the CPT code book for descriptions of modifiers 52, 53, 73, and 74). The AMA published a Colonoscopy Decision Tree, outlining coding decisions for incomplete procedures. Note the following examples:

Surgical Description	AMA Coding Guidance
Colonoscopy does not reach the splenic flexure	Code as sigmoidoscopy
Colonoscopy extends beyond the splenic flexure but does not reach the cecum	Code as colonoscopy with modifier 53 for diagnostic procedure or modifier 52 for therapeutic procedure

Coding Incomplete Colonoscopies for Physician Services

In the case of a colonoscopy, the procedure may be attempted, but circumstances may prevent the entire colon from being visualized (for instance, poor preparation). In this case, *CPT guidelines* instruct the coding professional to assign the colonoscopy code with modifier 53 for discontinued procedure (for physician services). See the note following the definition of Endoscopies (before code 45300).

Coding Incomplete Colonoscopies for Facility Services

For facility services coding of incomplete colonoscopies requiring anesthesia, CMS Transmittal 442 (January 2005) instructs the coding professional to append modifiers 73 (Discontinued Prior to Anesthesia) or 74 (Discontinued After Anesthesia) as appropriate.

Further clarification of the use of modifiers 52, 73, and 74 can be found in the CMS Manual.

Screening Colonoscopy (Medicare Guidelines)

Medicare covers colorectal cancer screening test/procedures for the early detection of colorectal cancer when coverage conditions are met. Among the screening procedures covered are screening colonoscopies with the following HCPCS (Level II) codes:

Screening colonoscopy is one example of a procedure with payer-specific guidelines.

- G0105   Colorectal cancer screening; colonoscopy on individual at high risk
- G0121   Colorectal screening; colonoscopy on individual not meeting criteria for high risk

These codes are to be assigned instead of 45378 (Diagnostic Colonoscopy) when there is no need for a therapeutic procedure (for example, polypectomy). Claims processing and payment of incomplete screening colonoscopies can be found in CMS Transmittal AB-03-114 (August 2003).

Biopsies and Lesion Removal

When performing a GI endoscopy, the physician may encounter one or many lesions. Biopsies of some or all lesions may be taken. Lesion removal may be performed after a biopsy or without a biopsy. Therefore, the following guidelines should be applied:

- When a biopsy of a lesion is taken and the remaining portion of the *same* lesion is excised during the same operative episode, assign a code for the excision only (*CPT Assistant,* February 1999).
- When one lesion is biopsied and a *different* lesion is excised, assign a code for the biopsy and a code for the excision. This rule is applicable unless the excision code narrative includes the phrase with or without biopsy. In this case, only the excision code is assigned. It would be appropriate to append the biopsy code with modifier 59, Distinct Procedural Service.
- Biopsy codes use the terminology with biopsy, single or multiple. These codes are to be used only once, regardless of the number of biopsies taken.

Exercise 4.24 Digestive System—Endoscopy

Answers to odd-numbered questions can be found in appendix C of this book. The answers to even-numbered questions are located in the instructor materials and are available to approved instructors.

Assign appropriate CPT code(s) for the following procedures. Assign only CPT surgical codes (no E/M codes) and append any applicable modifiers.

1. Flexible esophagoscopy, inserted in the mouth with biopsy of a small lesion in the esophagus and a snare removal of a polyp from another area of the esophagus

   Code(s): _____

2. Proctosigmoidoscopy with removal of two polyps with the use of hot biopsy forceps

   Code(s): _____

3. Laparoscopic insertion of LINX magnetic esophageal sphincter augmentation device for a patient with GERD

   Code(s): _____

4. ERCP with removal of biliary stent

   Code(s): _____

5. Endoscope was inserted through the anus and progressed to the transverse colon but due to a poor prep, the diagnostic procedure could not be complete. Code for the physician's services.

   Code(s): _____

6. Laparoscopic pyloroplasty

Code(s): _____

7. Flexible sigmoidoscopy with laser removal of polyp in the rectum

Code(s): _____

Exercise 4.25   Digestive System—Operative Reports

Answers to odd-numbered questions can be found in appendix C of this book. The answers to even-numbered questions are located in the instructor materials and are available to approved instructors.

Operative Report #1

Operative Note

Procedure: EGD with foreign body removal

Clinical Note: This patient is a 47-year-old man who experienced acute odynophagia after eating a meal consisting of fish. The patient felt a foreign body-like sensation in his proximal esophagus. He was evaluated with lateral cervical spine films and soft-tissue films without any evidence of perforation.

Findings: After obtaining informed consent, the patient underwent flexible endoscopy. He was premedicated without any complication. Under direct visualization, an Olympus Q20 was introduced orally and the esophagus was intubated without any difficulty. The hypopharynx was carefully reviewed, and no abnormalities were noted. There were no foreign bodies and no lacerations to the hypopharynx. The proximal esophagus was normal. No active bleeding was noted. The endoscope was advanced farther into the esophagus, where careful review of the mucosa revealed no foreign bodies and no obstructions. However, the gastroesophageal junction did show a very small fish bone, which was removed without any complications. The endoscope was advanced into the stomach, where partially digested food was noted. The duodenum was normal. The endoscope was then removed. The patient tolerated the procedure well, and his postprocedural vital signs are stable.

(Continued on next page)

Exercise 4.25 (Continued)

Assign only CPT surgical codes (no E/M codes) and append any applicable modifiers.

Code(s): _____

Operative Report #2

Operative Report

Procedure: Colonoscopy

Instrument Used: Olympus CF100L

Indications: The patient has a family history of carcinoma of the colon and colonic polyps.

The digital and anal examinations were normal. The colonoscope was inserted to the cecum. Preparation was good. Eight to 10 very sessile and diminutive polyps were identified, all but one located in the rectum. The other polyp was located in the proximal transverse colon. All were coagulated and removed with the hot biopsy forceps. No other mucosal lesions were identified.

Pathology Report

Results of Gross Examination:
1. The specimen labeled biopsy of polyp, transverse colon, consists of a pale tan, slightly firm tissue measuring 0.2 cm in greatest diameter; completely submitted.
2. The specimen labeled biopsy of polyp, rectum, consists of six pieces of slightly firm pinkish-tan tissue ranging from 0.2 to 0.3 cm in greatest diameter; completely submitted.

Results of Microscopic Examination:
No high-grade dysplasia or malignant change is seen in the colorectal polyps.
Pathological Diagnosis:
1. Biopsy of polyp, transverse colon: Hyperplastic polyp
2. Biopsy of polyp, rectum: Hyperplastic polyp

Assign only CPT surgical codes (no E/M codes) and append any applicable modifiers.

Code(s): _____

Operative Report #3

Operative Report

Preoperative Diagnosis: Residual inflammatory changes

Postoperative Diagnosis: See below

Operation: Flexible sigmoidoscopy

The sigmoidoscope was inserted into the rectum and eventually advanced up to a level 60 cm from the anus. The mucosa throughout the colon and rectum were examined and appeared completely normal with no inflammation, ulceration, or exudate. There was no bleeding. I did not see any narrowed areas, polyps, or masses. I did see a few sigmoid diverticula.

With the exception of a few sigmoid diverticula, the examination up to a level of 60 cm from the anus was noted to be normal. The previous inflammatory changes have completely subsided.

Assign only CPT surgical codes (no E/M codes) and append any applicable modifiers.

Code(s): _____

Treatment of Hemorrhoids

There are a variety of CPT codes dedicated to the treatment of hemorrhoids. Hemorrhoids are swollen and inflamed veins in the anus and rectum. They may result from straining during bowel movements or the increased pressure on these veins during pregnancy. It is important to note that several codes in this section are not in numerical order. The symbol (#) identifies codes that are resequenced. Treatments are discussed in the following sections.

Incision of External Thrombosed Hemorrhoid (46083)

An incision is made over the thrombus, and the clot and diseased hemorrhoid plexus are removed in one piece.

Rubber Band Ligation (46221)

Hemorrhoidectomy, by simple ligature (without incision or excision), is a treatment for internal hemorrhoids that is sometimes referred to as banding. The physician attaches tiny rubber bands to the base of hemorrhoids. With their circulation cut off, the hemorrhoids painlessly fall away after 7 to 10 days and are expelled with stool. The code is only assigned once per operative session regardless of how many hemorrhoids the physician bands at a time.

Destruction of Internal Hemorrhoid(s) by Thermal Energy (46930)

Methods for this procedure include cautery, radiofrequency, and infrared coagulation. Infrared coagulation involves a small probe with a light source that coagulates the veins above the hemorrhoid, causing it to shrink and recede.

Suture Ligation (46945–46946)

Suture ligation differs from hemorrhoidectomy by simple ligature in that the physician isolates the hemorrhoid and ties suture material to its base. For accurate code selection, documentation must support the number of columns or groups ligated.

Hemorrhoidectomy (46250–46262)

The surgical excision codes are differentiated by whether the hemorrhoids were internal, external, or both. In addition, codes are distinguished by the number of columns or groups (single vs. multiple).

Destruction by Cryosurgery (46999)

Coders are instructed to report an unlisted code of 46999 for destruction of hemorrhoids by cryosurgery.

Percutaneous Biliary Procedures

A range of procedures codes (47531–47544) pertain to the biliary system. The biliary system consists of organs and structures that secrete and transport bile, including the liver, gallbladder, and bile ducts. The codes focus on placement (with subsequent codes for removal or exchange) of stents or catheters for biliary drainage. This procedure is most commonly performed for blocked bile ducts, which may be caused by a number of conditions including cancer, infection, cirrhosis, or trauma. Typically, the interventional radiologist uses guidance to place the drainage tube through the skin into one of the bile ducts in the liver to allow the bile to drain. This procedure is called percutaneous transhepatic cholangiogram (PTC).

Placement of Biliary Drains

The CPT codes for placement of biliary drainage catheters differentiate between external and internal-external (47533, 47534).

External: Under guidance, the surgeon passes a needle into one of the bile ducts. The needle is exchanged over a guidewire for a catheter and the catheter is position. The patient will have an external catheter that is attached to a drainage bag.

Internal-External: One end of the catheter will rest in the small intestine and the other end will drain into an external collection bag. This method allows bile to flow in two directions, internally and externally.

Placement of Biliary Stents

For treatment of the biliary obstruction, the surgeon can elect to insert biliary stents (thin, tube-like structure) to support a narrowed part of the bile duct and to prevent reformation of the stricture. The codes (47538–47540) are differentiated by new vs. existing access and if placement of a separate biliary drainage catheter was necessary.

Hernia Repairs

An abdominal hernia occurs when internal organs, such as the intestines, break through a hole or tear in the musculature of the abdominal wall. This protrusion produces a bulge that can be seen or felt. Symptoms include burning and pain with activity.

Codes 49491 through 49659 describe procedures related to hernia repair. To assign these codes accurately, the coding professional must be able to specify the type and/or site of the hernia, the history of the hernia, the age of the patient, and the clinical presentation of the hernia.

The following terms are used to describe the type and/or location of different hernias:

- *Inguinal hernia:* A common herniation of the inguinal canal in the groin area
- *Lumbar hernia:* A rare herniation in the lumbar region of the torso
- *Incisional hernia:* A herniation at the site of a previous surgical incision
- *Femoral hernia:* A common herniation in the femoral canal in the groin area
- *Epigastric hernia:* A herniation above the navel
- *Umbilical hernia:* A herniation at the navel
- *Spigelian hernia:* A herniation usually above the inferior epigastric vessel along the outer border of the rectus muscle

Some codes provide historical information specifying whether the hernia is an *initial* repair (first surgical repair of the hernia) or a *recurrent* repair (hernia has been surgically repaired previously). Other codes differentiate patients by age: any age, younger than 6 months, 6 months to younger than 5 years, or 5 years or older. Finally, a number of terms are used to describe the clinical presentation of hernias. These include:

- *Reducible:* The protruding organs can be returned to normal position by surgical (not medical) manipulation.
- *Sliding:* The colon or cecum is part of the hernia sac (in some cases, the urinary bladder also may be involved).
- *Incarcerated:* The hernia cannot be reduced without surgical intervention.
- *Strangulated:* The hernia is an incarcerated hernia in which the blood supply to the contained organ is reduced. A strangulated hernia presents a medical emergency.

The following example illustrates how the different variables describing hernias can be represented in a specific code assignment:

Example:

49550 Repair initial femoral hernia, any age; reducible
49553 incarcerated or strangulated

Traditional Hernia Repair (49491–49611)

A physician may perform one of three common types of repairs. The first type is the traditional or conventional repair. Under general anesthesia, the physician pushes the bulging tissue back into the abdominal cavity. The defect is closed by pulling together and stitching the surrounding muscles and ligaments. A recovery period of four to six weeks is usually needed.

Use of Mesh (49568)

The second type of herniorrhaphy uses mesh rather than stitches to repair the abdominal defect. Because stitches are not used, the patient experiences less postoperative pain. Commonly used meshes are Marlex and Prolene. When

If an operative report documents a reducible ventral hernia repaired laparoscopically with insertion of mesh (figure 4.25), the code assignment would be 49652. Note that the use of mesh is included in the code description.

coding a mesh repair of an **incisional** or **ventral** hernia, code 49568, Implantation of mesh or other prosthesis for an open incisional or ventral hernia repair (or for closure of debridement for necrotizing soft tissue infection), must be assigned in addition to the repair code. The use of mesh with other hernia repairs is not coded.

Laparoscopic Hernia Repair (49650–49659)

The third type of hernia repair is performed by a laparoscope. A laparoscopic repair is commonly performed to repair bilateral and recurrent hernias. Less discomfort and faster recovery are the main advantages of this approach. As with other endoscopies, a surgical laparoscopy includes a diagnostic laparoscopy. Figure 4.25 shows a laparoscopic ventral hernia repair.

Figure 4.25.   Laparoscopic ventral hernia repair

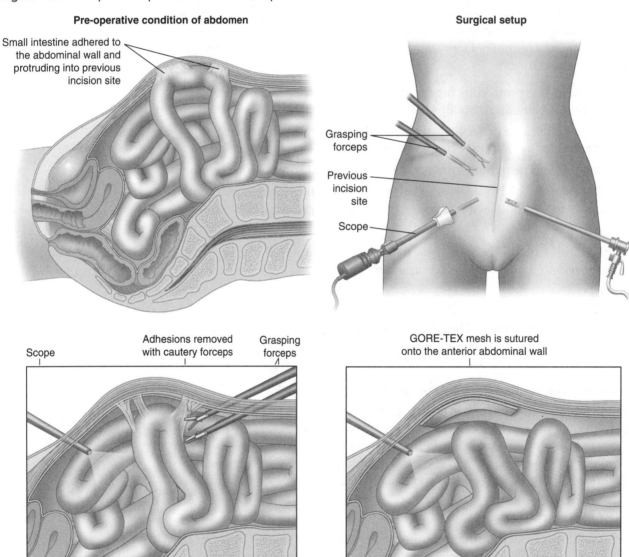

Pre-operative condition of abdomen

Small intestine adhered to the abdominal wall and protruding into previous incision site

Surgical setup

Grasping forceps

Previous incision site

Scope

Scope   Adhesions removed with cautery forceps   Grasping forceps

GORE-TEX mesh is sutured onto the anterior abdominal wall

Source: ©AHIMA.

Paraesophageal Hiatal Hernia Repair (43332–43337)

A paraesophageal hernia occurs when part of the stomach pushes through the opening in the diaphragm. The repair codes in this section are differentiated by the surgical technique used (laparotomy, thoracotomy, and thoracoabdominal incision) and by whether or not the procedure involved implantation of mesh. Figure 4.26 illustrates normal anatomy with a hiatal hernia.

Figure 4.26. Hiatal hernia

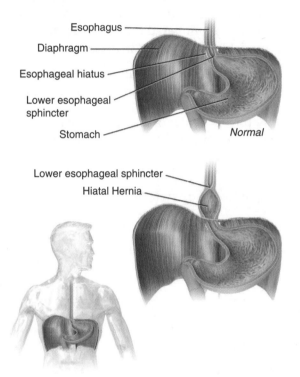

If documentation supports the repair of a hiatal hernia via thoracotomy (figure 4.26), the correct code would be 43334.

Source: Blaus, Bruce. "Hiatal Hernia." Digital Image. Wikimedia Commons. November, 2015. Accessed September, 2018. https://commons.wikimedia.org/wiki/File:Hiatal_Hernia.png.

Other Laparoscopic Procedures of the Digestive System

Laparoscopic procedures are minimally invasive, requiring less recovery time than traditional open procedures.

Laparoscopy was long used by gynecologists for the diagnosis of diseases of the ovary and uterus. Technological improvements, such as use of video cameras, have permitted procedures on the smallest of structures, and the use of laparoscopy has been extended to surgical procedures involving the appendix, colon, and other areas of the body.

In earlier editions of CPT, laparoscopic procedures were consolidated into one section. Laparoscopic procedures currently have their own headings in the various surgical sections.

For example, note the following sampling of laparoscopic procedures in the digestive system:

- 43280 Laparoscopic fundoplasty
- 44970 Laparoscopic appendectomy
- 45400 Laparoscopic proctopexy

Note: The format of CPT provides for an unlisted procedure code in each of the Laparoscopic code ranges. Because of the advancements of surgical practice and technology, it is common for unlisted procedures to be assigned for new procedures.

Exercise 4.26 Digestive System—Hernia Repairs

Answers to odd-numbered questions can be found in appendix C of this book. The answers to even-numbered questions are located in the instructor materials and are available to approved instructors.

Assign appropriate CPT code(s) for the following procedures. Assign only CPT surgical codes (no E/M codes) and append any applicable modifiers.

1. Initial herniorrhaphy for repair of an inguinal hernia and a unilateral hydrocelectomy of the spermatic cord (4-year-old patient)

   Code(s): _____

2. Laparoscopic repair of recurrent incisional hernia

   Code(s): _____

3. Diagnosis: recurrent inguinal hernia. Procedure: laparoscopic hernia repair

   Code(s): _____

4. Recurrent incarcerated inguinal hernia repair with implantation of mesh (56-year-old patient)

   Code(s): _____

5. Umbilical reducible herniorrhaphy (4-year-old patient)

   Code(s): _____

6. Initial repair of strangulated ventral hernia requiring mesh (49-year-old patient)

   Code(s): _____

7. Laparoscopic repair of paraesophageal hernia (no mention of mesh in documentation)

   Code(s): _____

Exercise 4.27 Digestive System—Operative Report

Answers to odd-numbered questions can be found in appendix C of this book. The answers to even-numbered questions are located in the instructor materials and are available to approved instructors.

Operative Report #1

Operative Report

Preoperative Diagnosis: Left inguinal hernia

Postoperative Diagnosis: Same

Procedure: Left initial inguinal hernia repair with mesh

Anesthesia: General

The patient is a 23-year-old man who presented with several weeks' history of pain in his left groin associated with a bulge. Examination revealed that his left groin did indeed have a bulge and his right groin was normal. We discussed the procedure as well as the choice of anesthesia.

After preoperative evaluation and clearance, the patient was brought into the operating suite and placed in a comfortable supine position on the OR table. Monitoring equipment was attached, and general anesthesia was induced. His left groin was sterilely prepped and draped, and an inguinal incision made. This was carried down through the subcutaneous tissues until the external oblique fascia was reached. This was split in a direction parallel with its fibers, and the medial aspect of the opening included the external ring. The ileo-inguinal nerve was identified, and care was taken to retract this inferiorly out of the way. The cord structures were encircled and the cremasteric muscle fibers divided. At this point, we examined the floor of the inguinal canal, and the patient did appear to have a weakness here. We then explored the cord. There was no evidence of an indirect hernia. A piece of 3×5 mesh was obtained and trimmed to fit. It was placed down in the inguinal canal and tacked to the pubic tubercle. It was then run inferiorly along the pelvic shelving edge until lateral to the internal ring and tacked down superiorly using interrupted sutures of 0-Prolene. A single stitch was placed lateral to the cord to recreate the internal ring. Details of the mesh were tucked underneath the external oblique fascia. The cord and the nerve were allowed to drop back into the wound, and the wound was infiltrated with

(Continued on next page)

Exercise 4.27 (Continued)

30 cc of half percent Marcaine. The external oblique fascia was then closed with a running suture of 0-Vicryl. Subcutaneous tissues were approximated with interrupted sutures of 3-0 Vicryl. The skin was closed with a running subcuticular suture of 4-0 Vicryl. Benzoin and Steri-Strips and a dry sterile dressing were applied. All sponge, needle, and instrument counts were correct at the end of the procedure. The patient tolerated the procedure well and was taken to the recovery room in stable condition.

Assign only CPT surgical codes (no E/M codes) and append any applicable modifiers.

Code(s): _____

Exercise 4.28 Digestive System Review

Assign appropriate CPT code(s) for the following procedures and indicate the index entries that were used to identify the codes. Assign only CPT surgical codes (no E/M codes) and append any applicable modifiers.

1. Infrared coagulation of internal hemorrhoids

    Code(s): _____

2. Laparoscopic gastric bypass and Roux-en-Y gastroenterostomy performed for obesity

    Code(s): _____

3. EGD (flexible, transoral) with balloon dilation of gastric outlet obstruction

    Code(s): _____

4. Under fluoroscopy, the physician percutaneously places an external biliary catheter into the bile duct for drainage.

    Code(s): _____

5. Colonoscopy with removal of polyp with a saline-left technique followed by a hot snare excision

    Code(s): _____

6. Laparoscopic aspiration of ovarian cyst

    Code(s): _____

7. Removal of a chicken bone from pharynx

Code(s): _____

8. Percutaneous replacement of gastrostomy tube requiring debridement of granulation tissue in order to insert the new tube

Code(s): _____

9. Anoscopy with removal of polyp via snare

Code(s): _____

10. Palatoplasty for cleft palate, soft

Code(s): _____

Urinary System

Learning Objectives

- Describe the organization and format for genitourinary endoscopy procedures.

- Identify the documentation requirements for coding treatment of urinary calculi.
- Define *bundled codes*.

The urinary subsection includes surgical procedures involving the kidney, ureter, bladder, and urethra. These codes are categorized first by body part involved and then by procedure performed, such as cystourethroscopy, percutaneous renal biopsy, transurethral resection of the prostate, and urethroplasty. Figure 4.27 provides an illustration of the urinary system.

Be careful to distinguish between *urethra* and *ureter* in the code descriptions.

Figure 4.27. Components of the urinary system

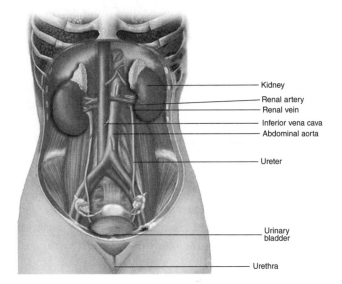

- Kidney
- Renal artery
- Renal vein
- Inferior vena cava
- Abdominal aorta
- Ureter
- Urinary bladder
- Urethra

Source: ©AHIMA.

Expansion of Minimally Invasive Procedures

Similar to the percutaneous placement of biliary stents and catheters, the urinary system also has several codes that highlight the expansion of minimally invasive procedures, commonly performed by interventional radiologists. CPT codes, such as 50432 (Percutaneous placement of nephrostomy catheter) and 50693 (Percutaneous placement of ureteral stent) describe procedures that can be performed, under guidance, through a small incision in the skin.

Urodynamics

Urodynamics is the investigation of the function of the lower urinary tract (the bladder and urethra) using physical measurements, such as urine pressure and flow rate, as well as clinical assessments. Codes 51725 through 51798 describe urodynamic procedures that may be reported separately or in combination when more than one procedure is performed. Modifier 51 should be reported when multiple procedures are performed (modifier 51 is for physician use only) if required by the payer. These procedures are performed either by the physician or under his or her direction. The following services/supplies are considered part of the procedure and should not be reported separately: instruments, equipment, fluids, gases, probes, catheters, technicians' fees, medications, gloves, trays, tubing, and other sterile supplies.

If the physician is providing only the professional component (that is, the supervision and interpretation), modifier 26 also should be reported for physician services.

The following definitions (Rogers 2004) describing the various urodynamic procedures will help the coding professional assign the appropriate CPT code:

- *Cystometrogram:* An examination performed to determine the capacity of the urinary bladder. A simple cystometrogram is the measurement of the bladder's capacity, sensation of filling, and intravesical pressure. A complex cystometrogram involves the measurement of the bladder's capacity, sensation of filling, and intravesical pressure using a rectal probe to distinguish between intra-abdominal pressure and bladder pressure.
- *Uroflowmetry:* An examination performed to determine the functional capacity of the urinary bladder. *Simple* uroflowmetry is the measurement of voiding time and peak flow. *Complex* uroflowmetry involves the measurement and recording of mean and peak flow and the time taken to reach peak flow during continuous urination.
- *Urethral pressure profile (UPP):* An examination that involves the recording of pressures along the urethra as a special catheter is slowly withdrawn.
- *Electromyography:* Studies performed to record muscle activity during voiding and to simultaneously record urine flow rate.

Genitourinary Endoscopies

In general, genitourinary endoscopies are categorized by body part involved—urethra, prostate, or ureter—and specific procedure performed, such as cystourethroscopy with biopsy of the bladder or urethra, transurethral incision of prostate, cystourethroscopy with ureteral meatotomy, and cystourethroscopy with insertion of indwelling ureteral stent. Cystourethroscopy, also known as cystoscopy, is an examination with a narrow, flexible tube-like instrument passed through the urethra to examine the bladder and urinary tract for structural abnormalities or obstructions, such as tumors or stones. Figure 4.28 shows an example of a cystoscopy procedure. If the physician documents that a diagnostic procedure was performed, the correct code assignment would be 52000 for Cystourethroscopy. An operative report that documents that a biopsy was performed during the cystoscopy, the correct code would be 52204, Cystourethroscopy with biopsy.

> If the urologist inserted the cystoscopy into the male patient for balloon dilation of a stricture in the ureteropelvic junction (figure 4.28), the code would be 52342.

Figure 4.28. Cystoscopy

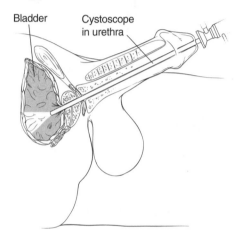

Source: ©AHIMA.

Treatment of Calculi

Urinary calculi are solid particles that can be found anywhere along the urinary tract and can cause pain, vomiting, and potentially obstruction. CPT includes a variety of codes pertaining to treatment of calculi (stones). The stone may be fragmented, manipulated, taken out, or a treated by a combination of these methods. Figure 4.29 depicts stones in the portion of the ureter that is exiting the bladder as well as a mid-ureteral stone and one that is in the ureteropelvic junction. Accurate coding requires documentation of both the anatomic site and the treatment (such as fragmentation or removal).

Bundled Codes

In some cases, CPT "bundles" several minor procedures under a main procedure description, such as code 52647. For example, if laser vaporization of the prostate were performed with meatotomy or dilation, codes for those minor procedures would be included in 52647 and would not warrant an additional code assignment.

Example:

52647 Laser vaporization of prostate, including control of postoperative bleeding, complete (vasectomy, meatotomy, cystourethroscopy, urethral calibration and/or dilation, internal urethrotomy and transurethral resection of prostate are included if performed)

Figure 4.29. Calculous urinary obstruction

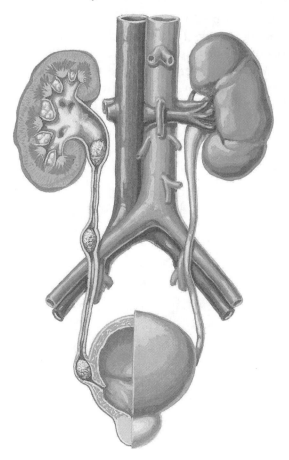

JOHN A.CRAIG—AD

Exercise 4.29   Urinary System—Cystoscopy

Answers to odd-numbered questions can be found in appendix C of this book. The answers to even-numbered questions are located in the instructor materials and are available to approved instructors.

Assign appropriate CPT code(s) for the following procedures. Assign only CPT surgical codes (no E/M codes) and append any applicable modifiers.

1. Cystoscopy for insertion of double-J ureteral stent

    Code(s): _____

2. Cystoscopy, left ureteroscopy with laser lithotripsy

    Code(s): _____

3. Cystoscopy with fulguration of 2.0-cm lesion of bladder

Code(s): _____

4. Cystoscopy with insertion of permanent urethral stent

Code(s): _____

5. Cystoscopy passes through the urethra to the bladder and manipulates the ureteral stone so that the patient may pass it on their own

Code(s): _____

6. Cystourethroscopy for removal of ureteral stent

Code(s): _____

Exercise 4.30   Urinary System—Operative Reports

Answers to odd-numbered questions can be found in appendix C of this book. The answers to even-numbered questions are located in the instructor materials and are available to approved instructors.

Operative Report #1

Operative Report

Preoperative Diagnosis: Right ureteral stone

Postoperative Diagnosis: Same

Procedure: Right ureteroscopy, stone extraction, stent

The patient was taken to the operating suite and placed in the dorsal lithotomy position, and then sterilely prepared and draped in the usual fashion. Cystoscope was then inserted into the urethra; it was normal. The prostate was nonobstructed, and the bladder was free of neoplasm, infection, or calculus. There was some edema of the right intramural ureter. A guide wire was introduced into the right ureteral orifice, and advanced to the right renal-collecting system without difficulty. A balloon was used to dilate the ureter, and a scope was introduced. The gravel was noted from the stone being fragmented from the balloon. This was washing out. The remainder of the ureter was examined and found to be free of neoplasm, perforation, or calculus. The stent was inserted. A string was kept attached. The patient was transferred to the recovery room in satisfactory condition.

(Continued on next page)

Exercise 4.30 (Continued)

Assign only CPT surgical codes (no E/M codes) and append any applicable modifiers.

Code(s) (physician services only): _____

Operative Report #2

Operative Report

Preoperative Diagnosis: Recurrent bladder cancer

Postoperative Diagnosis: Recurrent bladder cancer

Procedure: Cystoscopy with bladder biopsies and fulguration

Anesthesia: General

The patient has prior transitional cell carcinoma of the bladder and also carcinoma *in situ*. He has received MVAC therapy and BCG. Surveillance cystoscopy demonstrated erythema of the bladder wall. He is currently being admitted for cystoscopy, bladder biopsy, and fulguration. Procedure, reasons, risks, and complications were reviewed and consent was granted.

He was brought to the operating room under general anesthesia, placed in the dorsolithotomy position, and prepped and draped in a sterile manner. A #21 French cystoscope was inserted, urethra was normal, verumontanum intact. Prostate examination revealed evidence of prior transurethral resection and moderate outlet obstruction. There were erythematous areas throughout the bladder, and a 0.5-cm lesion was fulgurated. Both ureteric orifices were normal size, shape, and caliber with clear efflux. The erythematous areas were then biopsied with flexible biopsy forceps. After obtaining biopsies, the area was then fulgurated with a Bugbee electrode. Reinspection was carried out; no gross bleeding was noted. The bladder was drained, cystoscope was withdrawn, and the patient was transferred to the recovery room in satisfactory condition with all vital signs stable.

Pathology Report

Final Diagnosis: 1. Urothelial carcinoma in situ, focal

2. Chronic nonspecific cystitis

Assign only CPT surgical codes (no E/M codes) and append any applicable modifiers.

Code(s): _____

Exercise 4.31   Urinary System Review

Answers to odd-numbered questions can be found in appendix C of this book. The answers to even-numbered questions are located in the instructor materials and are available to approved instructors.

Assign appropriate CPT code(s) for the following procedures. Assign only CPT surgical codes (no E/M codes) and append any applicable modifiers.

1. Laparoscopic sling procedure for stress incontinence

    Code(s): _____

2. Under ultrasound guidance, the physician percutaneously inserts a ureteral stent. This was a new access and no nephrostomy catheter was needed.

    Code(s): _____

3. Cystoscopy with fulguration of 2.0-cm benign tumor

    Code(s): _____

4. Closure of ureterocutaneous fistula

    Code(s): _____

5. Needle renal biopsy

    Code(s): _____

6. Cystoscopy with ureteroscopy for removal of ureteral stone

    Code(s): _____

7. Cystourethroscopy with bilateral ureteral meatotomy

    Code(s): _____

8. Endoscopic injection of pyrolytic carbon coated beads (Durasphere) into the bladder neck for a patient with incontinence.

    Code(s): _____

9. Laparoscopic partial nephrectomy

    Code(s): _____

10. Cystotomy with excision of bladder diverticulum

    Code(s): _____

Male Genital System

Learning Objectives

- Differentiate between the removal of lesion codes for the penis.
- Describe the various methods for removing prostate tissue.

The codes in the male genital system subsection are used to report procedures on the penis, testis, epididymis, tunica vaginalis, scrotum, vas deferens, spermatic cord, seminal vesicle, and prostate gland. Figure 4.30 illustrates these structures.

Figure 4.30. The male genital system

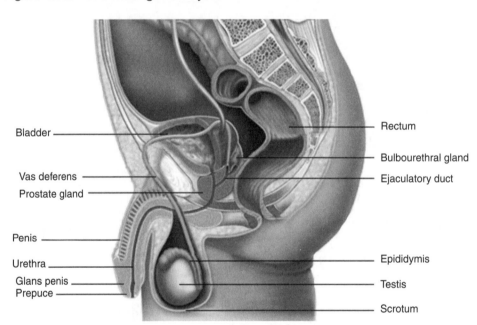

Source: ©AHIMA.

Removal of Lesions

Removal of lesions (for example, condyloma, papilloma, molluscum contagiosum, herpetic vesicle) of the penis is not located in the integumentary system subsection but, rather, in the male genital system (54050–54065) subsection. The code selection is determined by the method of removal. For destruction or excision of other lesions, reference the integumentary system subsection of the surgery section.

Prostatectomy

CPT is a terminology that describes surgical techniques of which prostatectomy is a good example.

The prostate gland lies under the bladder and surrounds the first part of the urethra, which carries urine to the penis. When the prostate becomes enlarged, it tends to obstruct the urethra and makes urination difficult. There are several methods for prostatectomy procedures, each involving a different approach: transurethral (most common), retropubic, and perineal. Transurethral resection of the prostate (TURP) (52601–52640) in the urinary system section uses a scope inserted through the urethra to remove the prostate tissue piece by piece (see figure 4.31). In the male genital subsection procedures described as perineal prostatectomy (55801–55815), the prostate is removed through an incision in the area between the scrotum and the anus. The suprapubic approach (55821) requires an incision in the front wall of the bladder. A retropubic prostatectomy (55831–55845) requires the surgeon to make an incision in the wall of the abdomen to directly reach the prostate. CPT also provides a code for laparoscopic retropubic radical prostatectomy (55866). In 2019, CPT added another technique for destruction of prostate tissue using radiofrequency-generated water vapor thermotherapy (53854). Category III codes include another technique called waterjet ablation (0421T).

Figure 4.31.   Benign prostate surgery: Transurethral

If the operative report described a TURP (figure 4.31), the code assignment would be 52601.

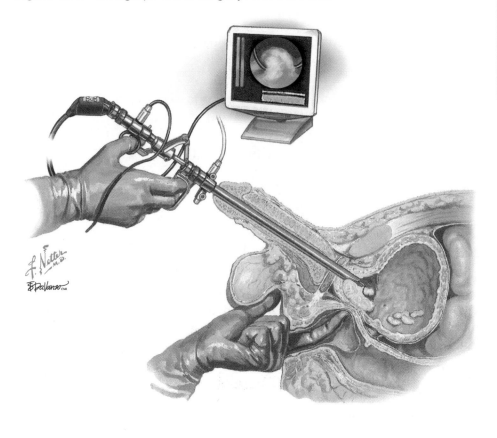

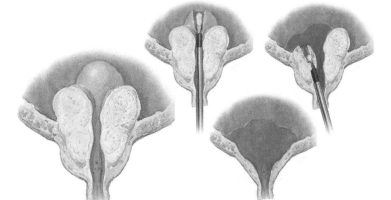

Exercise 4.32 Male Genital System

Answers to odd-numbered questions can be found in appendix C of this book. The answers to even-numbered questions are located in the instructor materials and are available to approved instructors.

Assign appropriate CPT code(s) for the following procedures. Assign only CPT surgical codes (no E/M codes) and append any applicable modifiers.

1. Laser destruction of four condylomas of the penis

   Code(s): _____

2. Incision and drainage of subcutaneous abscess of the penis

   Code(s): _____

3. Radical retropubic prostatectomy with bilateral pelvic lymphadenectomy

   Code(s): _____

4. For elective sterilization, the surgeon performs a vasectomy

   Code(s): _____

5. Clamp circumcision, newborn, with regional anesthesia

   Code(s): _____

Exercise 4.33 Male Genital System—Operative Reports

Answers to odd-numbered questions can be found in appendix C of this book. The answers to even-numbered questions are located in the instructor materials and are available to approved instructors.

Operative Report #1

Operative Report

Preoperative Diagnosis: Adenocarcinoma of the prostate

Postoperative Diagnosis: Same

Procedure: Transrectal ultrasound

Transperineal implant of I–125 seeds into the prostate

Anesthesia: General

The patient was brought to the cysto suite and placed in the lithotomy position at a 90-degree angle. General anesthesia was induced, and a Foley catheter was placed. The ultrasound probe was positioned in the rectum, and the appropriate reference points were identified and compared to his previous volumetric studies.

Under fluoroscopic and ultrasound guidance, 19 needles were inserted into the prostate based on a premeasured template. Approximately 70 seeds were placed.

A cystoscopic examination was performed at the end of the case, and no seeds were identified within the urinary bladder.

A Foley catheter was replaced into the bladder and will be removed later today. The appropriate postimplantation radiation and postoperative instructions were given. He tolerated the procedure well and was taken to the recovery room in satisfactory condition.

Assign only CPT surgical codes (no E/M codes) and append any applicable modifiers.

Code(s) for the physician's services: _____

Operative Report #2

Operative Report

Preoperative Diagnosis:	Chronic left orchialgia
	Chronic epididymitis
Procedure:	Left inguinal orchiectomy
Anesthesia:	Local standby; 0.25% Marcaine, 1% Xylocaine, 1/1 dilution. Total 25 cc used as inguinal block
Estimated Blood Loss:	Minimal

This is an 82-year-old man with chronic left gonadal pain due to chronic granulomatous epididymitis. This has failed to respond to conservative measures and has caused him marked discomfort in the left groin. As a result, we recommended that he consider outpatient orchiectomy. The risks and potential complications were discussed and informed consent obtained.

The patient was given Ancef IV as well as IV sedation and placed on the operating table in the supine position. The lower groin and abdomen were shaved, prepared, and draped in the standard fashion. The external inguinal ring was identified, and an area just distal to the external inguinal ring was anesthetized with the local anesthetic, and a small transverse incision was made down to the spermatic cord. The testis was then brought out through the inguinal incision after the spermatic cord blockade with local anesthetic. The testis was separated from the scrotum by incision in the

(Continued on next page)

Exercise 4.33   (Continued)

gubernaculum with needle tip Bovie. The spermatic cord was identified, dissected back to the external inguinal ring, and bisected with a curved Kelly clamp and then clamped and transected with Metzenbaum scissors. The spermatic cord was closed with suture ligature of 0 Vicryl and a free tie of 0 Vicryl proximal to this on each side of the spermatic cord. The incision was inspected for hemostasis. No further bleeding was noted, and the testis was delivered for pathologic evaluation. The Scarpa's fascia was closed with interrupted 2-0 Vicryl, and the skin was closed with a running 4-0 Vicryl subcuticular closure. Steri-Strips and four by fours were applied as a dressing. He was returned to the recovery room in stable condition. Estimated blood loss was minimal.

Assign only CPT surgical codes (no E/M codes) and append any applicable modifiers.

Code(s) for the physician's services: _____

Exercise 4.34   Male Genital System Review

Answers to odd-numbered questions can be found in appendix C of this book. The answers to even-numbered questions are located in the instructor materials and are available to approved instructors.

Assign appropriate CPT code(s) for the following procedures. Assign only CPT surgical codes (no E/M codes) and append any applicable modifiers.

1. Excision of spermatocele with epididymectomy

   Code(s): _____

2. Removal of condylomas of the penis with use of cryosurgery

   Code(s): _____

3. Laparoscopic orchiectomy

   Code(s): _____

4. Incision into abscess of scrotal wall to drain pus

   Code(s): _____

5. Biopsy and exploration of epididymis

   Code(s): _____

6. Laparoscopic retropubic radical prostatectomy

   Code(s): _____

7. Punch biopsy of prostate

   Code(s): _____

8. Waterjet ablation of prostatic tissue, transurethral

   Code(s): _____

9. Bilateral orchiopexy, inguinal approach with hernia repair

   Code(s): _____

10. One-stage distal hypospadias repair with simple meatal advancement

    Code(s): _____

Female Genital System

Learning Objectives

- Define *LEEP*.
- Differentiate between a laparoscopic and hysteroscopic procedure.
- Describe the documentation requirements for hysterectomy procedures.

The female genital system subsection of the CPT surgery chapter includes codes for various surgical repairs, dilation and curettage (D&C), and hysterectomies and hysteroscopies. This section also contains codes for maternity care and delivery. Figure 4.32 provides an illustration of the female reproductive system.

Colposcopy

Colposcopy is a visual examination of the women's genital area, including the cervix, vagina, and vulva. CPT code ranges 57420–57421 and 57452–57461 are differentiated by the area visualized and additional procedures, such as biopsy, performed during the endoscopy.

Loop Electrode Biopsy (57460) vs. Loop Electrode Conization of Cervix (57461)

A loop electrosurgical excision procedure (LEEP) uses a thin wire loop with electric current to remove a piece of tissue and control bleeding. Figure 4.33 depicts a LEEP in which the wire loop scrapes off tissue for a biopsy specimen to determine a pathological diagnosis. If this were performed via colposcopy with no mention of a portion of the endocervix/transformation zone being removed, the correct code would be 57460. If the loop electrode were used to

Figure 4.32. The female reproductive system

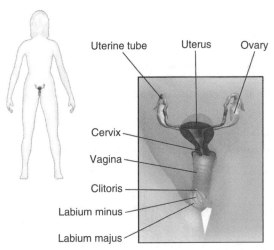

Uterine tube   Uterus   Ovary

Cervix

Vagina

Clitoris

Labium minus

Labium majus

Source: Blaus, Bruce. "Female Reproductive System" Digital Image. Wikimedia Commons. November, 2013. Accessed September, 2018. https://commons.wikimedia.org/wiki/File:Blausen_0399 _FemaleReproSystem_01.png.

Figure 4.33. Loop electrosurgical excision procedure (LEEP)

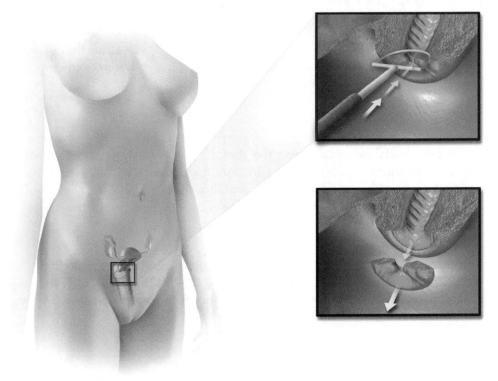

Source: Blaus, Bruce. "LEEP" Digital Image. Wikimedia Commons. June, 2017. Accessed September, 2018. https://commons.wikimedia.org/wiki/File:LEEP.png.

remove a cone-shaped section of tissue (conization) from the cervix, code 57461 would be reported.

Documentation within the health record should support the coding decision. For example, documentation to support code 57461 may include removal of a portion of the endocervix or transformation zone. If documentation is unclear, a physician query may be necessary.

Laparoscopy

In a laparoscopic procedure, the surgeon first inserts a needle through the navel and the abdomen is filled with carbon dioxide gas. The gas pushes the internal organs away from the abdominal wall to decrease the risk of injury to surrounding organs. Next, the surgeon makes a small incision in the abdominal area (navel is common) and inserts a tube with a tiny video camera (laparoscope) to visualize the inside of the pelvis and abdomen. Additional small cuts may be made if other instruments are needed such as a small probe for a clearer view. If defects or abnormalities are discovered, a diagnostic laparoscopy can become an operative laparoscopy. Figure 4.34 illustrates a laparoscopic procedure on a female patient.

> If the operative report stated that, during the laparoscopic procedure, both tubes and ovaries were resected, the code assignment would be 58661.

....

Figure 4.34.   Laparoscopy

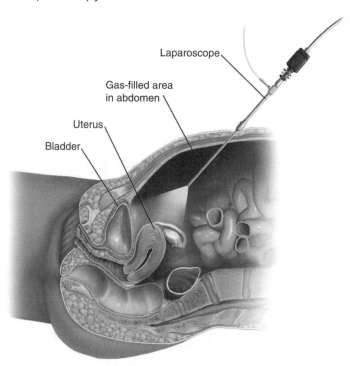

Laparoscope

Gas-filled area in abdomen

Uterus

Bladder

Source: Blaus, Bruce. "Laparoscopy" Digital Image. Wikimedia Commons. February, 2014. Accessed September, 2018. https://commons.wikimedia.org/wiki/File:Blausen_0602_Laparoscopy_02.png.

Hysteroscopy

A hysteroscope is a thin, telescope-like instrument that allows the physician to look inside the uterus. After insufflation of the uterine cavity with CO_2, the hysteroscope is inserted through the cervical canal and into the uterus. This direct visualization improves the accuracy of diagnosis and treatment. Accessory instruments that may be used with a hysteroscope procedure include scissors, forceps, lasers, and various electrodes. A D&C is commonly performed with a hysteroscopic biopsy or polypectomy. Therefore, no additional code is assigned to identify the D&C. Codes for hysteroscopies are included in the range 58555 through 58579. Figure 4.35 displays a hysteroscopy procedure.

If the surgeon performed a hysteroscopy for removal of a fibroid (figure 4.35), the correct code would be 58561.

Figure 4.35. Hysteroscopy

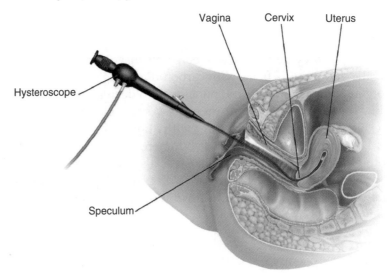

Source: Blaus, Bruce. "Hysteroscopy" Digital Image. Wikimedia Commons. November, 2015. Accessed September, 2018. https://commons.wikimedia.org/wiki/File:Hysteroscopy.png.

Hysterectomy

CPT bases the coding selection for hysterectomies on several decision-making pathways:

- Laparoscopic versus open
- Type of hysterectomy (such as vaginal, supracervical, abdominal)
- Weight of uterus
- Uterus removed with other structures such as tubes or ovaries

Laparoscopic Supracervical Hysterectomy (58541–58544)

This laparoscopic procedure removes the uterus but preserves the cervix. CPT codes differentiate between the weight of the uterus and whether or not the tubes and ovaries were removed.

Laparoscopic Vaginal Hysterectomy (58550–58554)

Laparoscopically assisted vaginal hysterectomy (LAVH) is a surgical procedure using a laparoscope to remove the uterus and/or fallopian tubes and ovaries through the vagina.

Laparoscopic Total Hysterectomy (58570–58573)

For this procedure, the uterus and the cervix both are removed entirely through the scope. The code selection provides for the weight of the uterus and whether or not the tubes and ovaries were removed.

Excisional (Open) Approach (58150–58294)

The excisional operation can be performed through the vagina (58260–58294) or through a conventional incision in the front wall of the abdomen (58150–58240).

Maternity Care and Delivery Subsection (Guidelines for Physician Services)

Along with codes for surgery and other procedures involving the female reproductive organs, the female genital system subsection includes CPT codes for maternity care and delivery services. Antepartum care includes initial and subsequent history, physical examination, recording of clinical information, and monthly visits up to 28-week gestation, biweekly visits to 36-week gestation, and weekly visits until the time of delivery. According to the CPT code book, any additional visits are to be coded separately using E/M codes. Health plans may have specific rules about the reporting of services beyond those included in the global service package that often accompanies maternity coverage. This may affect the reporting of services, particularly if more than one physician is required to care for the patient, as may occur with unexpected cesarean delivery.

Delivery services include admission to the hospital, admission H&P, management of uncomplicated labor, vaginal delivery (with or without episiotomy, with or without forceps), or cesarean delivery. Detailed guidance for reporting services is provided before code 59000.

Postpartum care codes include both hospital and office visit codes following either vaginal or cesarean delivery.

Some CPT codes address global care, and some are used to report only a portion of care.

Example:

CPT code 59425 is for antepartum care only, 4 to 6 visits. It may be used by a family practice physician who refers a patient in the second trimester of pregnancy to an obstetrician due to a high risk of complications.

Code 59510 would be reported by a physician providing global care for a cesarean delivery from start to finish.

Patients who attempt vaginal delivery after previous cesarean delivery or who successfully deliver vaginally after previous cesarean delivery have specific CPT codes assigned from the 59610 through 59622 range. These codes should always be used when they apply.

Exercise 4.35   Female Genital System

Answers to odd-numbered questions can be found in appendix C of this book. The answers to even-numbered questions are located in the instructor materials and are available to approved instructors.

Assign appropriate CPT code(s) for the following procedures. Assign only CPT surgical codes (no E/M codes) and append any applicable modifiers.

1. Laparoscopic fulguration of fallopian tubes

Code(s): _____

(Continued on next page)

Exercise 4.35 (Continued)

2. Laparoscopy with aspiration of ovarian cyst

Code(s): _____

3. D&C performed for a patient with diagnosis of incomplete abortion (8 weeks pregnant)

Code(s): _____

4. D&C performed for a patient with dysfunctional bleeding

Code(s): _____

5. Laparoscopic ablation of fibroids

Code(s): _____

6. Abdominal hysterectomy with salpingo-oophorectomy (uterus weight 270 g)

Code(s): _____

7. Laparoscopic vaginal hysterectomy (uterus 240 gr) with salpingo-oophorectomy

Code(s): _____

8. Total abdominal hysterectomy with bilateral salpingo-oophorectomy, omentectomy, dissection of pelvic lymph nodes with removal of a portion of the para-aortic lymph nodes, and debulking of ovarian tumors.

Code(s): _____

Exercise 4.36 Female Genital System—Operative Reports

Answers to odd-numbered questions can be found in appendix C of this book. The answers to even-numbered questions are located in the instructor materials and are available to approved instructors.

Operative Report #1

Operative Report

Preoperative Diagnosis:	Moderate dysplasia of the cervix
Postoperative Diagnosis:	Same
Procedure:	Loop electrosurgical excision procedure (LEEP)
Anesthesia:	General inhalation anesthesia per mask The patient was brought to the OR with IV fluids infusing and

placed on the table in the supine position. General inhalation anesthesia per mask was administered after acquisition of an adequate anesthetic level, and the patient was placed in the lithotomy position. The perineum was draped. A laser speculum was placed in the vaginal vault. The cervix was rinsed with a solution of acetic acid, and colposcopic examination of the cervix showed areas of wide epithelium across the anterior lip of the cervix, consistent with the previous biopsy showing moderate dysplasia. Using the 2-cm electrosurgical loop excision, the endocervical canal was cauterized with bipolar cautery to remove all diseased tissue. Then the conization procedure was completed. The speculum was removed. The patient was taken out of the lithotomy position. Her anesthesia was reversed. She was awakened and taken to the recovery room in stable condition. Sponge, instrument, and needle counts were correct times three. Estimated blood loss was less than 25 cc.

Assign only CPT surgical codes (no E/M codes) and append any applicable modifiers.

Code(s) for the physician's services: _____

Operative Report #2

Operative Report

Preoperative Diagnosis: Dysfunctional uterine bleeding, failed hormonal therapy

Postoperative Diagnosis: Same

Procedure Performed: Diagnostic hysteroscopy

Fractional dilation and curettage

The patient is a 35-year-old Gravida V Para IV AB I female from the Towne Health Center. She has been bleeding the majority of each month over the past 4 months. She has been tried on Ortho-Novum 7/7 to control the bleeding, but this has been of no help. The patient is here for the above procedure.

Description of Procedure: With the patient under satisfactory general anesthesia in the dorsal lithotomy position, a pelvic examination revealed a cervix that came down to the introitus, constituting a second-degree uterine prolapse. The patient had many hymenal tags on both the right and left side. A large speculum was placed inside the vagina. The anterior lip of the cervix was grasped with a single-toothed tenaculum. The cervix was sounded to 8.5 cm. The endocervical canal was now serially

(Continued on next page)

Exercise 4.36 (Continued)

dilated. Using the hysteroscope and lactated Ringer's solution as a distending solution, the hysteroscope was passed through the internal os into the uterine cavity. Inspection of the uterine contents revealed both right and left ostia identified. Some lining was on the floor of the uterus and some on the roof. The fundus was devoid of any lining. There were no submucosal fibroids and no submucosal septa. The hysteroscope was removed, and the next procedure was fractional dilation and curettage. Using a Kevorkian-Younge curette, the endocervical canal was curetted and the cervical canal was further dilated using a medium-sized curette. The endometrial cavity was curetted with moderate curettings obtained. These were sent for pathological diagnosis. The patient tolerated the procedure fairly well and was escorted to the recovery room in satisfactory condition.

Assign only CPT surgical codes (no E/M codes) and append any applicable modifiers.

Code(s) for the physician's services: _____

Exercise 4.37 Female Genital System Review

Answers to odd-numbered questions can be found in appendix C of this book. The answers to even-numbered questions are located in the instructor materials and are available to approved instructors.

Assign appropriate CPT code(s) for the following procedures. Assign only CPT surgical codes (no E/M codes) and append any applicable modifiers.

1. Colposcopy of the vagina with biopsy

   Code(s): _____

2. Vulvectomy, partial removal of skin and superficial subcutaneous tissues

   Code(s): _____

3. Laparoscopy with fulguration of peritoneal lesions

   Code(s): _____

4. Patient desires elective sterilization. Surgeon performs laparoscopic coagulation of the fallopian tubes.

   Code(s): _____

5. Laparoscopic ablation of fibroids

   Code(s): _____

6. Biopsy of two lesions, one from labia minora and another from the vaginal orifice, which required suture closure

Code(s): _____

7. Laparoscopic vaginal hysterectomy with bilateral salpingo-oophorectomy (uterus weighing 280 g)

Code(s): _____

8. Hysteroscopy with polypectomy and D&C

Code(s): _____

9. Laparoscopic total hysterectomy with bilateral salpingo-oophorectomy (uterus weighing 280 g)

Code(s): _____

10. Endometrial cryoablation with ultrasonic guidance

Code(s): _____

Endocrine System

Learning Objective

- Apply CPT coding principles and guidelines to successfully assign codes.

The endocrine system functions in the regulation of body activities. This ductless system acts through chemical messengers called hormones that influence growth, development, and metabolic activities. There are no specific coding guidelines applicable to this subsection, but knowledge of anatomy, physiology, and medical terminology is necessary for accurate code assignment.

Exercise 4.38   Endocrine System Review

Answers to odd-numbered questions can be found in appendix C of this book. The answers to even-numbered questions are located in the instructor materials and are available to approved instructors.

Assign appropriate CPT code(s) for the following procedures and indicate the index entries that were used to identify the codes. Assign only CPT surgical codes (no E/M codes) and append any applicable modifiers.

1. Excision of thyroglossal duct cyst

Code(s): _____

(Continued on next page)

Exercise 4.38   (Continued)

2. Parathyroidectomy

Code(s): _____

3. Patient had a previous surgery for removal of part of thyroid; she now has a bilateral thyroidectomy for remaining tissue

Code(s): _____

4. Laparoscopic hemithyroidectomy

Code(s): _____

5. Aspiration of thyroid cyst

Code(s): _____

6. Laparoscopic adrenalectomy, complete

Code(s): _____

Nervous System

Learning Objectives

- Differentiate between laminotomy and laminectomy.

- Describe the documentation requirements for coding spinal injection procedures

Coding for spine surgeries can be considered complex. Advanced coding practice and education helps coding professionals become more confident in this specialty area.

The nervous system subsection of the CPT surgery chapter includes the procedures that involve the brain, spinal cord, and peripheral nerves. The CPT codes for procedures performed to manage pain, such as nerve blocks and epidural procedures, also are part of this subsection. Examples of procedures in this subsection include major brain operations such as craniectomies and craniotomies, as well as relatively minor spinal injections and catheter insertions into the nerves and the spinal cord. Figure 4.30 reveals the anatomy of the spine.

Laminotomy and Laminectomy

If the documentation stated that the patient suffered from a herniated lumbar disc at L3-L4, and therefore a hemilaminectomy with partial facetectomy was performed to relieve the pressure on the nerve root, the code would be 63030.

Laminectomy is surgery to remove the lamina (back part of the vertebra) that covers the spinal canal. Figure 4.36 displays the anatomic structures and surgical procedures associated with lumbar laminectomy. The procedure is used to relieve pressure on the spinal cord or nerves. Pressure is often caused by stenosis or a herniated disk. Decompression is accomplished by removing bony overgrowths or tissues that are pressing on the spine. Laminotomy is the removal a small portion of the lamina, usually on one side. The CPT codes for surgical procedures involving the spine are based on the surgical approach, the anatomic location of the precipitating condition, and the specific procedures performed.

Figure 4.36. Lumbar laminectomy

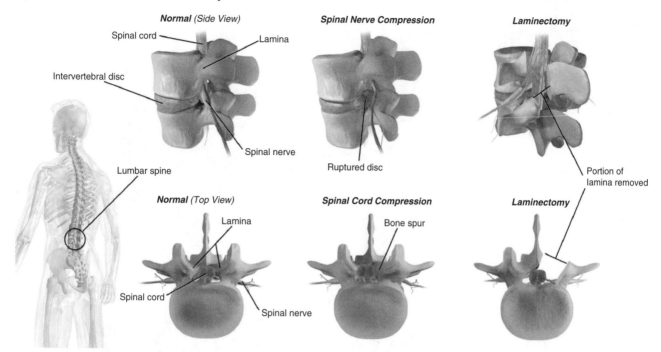

Source: Blaus, Bruce. "Lumbar Laminectomy." Digital Image. Wikimedia Commons. November, 2015. Accessed September, 2018. https:// commons.wikimedia.org/wiki/File:Lumbar_Laminectomy.png.

Spinal Injections

Spinal injections, or infusions, are coded according to the site of the injection and the substance injected. Spinal injections deliver medications through a needle placed into a structure or space in the spine to allow the physician to identify the source of pain or to reduce it. Typical medications used include local anesthetics and corticosteroids. Local anesthetics numb the nerves and corticosteroids help reduce inflammation.

To accurately assign codes for these procedures, coding professionals must abstract documentation from the operative report to determine the following:

- Approach (such as epidural, transforaminal, or facet)
- Injection site (such as cervical or lumbar)
- Substance injected (such as neurolytic, steroid, or anesthetic)
- Number of levels being treated

For example, a single interlaminar epidural steroid injection into the lumbar spine would be assigned CPT code 62322 If the same epidural lumbar (single level) injection was inserted transforaminal the correct CPT code would be 64483. Figure 4.37 illustrates a facet joint injection.

> Radiofrequency ablations are reported with destruction codes beginning with 64633.

If the operative note described a facet joint steroid injection L2-L3 (figure 4.37), the correct code would be 64493.

Figure 4.37. Facet joint injection

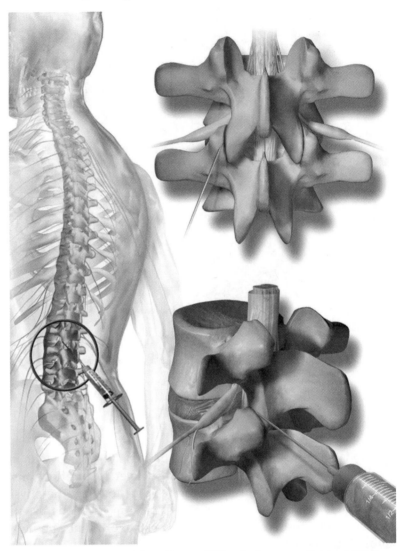

Source: Blaus, Bruce. "Hysteroscopy" Digital Image. Wikimedia Commons. October, 2013. Accessed September, 2018. https://commons.wikimedia.org/wiki/File:Blausen_0391_FacetJointInjection.png.

Exercise 4.39   Nervous System

Answers to odd-numbered questions can be found in appendix C of this book. The answers to even-numbered questions are located in the instructor materials and are available to approved instructors.

Assign appropriate CPT code(s) for the following procedures. Assign only CPT surgical codes (no E/M codes) and append any applicable modifiers.

1. Patient with chronic pain receives a nerve block; ropivacaine (anesthetic agent) injected into the branch of sciatic nerve

   Code(s): _____

2. The physician performs a neuroplasty of the left ring finger.

Code(s):_____

3. Cervical epidural spinal injection of phenol (neurolytic substance)

Code(s):_____

4. Neurorrhaphy of digital nerves of right thumb and ring finger

Code(s):_____

5. Endoscopic removal of acoustic neuroma

Code(s):_____

6. Insertion of a subcutaneous Ommaya reservoir under the scalp for delivery of chemotherapy

Code(s):_____

7. Lumbar laminectomy at L4-L5 for decompression of the spinal cord.

Code(s):_____

8. The patient has chronic lumbar back pain. Using radiofrequency ablation, the spinal nerve root at L3-L4 was destroyed.

Code(s):_____

Exercise 4.40   Nervous System—Operative Report

Answers to odd-numbered questions can be found in appendix C of this book. The answers to even-numbered questions are located in the instructor materials and are available to approved instructors.

Operative Report #1

Operative Report

Preoperative Diagnosis: C5–C6 disc herniation

Postoperative Diagnosis: Same

Procedure: Anterior cervical discectomy

This 45-year-old man presents with a 6-month history of neck pain, right shoulder pain, right intra-scapular pain, and pain radiating on the outer aspect of the right arm. He was found to have wasting of the supraspinatus and infraspinatus muscles, and EMG confirmed a C-6 radiculopathy.

MRI scan showed a lateral disc herniation at the level of C5–C6. The patient tried initial conservative measures, which did not help him; hence, recommendation of

(Continued on next page)

Exercise 4.40   (Continued)

surgery was made. The risks and benefits included infection, hemorrhage, injury to the nerve roots, paralysis, injury to the spinal cord with paralysis, failure to improve, or even death. The patient fully understands and agrees to go ahead with the procedure.

The patient was anesthetized and positioned supine with a shoulder support, and the neck was prepared and draped in the usual manner. Midcervical crease incision was marked, both 4 cm. Incisions were placed transversely and the skin was sharply cut, and then the platysma was cut in the line of incision. The cervical fascia was dissected. Then we entered the plane between the trachea and the carotid sheath by blunt dissection reaching the prevertebral space. The prevertebral fascia was incised longitudinally. The disc bulge at C5–C6 was easily identified, and a spinal needle placed confirmed the position to be at C5–C6. The anterior osteophytes were prominent. They were removed and then we entered the disc space. The disc space itself had collapsed, and there was only desiccated disc material. We curetted out the disc and the cartilage plate, and the vertebral spreader was put in. More disc was removed from the lateral parts of the disc extending toward the uncus on both sides. As we moved posteriorly toward the ligament, there was subligamentous disc herniation to the right side. It was removed, and the ligament was reached. The ligament was lifted with a blunt hook and opened with micropunches. Using a Midas Rex drill, the posterior parts of the bone in this region were drilled doing a right foraminotomy on the right, and the nerve root was decompressed. A no-free fragment was identified inside the canal, and the entire ligamentum disc was removed over the nerve root. The bone was punched in those corners to give adequate space. The ligament was cut across the width of the space, and on the left side also foraminotomy was done removing the osteophytes in the corner and decompressing the nerve root. After we were satisfied with the decompression, the space was irrigated with antibiotic solution and hemostasis was achieved with some Gelfoam powder, and the wound was thoroughly irrigated. Hemostasis was achieved in the muscle plane, and closure was done with 3-0 Vicryl for the platysma and subcutaneous layer, and the skin was closed with 4-0 subcuticular Vicryl. Dressings were applied in the usual manner with Steri-Strips, Telfa gauze, and Tegaderm. The patient was reversed from anesthesia and had an uneventful recovery. He was moving all the limbs well and was transferred in stable condition to the recovery room.

Assign only CPT surgical codes (no E/M codes) and append any applicable modifiers.

Code(s): _____

Exercise 4.41   Nervous System Review

Answers to odd-numbered questions can be found in appendix C of this book. The answers to even-numbered questions are located in the instructor materials and are available to approved instructors.

Assign appropriate CPT code(s) for the following procedures. Assign only CPT surgical codes (no E/M codes) and append any applicable modifiers.

1. Creation of ventricular peritoneal (VP) shunt for a patient with hydrocephalus

   Code(s):_____

2. Glycerol rhizotomy of trigeminal nerve

   Code(s):_____

3. Excision of neuroma of peripheral nerve of foot

   Code(s):_____

4. Patient with severe back pain requires a single interlaminar epidural steroid injection, L5–S1 interspace with imaging

   Code(s):_____

5. Laminectomy and excision of intradural lumbar lesion

   Code(s):_____

6. Craniotomy for evacuation of supratentorial subdural hematoma

   Code(s):_____

7. Removal of implanted spinal neurostimulator pulse generator

   Code(s):_____

(Continued on next page)

Exercise 4.41   (Continued)

8. Sciatic neuroplasty, leg

Code(s): _____

9. Vagus nerve block injection—Naropin (anesthetic agent)

Code(s): _____

10. Suture repair of posterior tibial nerve

Code(s): _____

Eye and Ocular Adnexa

Learning Objectives

- Differentiate between extracapsular and intracapsular cataract extraction procedures.

- Describe documentation requirements for coding strabismus surgery.

The eye and ocular adnexa subsection includes procedures involving the eyeball, anterior and posterior segment, ocular adnexa, and conjunctiva (figure 4.38 shows the structure of the eye). The codes are categorized first by body part involved and then by type of procedure, such as retinal and choroid repair, conjunctivoplasty, cataract removal, and removal of foreign body.

Figure 4.38.   Anatomy of the eye

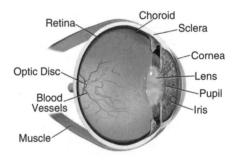

Source: Blaus, Bruce. "Hysteroscopy" Digital Image. Wikimedia Commons. October, 2013. Accessed September, 2018. https://commons.wikimedia.org/wiki/File:Blausen_0388_EyeAnatomy_01.png.

Cataract Extraction

The note at the beginning of the cataract extraction subsection (66830–66986) identifies the following procedures as part of the extraction: lateral canthotomy, iridectomy, iridotomy, anterior capsulotomy, posterior capsulotomy, use of viscoelastic agents, enzymatic zonulysis, use of other pharmacologic agents, and subconjunctival or sub-Tenon injections. When performed as part of the cataract extraction, these procedures should not be coded separately because they are incorporated into the bigger procedure of the cataract removal.

The two types of cataract extraction are extracapsular and intracapsular. Extracapsular extraction, which includes removal of the lens material without removing the posterior capsule, is reported with codes 66840 through 66852, 66940, 66982, and 66984. Intracapsular extraction, which involves removal of the entire lens including the capsule, is reported with codes 66920, 66930, and 66983.

Codes 66982, 66983, and 66984 describe cataract extraction with insertion of intraocular lens (IOL) prosthesis during the same operative episode. Insertion of IOL prosthesis performed during a subsequent encounter is reported with code 66985.

Exercise 4.42   Eye and Ocular Adnexa—Operative Report

Answers to odd-numbered questions can be found in appendix C of this book. The answers to even-numbered questions are located in the instructor materials and are available to approved instructors.

Operative Report #1

Operative Report

Preoperative Diagnosis:	Cataract of the left eye
Postoperative Diagnosis:	Cataract of the left eye
Operative Procedure:	Phacoemulsification of cataract of the left eye with lens implantation
Complications:	None

The patient is a 77-year-old woman with a history of decreasing vision to a level of 20/100 in her left eye. Slit lamp examination showed a nuclear sclerotic cataract. Fundus examination view appeared to be normal. The patient requested removal of the cataract for improvement in her vision.

Procedure: The patient was brought to the OR and placed on the operating table in the supine position. A small amount of Brevital was given intravenously for relaxation, and then a local anesthetic using 0.75% Marcaine in a peribulbar manner and a modified Van Lint manner was administered. After obtaining proper anesthetic effect, the eye was prepared and draped in the usual manner. A blepharostat was placed between the lids of the eye, and a bridle suture using 4-0 silk was placed through the superior rectus tendon. A peritomy was performed from the

(Continued on next page)

Exercise 4.42   (Continued)

2 to 10 o'clock position superiorly with cautery used to obtain hemostasis. A 3.5-mm grooved incision was placed tangent to the limbus, approximately 2 mm posterior to the surgical limbus, and a scleral tunnel was formed anteriorly toward clear cornea. A stab incision was made at the 2 o'clock position in the limbus with a #75 Beaver blade, forming an irrigating peritomy site, and the anterior chamber was entered at the base of the scleral tunnel, using a #55 Keratome blade. Healon was instilled in the anterior chamber, and then an irrigating cystotome blade was used to perform a smooth capsulorrhexis opening of the anterior capsule. A balanced salt solution was used to perform hydrodissection, and the phacoemulsification tip was used to break up and remove the nucleus of the lens. The remaining cortical material was removed from the eye using the irrigation-aspiration tip. The posterior capsule of the lens was polished using a Kratz scratcher. The wound was extended very slightly, and then a 6-mm folding posterior chamber lens was placed in the eye with the lens within the capsular bag. Excess Healon was removed from the eye using the irrigation-aspiration tip.

The corneosclera was tested and found to be watertight and free of any iris incarceration. The conjunctiva was repositioned to its original site and tacked down using bipolar cautery. A collagen shield, which had been soaked in a suspension of Tobradex eyedrops, was then placed over the cornea, and one drop of Timoptic was instilled on the conjunctiva. The blepharostat and the bridle suture were removed from the eye, and a dry dressing and Fox shield were placed over the eye. The patient tolerated the procedure well and left the OR in good condition. She was instructed to leave the eye dressing intact for the remainder of the day and to return to the office the following day for follow-up care and instructions.

Assign only CPT surgical codes (no E/M codes) and append any applicable modifiers.

Code(s): _____

Strabismus Surgery

Strabismus is a condition in which there is abnormal deviation of one eye in relation to the other. Surgical correction is performed on the muscles that regulate the movement of the eyeball. CPT codes from the series 67311 through 67318 require documentation of the number and types of muscles involved in the procedure. The procedure descriptions are considered to be unilateral. Note the following definitions:

- *Extraocular muscles:* Six extraocular muscles are attached to each eye, two horizontal and four vertical.

- *Horizontal muscles:* Two horizontal extraocular muscles—lateral rectus and medial rectus—move the eye from side to side.

- *Vertical muscles:* Four vertical extraocular muscles—inferior rectus, superior rectus, inferior oblique, and superior oblique—move the eye up and down. Figure 4.39 depicts the superior and inferior rectus muscles.

Figure 4.39. Movement of the eye

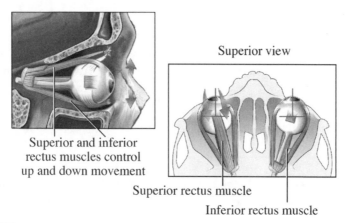

Source: ©AHIMA.

Exercise 4.43   Eye and Ocular Adnexa Review

Answers to odd-numbered questions can be found in appendix C of this book. The answers to even-numbered questions are located in the instructor materials and are available to approved instructors.

Assign appropriate CPT code(s) for the following procedures. Assign only CPT surgical codes (no E/M codes) and append any applicable modifiers.

1. With the use of a slit lamp, the physician removes a piece of metal from the patient's cornea.

   Code(s): _____

2. Strabismus correction involving the lateral rectus muscle

   Code(s): _____

(Continued on next page)

Exercise 4.43 (Continued)

3. Excision of 0.5-cm lesion of conjunctiva

   Code(s): _____

4. Orbitotomy of right eye to remove a piece of glass

   Code(s): _____

5. Incisional biopsy of left upper eyelid including lid margin

   Code(s): _____

6. Excisional transverse blepharotomy with one-fourth lid margin rotation graft

   Code(s): _____

7. Repair of left blepharoptosis using superior rectus technique with fascial sling

   Code(s): _____

8. Patient is experiencing pain along the lower right eyelash line. The surgeon diagnoses trichiasis and uses cryosurgery to destroy the follicles.

   Code(s): _____

9. Ectropion repair using absorbable sutures

   Code(s): _____

10. Patient has severe diabetes with retinopathy. The surgeon performs laser photocoagulation to resolve the leaking microaneurysms in the left retina.

    Code(s): _____

Auditory System

Learning Objectives

- Describe a tympanostomy procedure.

- Differentiate between tympanostomy and myringotomy for insertion of ventilating tubes.

The auditory system subsection includes codes for procedures performed on the inner, outer, and middle ear (figure 4.40 depicts the structure of the ear). Diagnostic services such as audiometry and vestibular testing, however, are found in the medicine section of CPT. Surgical procedures are found in the code range from 69000 through 69979 and have no specific coding guidelines designated that impact code assignment.

Figure 4.40. Structure of the ear

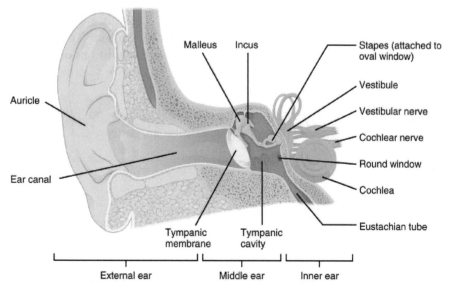

Source: OpenStax College. "The Structures of the Ear." Digital Image. Wikimedia Commons. May, 2016. Accessed October, 2017. https://commons.wikimedia.org/wiki/File:1404_The_Structures_of_the_Ear.jpg.

One of the most commonly performed auditory surgical procedures is the tympanostomy for insertion of ventilating tubes for children with chronic ear infections. Under direct visualization with a microscope, the physician makes an incision in the eardrum (tympanum). The physician also may remove fluid from the middle ear. A ventilating tube is inserted through the opening in the tympanum. Coding professionals may be confused by the terminology when the physicians state that they performed a myringotomy for insertion of ventilating tubes. For coding purposes, this describes a tympanostomy (code 69433 or 69436).

Exercise 4.44   Auditory System—Operative Report

Answers to odd-numbered questions can be found in appendix C of this book. The answers to even-numbered questions are located in the instructor materials and are available to approved instructors.

Operative Report #1

Operative Report

Preoperative Diagnosis: Bilateral otitis media

Postoperative Diagnosis: Same

Procedure: Bilateral myringotomy with tubes

The patient was brought to the operating room, placed in a supine position, and given a general anesthesia. Myringotomies were performed bilaterally in the anterior-superior quadrant of each tympanic membrane. The left middle ear cavity contained a

(Continued on next page)

Exercise 4.44   (Continued)

mucopurulent material; the right middle ear cavity contained a thick mucoid material. Tympanostomy tubes were placed bilaterally without difficulty. The patient tolerated the procedure well and was discharged to the recovery area.

Assign only CPT surgical codes (no E/M codes) and append any applicable modifiers.

Code(s): _____

Exercise 4.45   Auditory System Review

Answers to odd-numbered questions can be found in appendix C of this book. The answers to even-numbered questions are located in the instructor materials and are available to approved instructors.

Assign appropriate CPT code(s) for the following procedures and indicate the index entries that were used to identify the codes. Assign only CPT surgical codes (no E/M codes) and append any applicable modifiers.

1. Labyrinthectomy with mastoidectomy

   Code(s): _____

2. Under general anesthesia, a surgeon removes a pebble from the left external auditory canal of a 1-year-old child.

   Code(s): _____

3. Tympanomastoidectomy with ossiculoplasty

   Code(s): _____

4. The surgeon inserted cochlear implants in both ears

   Code(s): _____

5. Drainage of external left ear hematoma requiring an extensive amount of time

   Code(s): _____

Chapter 4 Review: Coding for Facility

Answers to odd-numbered questions can be found in appendix C of this book. The answers to even-numbered questions are located in the instructor materials and are available to approved instructors.

Assume that the following procedures were performed in either the outpatient department or the emergency department of Central Hospital. Assign the appropriate CPT code(s) and modifiers that the hospital would submit to payers for reimbursement.

1. Incision and drainage of complicated parotid gland abscess

    Code(s): _____

2. Layered (intermediate) wound repair of a 3-cm laceration of the hand and an intermediate repair of 5.0 cm of arm

    Code(s): _____

3. Colposcopy of cervix with biopsy

    Code(s): _____

4. Mediastinoscopy with biopsy of mediastinal adenoma

    Code(s): _____

5. Insertion of breast implant, following mastectomy that was performed previously

    Code(s): _____

6. Bilateral tympanostomy with insertion of ventilating tube, performed under general anesthesia

    Code(s): _____

7. Closed treatment of distal phalangeal fracture of right thumb without manipulation

    Code(s): _____

8. Open lumbar laminectomy for decompression of the spinal cord, L3–L4

    Code(s): _____

9. Placement of central venous catheter via basilic vein in 50-year-old patient for hemodialysis

    Code(s): _____

10. Cystourethroscopy with fulguration of bladder tumor (3.0 cm)

    Code(s): _____

(Continued on next page)

11. Repair of bilateral, strangulated, initial inguinal hernia in a 10-year-old patient

    Code(s): _____

12. Diagnosis: Mass of chest area. The surgeon made an elliptical incision encompassing the whole mass (6.5 cm × 3 cm × 1.5 cm) dissecting laterally deep to the subcutaneous tissue. Pathology report reveals inflamed epidermal cyst.

    Code(s): _____

13. Drainage of abscess of left thumb and second finger

    Code(s): _____

14. Patient has a large obstructing mass of the left glottis and subglottis. A direct laryngoscopy with biopsy was performed to reveal squamous cell carcinoma.

    Code(s): _____

15. Repair of oval window fistula

    Code(s): _____

16. Full-thickness wedge skin biopsies of suspicious tissue of the arm and hand.

    Code(s): _____

17. Excision of 2-mm papilloma of the penis

    Code(s): _____

18. Arthroscopy of the left elbow with removal of loose body

    Code(s): _____

19. Physician extracts a small amount of amniotic fluid from the OB patient for diagnostic purposes.

    Code(s): _____

20. Diagnosis: Chronic menometrorrhagia, uterine leiomyomata, and left Bartholin's gland cyst Procedure: Operative hysteroscopy with resection of submucous myomas and left Bartholin's gland cystectomy

    Code(s): _____

Chapter 4 Review: Coding for Physician Services

Answers to odd-numbered questions can be found in appendix C of this book. The answers to even-numbered questions are located in the instructor materials and are available to approved instructors.

Assume that the following procedures were performed by physicians in the surgery department of a hospital. Assign the appropriate CPT codes and modifiers for the physician services only.

1. Craniectomy for excision of cerebellopontine angle tumor, a complex procedure that required the services of two neurosurgeons

    Code(s) for physician #1: _____

    Code(s) for physician #2: _____

2. The surgeon performed an anterior-to-posterior (total) intranasal endoscopic ethmoidectomy with sphenoidotomy

    Code(s): _____

3. Arthroscopy of the left shoulder with complete synovectomy

    Code(s): _____

4. Closed treatment of distal fibular fracture without manipulation; the patient was in the postoperative period for an arthroscopy of the shoulder performed 2 weeks ago; the same physician performed both surgeries

    Code(s): _____

5. Endoscopic retrograde cholangiopancreatography (ERCP) with endoscopic retrograde insertion of stent into pancreatic duct

    Code(s): _____

6. Laparoscopic resection of cystic duct

    Code(s): _____

7. Bilateral probing of lower nasolacrimal ducts with irrigation under general anesthesia

    Code(s): _____

8. Laparoscopy with removal of tubes and ovaries; the operative report indicates that the procedure was extremely difficult to perform and took two hours longer to complete than usual

    Code(s): _____

9. Total abdominal colectomy with continent ileostomy

    Code(s): _____

(Continued on next page)

Chapter 4 Review   (Continued)

10. Insertion of permanent cardiac pacemaker with right atrial and ventricular transvenous electrodes; at a university hospital. The surgeon performed procedure but not the preoperative or postoperative care.

Code(s): _____

11. Microdermabrasion of the epidermis to remove tattoo of arm

Code(s): _____

12. The surgeon performs a colonoscopy that extends to the first portion of the ascending colon before being stopped due to equipment failure.

Code(s): _____

13. Thoracoscopic repair of pectus excavatum

Code(s): _____

14. Direct laryngoscopy with injection of botulinum toxin for treatment of laryngeal dystonia

Code(s): _____

15. Hemorrhoidectomy, single column group, internal and external hemorrhoids with fissurectomy

Code(s): _____

16. Laparoscopic rectopexy for patient with prolapse

Code(s): _____

17. Epidural steroid injection into the lumbar spine by interlaminar approach under fluoroscopic guidance

Code(s): _____

18. Excision of rectal tumor transanal endoscopic approach

Code(s): _____

19. Flexible laryngoscopy with use of microscope for injection of vocal cord with polytetrafluoroethylene (PTFE)

Code(s): _____

20. Cystourethroscopy with ureteroscopy with lithotripsy and insertion of double J ureteral stent

Code(s): _____

Radiology

5

Learning Objectives

- Describe the use of a hospital chargemaster for radiological services.
- Define the term *bundling* in relationship to radiology coding.
- State the meaning of the phrase "supervision and interpretation" as it applies to radiological services.
- Identify the subsections in Radiology.
- Differentiate between technical components and professional components.
- Define *contrast*.
- Given a procedural statement or radiology report, assign correct CPT codes.

The radiology section of CPT includes the following subsections:

Subsections
Diagnostic Radiology (Diagnostic Imaging)
Diagnostic Ultrasound
Radiologic Guidance
Breast, Mammography
Bone/Joint Studies
Radiation Oncology
Nuclear Medicine

It is important to understand the differences between the subsections and not to assign codes based on the area of the body being treated or studied. Some of the subsections contain instructions that are unique to them, and notes are included throughout each subsection to explain important instructions, such as the definitions of A-mode, M-mode, or B-scan ultrasounds.

Many of the conventions and guidelines discussed in earlier chapters of *Basic Current Procedural Terminology* (CPT) and *Healthcare Common Procedure Coding System* (HCPCS) also apply to this chapter. Specific conventions pertinent to the radiology section are included in this chapter.

Links to the Society of Interventional Radiology and Centers for Medicare and Medicaid Service's (CMS's) MedLearn that are pertinent to the discussion in this chapter are located in the web resources at the back of this book.

Hospital Billing and Radiology Code Reporting

When reporting radiological procedures, most hospitals use a computer program called a chargemaster. The chargemaster contain a computer-generated list of CPT and HCPCS codes, abbreviated definition descriptions, charges, and sometimes other information used by any given hospital, physician office, or clinic (see table 5.1 for an example excerpt from a radiology chargemaster). In addition, the file contains a revenue code (defined by CMS), which is assigned to each procedure, service, or supply to indicate the location or type of service provided to a patient. For example, in table 5.1, revenue code 320 describes Radiology-Diagnostic-General Classification. Whenever a radiologic procedure is ordered and performed, the computer automatically assigns the CPT code. Assigning CPT codes for routine services (such as, chest x-ray, EKG, CBC) is systematic and does not require decision-making from the coding professional. The chargemaster is known by several other names, including charge description master (CDM), standard charge file, service item master, or charge compendium. In most cases, each ancillary department is responsible for maintaining its codes in the chargemaster. Requests for input, however, often are made to coding professionals.

Table 5.1.   Example excerpt from radiology chargemaster

Charge Seq Number	Revenue Center*		Description	CPT Code
DEPT 721 RADIOLOGY—DIAGNOSTIC				
1700004 999	320	X RAY	NO CHARGE	
1701101 999	320	X RAY	MANDIBLE	70110
1701309 999	320	X RAY	MASTOIDS STENVERS LAWS	70130
1701341 999	320	X RAY	INT AUD CANAL	70134
1701341 999	320	X RAY	FACIAL BONES	70150
1701903 999	320	X RAY	OPTIC FORAMINA	70190
1702000 999	320	X RAY	ORBITS	70200
1702208 999	320	X RAY	SINUSES	70220
1702406 999	320	X RAY	SELLA TURCICA	70240
1702604 910	320	X RAY	SKULL	70260
1703305 999	320	X RAY	TEMPMAND JT BI	70330
1703552 999	320	X RAY	DENTAL PANOREX	70355
1703602 999	320	X RAY	NECK FOR SOFT TISSUE	70360
1703800 999	320	X RAY	SALIVARY GLAND	70380

*73010320 = MDLAB, 910 = ER, 920 = OUTP, 921 = OUTP, 999 = INP

Periodic review of these systems is mandatory for correct reimbursement and data quality control. The wrong code attached to a procedure can result in significant revenue loss or overpayment for a hospital or large clinic. Inappropriate unbundling of codes can result in fraudulent charges to insurance companies, so the accuracy of any automated coding via a chargemaster program is an important data quality concern.

Physician Billing

When a radiology service is performed in a physician's office or a freestanding center owned by the radiologist, the Medicare Part B carrier would pay the radiologist for both the professional component (modifier 26) and the technical component (modifier TC). Payment for the technical component covers the cost for personnel, equipment, and supplies involved in the nonphysician portion of the services. Because many physicians do not have radiological equipment in their offices, they usually refer patients who need radiological procedures to the local hospital or a freestanding radiological center. In such cases, coding and billing professionals for referring physicians do not assign radiology codes unless the physicians or facilities provide supervision and interpretation. Usually, radiological procedures are reported by radiologists associated with a hospital, clinic, or freestanding radiology center. Individuals providing billing services for radiologists and radiation oncologists must have a thorough understanding of radiological procedures, ultrasound procedures, nuclear medicine procedures, and radiation therapy.

In some cases, hospitals employ radiologists and report both technical and professional components of procedures or, when available, CPT codes representing complete procedures or CPT codes without modifiers. Revisions have been made to CPT that has created fewer complete procedures and more procedures where the professional and technical components are reported using separate codes. The Medicare Physician Fee Schedule database contains a list of codes that have been approved for splitting.

Radiological Supervision and Interpretation

Many codes in the radiology section of CPT include the term *radiological supervision and interpretation* in their description. These codes are used to describe the radiological portion of a procedure that two physicians often perform. In situations where one physician performs the procedure and also provides the supervision and interpretation, two codes are reported: a radiological code and a code from another section of the CPT code book, such as surgery. This is often referred to as a complete procedure.

Example:

Unilateral lymphangiography of the extremity—complete procedure. The physician submits codes 75801 and 38790. Code 75801 identifies the radiological procedure, including interpretation of the results, and code 38790 identifies the injection provided for the lymphangiography.

It should be noted that the radiological supervision and interpretation codes do not apply to the radiation oncology subsection.

Some radiological supervision and interpretation services are **bundled** with the surgical procedure. For example:

37192	Repositioning of intravascular vena cava filter, endovascular approach including vascular access, vessel selection, and radiological supervision and interpretation, intraprocedural roadmapping, and imaging guidance (ultrasound and fluoroscopy), when performed.

Modifiers in the Radiology Section

A complete listing of modifiers is in appendix A of the CPT code book. Some of the common modifiers used with the radiology section follow:

22 **Increased Procedural Services**: This modifier is intended for physician use only when the service provided is greater than that usually required for the listed procedure. The CPT code book states that modifier 22 may be reported with computerized tomography codes when additional slices are required or when a more detailed examination is necessary.

26 **Professional Component**: In circumstances where a radiological procedure includes both a physician/qualified healthcare professional (professional) component and a technical component, modifier 26 may be reported to identify the physician/qualified healthcare professional (professional) component. The professional component includes supervising the procedure, reading and interpreting the results, and documenting the interpretation in a report. This service can be provided by the physician who ordered the procedure or by the radiologist on staff at the hospital or freestanding radiology clinic. The technical component includes performance of the actual procedure and expenses for supplies and equipment. Usually, this service is provided by a radiologic technician at a hospital or a freestanding radiology clinic. The physician/healthcare professional reports the professional component by attaching modifier 26 to the appropriate radiologic procedure. The freestanding radiology clinic reports the technical component by attaching modifier TC (technical component) to the same procedure. Modifier TC is a Level II HCPCS modifier that may not be recognized by all payers.

Example:

Code 74220, Radiologic examination of the esophagus. The radiologist should report 74220–26 representing the work performed, and the clinic should report 74220–TC.

When reporting a code that includes "radiologic supervision and interpretation" in the description, modifier 26 should not be appended to the procedure code. Because the radiologic supervision and interpretation code already describes the professional component, the modifier is unnecessary.

Example:

Cervical myelography with the physician providing only the supervision and interpretation of this procedure. The physician should report as follows: 72240, Myelography, cervical, radiological supervision and interpretation.

In this example, modifier 26 is inappropriate because the descriptor for code 72240 already indicates that the physician provided only supervision and interpretation of the procedure.

51 **Multiple Procedures**: Modifier 51 (for physician use only) may be reported to identify that multiple radiological procedures were performed on the same day or during the same radiological episode by the same provider. The first procedure listed should identify the major procedure or the one that is most resource intensive.

52 **Reduced Services**: Modifier 52 may be reported by hospitals or physicians/qualified healthcare professional to indicate that a radiological procedure has been partially reduced or eliminated at the discretion of the physician.

The CPT code book states that modifier 52 may be reported with computerized tomography codes for a limited study or a follow-up study.

53 **Discontinued Procedure**: Modifier 53 is appropriate in circumstances where the physician/qualified healthcare professional elected to terminate or discontinue a diagnostic procedure, usually because of risk to the patient's well-being. Modifier 73 or 74 would be used for hospital reporting.

Example:

A patient planned to have urography with KUB, which would be reported with code 74400. Because the patient fainted during the procedure, it was discontinued before completion. The physician should report 74400–53.

59 **Distinct Procedural Services**: Modifier 59 may be used by both hospitals and physicians to identify that a procedure or service was distinct or independent from other services provided on the same day. Modifier 59 is appropriate for procedures that have been performed together because of specific circumstances, although they usually are not integral to one another or not performed together.

Example:

A patient is seen in radiology for a single cervical spine x-ray (72020) due to an injury. Later in the day, the patient returns complaining of severe pain. The physician orders a complete examination with six views (72052). Codes 72020 and 72052–59 should be reported.

GH Diagnostic Mammogram Converted from Screening Mammogram on the Same Day

RT/LT Modifiers: Modifiers RT and LT are Level II HCPCS modifiers that should be reported to identify laterality (left and right) when the CPT code description is unilateral.

Example:

CT scan of the left forearm would be reported as 73200-LT

CPT Assistant (June 2006) states that modifier 50 (bilateral procedure) is generally not recommended when bilateral radiology examinations are reported. Many payers prefer that the radiology code is listed twice on the claim form. It is important to note that some third-party reporting guidelines may differ.

TC Technical Component: HCPCS Level II Modifier that indicates only the technical component was provided.

Diagnostic Radiology (Diagnostic Imaging)

Codes 70010 through 76499 describe diagnostic radiology services and are subdivided first by anatomic site and then by specific type of procedure performed:

- *X-ray:* An x-ray is a test that uses radiation to take pictures inside the body.
- *Computed tomography (CT) scan:* The CT scan can produce detailed pictures of slices of body structures and organs. Figure 5.1 illustrates a CT scan. For some types of CT scans, a dye substance (ingested or introduced via IV) is used to make the structures more easily seen. For example, the dye (contrast material) can be used to check blood flow or help to visualize tumors. Combination CPT codes are provided for CT scans of the abdomen and pelvis performed during the same session. Coding professionals are to reference the table (before code 74176) that outlines the stand-alone codes when the procedures are performed during the same session.

Example:

Patient has a CT scan of the abdomen and pelvis *(without contrast)*; the correct code assignment is 74176.

- *Magnetic resonance imaging (MRI) scan:* In this test, images are obtained with the use of high-powered magnets and radio waves.
- *Magnetic resonance angiography (MRA) scan:* This test uses a magnetic field and radio waves to provide pictures of blood vessels. In many situations, MRAs can provide information that cannot be obtained from many of the other types of tests (for example, CT scans).

These radiology procedures may be found in the alphabetic index of the CPT code book by referencing the following main entries: x-ray, CT scan, Magnetic Resonance Imaging, and Magnetic Resonance Angiography. They also may be referenced under the specific site with a subterm identifying the specific procedure.

If the procedure were described as a CT scan, without contrast of the right lower extremity (figure 5.1), the correct code would be 73700-RT.

Figure 5.1. Computed tomography (CT) scan

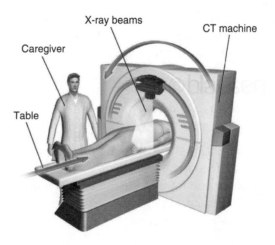

Source: Blausen Medical Communications, Inc. "CAT Scan." Digital Image. Wikimedia Commons. 1997–2013. Accessed September, 2018. https://commons.wikimedia.org/wiki/File:Blausen_0205_CATScan_01.png.

Contrast Material

The CPT code book differentiates between radiologic procedures with and without contrast material. Contrast material consists of radiopaque substances that obstruct the passage of x-rays and cause the areas containing the material to appear white on the x-ray film, thus outlining the contour of body structures and permitting the identification of abnormal growths. Contrast material may be administered orally or intravenously. Examples of contrast agents include barium or Gastrografin, iohexol, iopamidol, ioxaglate, Hypaque, and Renografin. Commonly performed radiologic examinations using contrast material include barium enema, angiography, cystogram, endoscopic retrograde cholangio-pancreatogram, fistulogram, intravenous pyelogram, excretory urogram, lymphangiography, oral cholecystogram, retrograde pyelogram, and voiding cystourethrogram.

CT scans also may be performed with or without contrast material. Although this radiological procedure can scan any body part, it is most helpful in evaluating the brain, lung, mediastinum, retroperitoneum, and liver.

When coverage requirements are met, reimbursement for the supply of contrast media may be obtained by reporting the appropriate HCPCS code.

MRI scans are almost equal to CT scans, although they are considered superior for scanning the brain, spinal cord, soft tissues, and adrenal and renal masses. This radiological procedure is contraindicated for patients who have metallic objects in their bodies such as pacemakers, shrapnel, cochlear implants, metallic eye fragments, and vascular clips in the central nervous system. Contrast material also can be used when performing MRI scans. Gadolinium (gadopentetate dimeglumine) is the contrast agent most often used.

Exercise 5.1   Diagnostic Radiology

Answers to odd-numbered questions can be found in appendix C of this book. The answers to even-numbered questions are located in the instructor materials and are available to approved instructors.

Assign the appropriate codes for the following procedure(s). Append modifiers if applicable.

1. MRI of knee with contrast

   _____

2. Diagnostic CT scan of the colon with and without contrast

   _____

3. X-ray of pelvis, AP

   _____

4. Thoracic myelography, radiological supervision and interpretation only

   _____

5. Cystography, three views, supervision and interpretation only

   _____

6. CT scan of lumbar spine with contrast

_____

7. CT scan of the abdomen and pelvis (with contrast)

_____

8. Upper GI x-ray exam with KUB

_____

9. CT of the thorax with contrast material

_____

10. Single view chest x-ray

_____

Interventional Radiology

Interventional radiology is the branch of medicine that diagnoses and treats diseases using percutaneous or minimally invasive techniques with the use of imaging guidance. Assigning codes for interventional radiology requires advanced study and thorough knowledge of anatomy and physiology. Suggested references are provided in this book.

Diagnostic Ultrasound

The subsection of diagnostic ultrasound includes codes 76506 through 76999, which are subdivided by anatomic site. The diagnostic ultrasound codes can be found in the alphabetic index of the CPT code book by referencing the main entries of Ultrasound or Echography. Diagnostic ultrasound involves the use of ultrasonic waves, or high-frequency sound waves, to visualize internal structures of the body. Ultrasounds are commonly performed for evaluation of the abdomen, the pelvis (for both gynecologic and obstetric diagnoses), and the heart.

Four types of diagnostic ultrasounds are recognized:

- _An A-mode ultrasound_ is a one-dimensional ultrasonic measurement procedure.
- _An M-mode ultrasound_ is a one-dimensional ultrasonic measurement procedure with movement of the trace to record amplitude and velocity of moving echo-producing structures.
- _A B-scan ultrasound_ is a two-dimensional ultrasonic scanning procedure with a two-dimensional display.
- _A real-time scan_ is a two-dimensional ultrasonic scanning procedure with display of both two-dimensional structure and motion with time.

The medicine section of the CPT code book includes ultrasounds such as Ultrasound of the heart (echocardiography), 93303–93355.

Complete vs. Limited Examination

Several CPT descriptions require the coding professional to differentiate between "complete" and "limited." For those anatomic regions that have "-complete" or "limited" ultrasound codes, the elements that comprise the examination are contained in the notes preceding the codes. For example, the note referenced before CPT code 76700 describes a complete examination of the abdomen as real time scans of the liver, gallbladder, common bile duct, pancreas, spleen, kidneys, and the upper abdominal aorta and inferior vena cava including any demonstrated abdominal abnormality.

Exercise 5.2   Diagnostic Ultrasound

Answers to odd-numbered questions can be found in appendix C of this book. The answers to even-numbered questions are located in the instructor materials and are available to approved instructors.

Assign the appropriate codes for the following procedure(s). Append modifiers if applicable.

1. Saline infusion hysterosonography with color flow Doppler

_____

2. Limited ultrasound of pregnant uterus to determine a fetal position

_____

3. Bilateral ultrasound of breast (real time imaging)

_____

4. Ultrasound of kidney, complete

_____

5. Ultrasound of scrotum

_____

Guidance Procedures

CPT includes codes that permit the radiologist to report imaging supervision and interpretation during guidance procedures. For example, a surgeon performs a diagnostic amniocentesis while the radiologist assists with the ultrasound guidance portion of the procedure. The following displays the coding assignment for each of the physicians:

Surgeon Reporting	Radiologist Reporting
59000 Amniocentesis, diagnostic	76946 Ultrasonic guidance for amniocentesis, imaging supervision and interpretation

Radiation Oncology

The radiation oncology codes (77261–77799) describe the therapeutic use of radiation to treat diseases, especially neoplastic tumors. Radiation therapy may be used as primary therapy to treat certain types of malignancies, such as early stages of Hodgkin's disease. It also may be used:

- As adjuvant treatment in small-cell lung cancer and head and neck cancers
- As palliative treatment to alleviate pain caused by metastasis to bone
- To control bleeding caused by gynecologic malignancies
- To relieve obstruction and compression from advanced lung cancer, brain lesions, and spinal cord lesions

The most common type of radiation used in the treatment is electromagnetic radiation with x-rays and gamma rays. X-rays are photons generated inside a machine; gamma rays are photons emitted from a radioactive source. Radiation is measured in units known as the radiation-absorbed dose (rad) or the gray (Gy). The Gy is equal to 100 rad.

The delivery of radiation therapy may be external or internal. *External radiation therapy* involves delivery of a beam of ionizing radiation from an external source through the patient's skin toward the tumor region. *Internal radiation therapy*, also known as brachytherapy, involves applying a radioactive material inside the patient or in close proximity. This material may be contained in various types of devices, including tubes, needles, wires, seeds, and other small containers. Common radioactive materials used in brachytherapy include radium-226, cobalt-60, cesium-137, and iodine-125. Three types of brachytherapy are recognized in the CPT code book:

- *Interstitial brachytherapy* involves placing a radiation source directly into tissues.
- *Intracavitary (intraluminal) brachytherapy* utilizes radiation source(s) placed in special devices and then implanted in body cavities, such as vagina, uterus, bronchus, or esophagus. Code selection is based on the number of radioactive sources used to produce the localized dose of radiation.
- *Surface application brachytherapy* uses radioactive material that is contained on the surface of a plaque or mold and applied directly or close to the surface of the patient.

Radiation Consultation (Clinical Management), Clinical Treatment Planning, and Radiation Treatment Delivery

Radiation oncology involves a variety of specialized planning, management, and treatment delivery services that physicians provide to patients throughout the course of radiation therapy. Accurate coding in these areas requires careful attention to the type, level, and extent of services provided.

Consultation: Clinical Management

Radiation oncologists often provide consultative services before a treatment plan is developed for the patient. Such treatment planning consultations should be reported with the appropriate E/M, medicine, or surgery code.

Clinical Treatment Planning

The planning that occurs before treatment involves a complex decision-making process that includes interpretation of testing, choice of treatment modality, selection of treatment devices, and so forth. Codes for treatment planning (77261–77263), simulation-aided field setting (77280–77299), and medical radiation physics, dosimetry, treatment devices, and special services (77300–77370) often require the coding professional to distinguish between "simple," "intermediate," and "complex." The definitions for each are provided in the Notes section before the CPT codes. For example, *simple* therapeutic radiology treatment planning requires a single treatment area of interest encompassed in a single port or simple parallel opposed ports with simple or no blocking.

Stereotactic Radiation Treatment

Stereotactic radiotherapy (77371–77373) uses multiple small fractions of radiation as opposed to one large dose. Stereotactic radiotherapy is frequently used to treat tumors in the brain as well as other parts of the body.

Radiation Treatment Delivery

Codes 77401 through 77425 describe the technical component of delivering the radiation treatment, as well as the various energy levels administered. To assign the appropriate code, the following information is needed:

- Number of treatment areas involved
- Number of ports involved
- Number of shielding blocks used
- Total million electron volts (MeV) administered

Two codes (77424–77425) are provided to report delivery of intraoperative radiation treatment.

Neutron Beam Treatment Delivery

This code selection (77422–77423) identifies a specialized form of radiation therapy that is often used to treat inoperable tumors or tumors that are resistant to other types of conventional radiation therapy.

Radiation Treatment Management

The actual management of radiation treatment services is reported in units of five fractions or treatment sessions, regardless of the actual time period in which the services are furnished. The services need not be furnished on consecutive days. Multiple fractions representing two or more treatment sessions furnished on the same day may be counted as long as there has been a distinct break in therapy sessions and the fractions are of the character usually furnished on different days.

Hyperthermia Treatment

Hyperthermia involves the use of heat to raise the temperature of a specific area of the body to increase cell metabolism and destroy cancer cells. Usually, it is performed as an adjunct to radiation therapy or chemotherapy. The hyperthermia codes (77600–77615) in the CPT code book include external, interstitial, and intracavitary treatment. If administered at the same time, radiation therapy should be reported separately.

Codes 77600 through 77615 include management during the hyperthermia treatment and follow-up care for three months after completion.

Clinical Brachytherapy

Clinical brachytherapy uses natural or manufactured radioactive elements that are applied in or around a particular treatment field. A therapeutic radiologist supervises the use of radioactive elements and interprets appropriate dosage. When the services of a surgeon are needed, modifiers 66 or 62 may be reported to ensure that both physicians are reimbursed.

Codes 77750 through 77799 include admission to the hospital and daily visits by the physician. The codes differentiate between interstitial and intracavitary brachytherapy, and are subdivided further to identify the number of sources/ribbons applied: simple, intermediate, or complex. The CPT code book includes definitions for each of these levels (in the context of clinical brachytherapy, the term *sources* refers to intracavitary or permanent interstitial placement of radioactive material, and the term *ribbons* refers to temporary interstitial placement of radioactive material).

Nuclear Medicine

Nuclear medicine involves the administration of radioisotopes, which are radioactive elements that diagnose diseases. The radioactive isotope deteriorates spontaneously and emits gamma rays from inside the body that enable the physician to view internal abnormalities. Some radioisotopes are selectively absorbed by tumors or specific organs in the body, making them visible on the scan.

Nuclear medicine procedures are organized in codes 78012 through 79999 according to body systems, such as the cardiovascular system. The provision of radium or other radioelements is not included in the services listed in this section. These procedures may be found in the alphabetic index of the CPT code book by referencing Nuclear Imaging or Nuclear Medicine.

Some of the more common diagnostic nuclear medicine scans include the following:

- *Bone scans* are performed as part of metastatic workups to identify infections such as osteomyelitis, to evaluate hip prostheses, to distinguish pathologic fractures from traumatic fractures, and to evaluate delayed union of fractures.
- *Cardiac scans* are performed for diagnosis of myocardial infarction, stress testing, ejection fraction, measurement of cardiac output, and diagnosis of ventricular aneurysms.
  - The thallium 201 scan examines myocardial perfusion, with normal myocardium appearing as "hot" and ischemic or infarcted areas appearing as "cold."
  - The technetium 99m pyrophosphate scan identifies recently damaged myocardial tissue and is most sensitive 24 to 72 hours after an acute myocardial infarction.
  - The technetium 99m ventriculogram scan identifies abnormal wall motion, cardiac shunts, size and function of heart chambers, cardiac output, and ejection fraction. The multigated acquisition (MUGA) scan is another form of this type of study.

- *Hepatobiliary scans,* or hydroxyiminodiacetic acid (HIDA) scans, are performed for diagnosis of biliary obstruction, acute cholecystitis, or biliary atresia.

- *Lung scans* (ventilation-perfusion [V/Q] scans) can reveal pulmonary disease, chronic obstructive pulmonary disease, and emphysema. When performed along with chest x-rays, these scans are important tools in evaluating pulmonary emboli.

- *Renal scans* are performed to evaluate the overall function of the kidneys.

- *Thyroid scans* are most commonly performed with technetium 99m pertechnetate and are useful in detecting nodules.

Chapter 5 Review

Answers to odd-numbered questions can be found in appendix C of this book. The answers to even-numbered questions are located in the instructor materials and are available to approved instructors.

Assign the appropriate codes for the following procedure(s). Include CPT modifiers and HCPCS Level II modifiers when applicable.

1. Radiological examination (x-ray) of the forearm, anteroposterior (AP), and lateral views. What code(s) should be submitted on the claim form if the physician provided only the supervision and interpretation (professional component) for this procedure?

   _____

2. MRI of the cervical spine with contrast material. The MRI is performed at an independent radiology facility, and the facility sends the images to an independent radiologist who will read and write a report of the findings. What code(s) should be submitted on the claim form for the radiologist to receive payment?

   _____

3. Physician performed the radiological supervision and interpretation for cystography (three views).

   _____

4. CT scan of the abdomen with contrast and the pelvis without contrast (same session).

   _____

5. High density barium enema with KUB (using air contrast).

   _____

6. Intracavitary placement of four radioelement sources.

   _____

(Continued on next page)

Chapter 5 Review   (Continued)

7. CT scan of the head with contrast material. The scan was performed at an independent radiology facility, and it was sent to an independent radiologist who reads and writes the report of the findings. What code(s) and modifier should the independent radiology facility report on the claim it submits?

   _____

8. Bilateral diagnostic mammography using computer-aided detection.

   _____

9. Radiologist provided radiological supervision and interpretation for ultrasonic guidance for pericardiocentesis.

   _____

10. Whole body bone marrow scan (nuclear medicine).

    _____

11. Screening ultrasound of abdominal aorta for aneurysm (real time with imaging).

    _____

12. Gastric emptying imaging study (nuclear medicine) with small bowel transit.

    _____

13. Delivery of radiation therapy to single area with single port and simple blocks–13 MeV.

    _____

14. Renal scan with vascular flow and function study (nuclear medicine) without pharmacologic intervention.

    _____

15. X-ray of clavicle.

    _____

16. Myocardial perfusion imaging tomographic (SPECT) (nuclear medicine) single study performed at rest.

    _____

17. Thoracic myelogram (S&I).

    _____

18. Needle biopsy of the lung with ultrasound guidance. (*Assign codes for surgical procedure and guidance.*)

    _____

19. X-ray of the knee, 2 view.

_____

20. A patient is known to have a mass in the temporal retina. A diagnostic ophthalmic B-scan ultrasound is performed along with a quantitative A-scan.

_____

Assign the appropriate CPT codes to the following reports. Assume that you are coding for the professional and technical component.

21. RENAL ULTRASOUND

History: Pyelonephritis

Findings: The right kidney measures 11.1 cm and left measures 11.5. Both kidneys are normal in echo texture and smooth in contour. There is no mass, calcification, or evidence of hydronephrosis. There is no perinephric fluid collection or abscess. There is no evidence of focal nephronia.

There is a cyst in the upper pole of the right kidney. This measures just under 2 cm. It has typical ultrasound characteristics of a benign renal cyst.

_____

22. AP PELVIS AND LEFT HIP X-RAYS

There is generalized demineralization of the bone.

There is an intertrochanteric fracture of the left hip with moderate angulation and displacement present.

There is a free fracture fragment of the lesser trochanter.

_____

23. KUB, UPPER GI X-RAY SERIES

A preliminary KUB study reveals a large amount of fecal matter present in the colon. Staples are seen in the right upper quadrant.

A barium swallow reveals a normal filling of the esophagus. The stomach is high and transverse in type. There is a small sliding hiatal hernia and there is small gastroesophageal reflux. The duodenal bulb fills without ulceration. The stomach empties well.

Opinion: Small sliding hiatal hernia with intermittent gastroesophageal reflux

_____

24. PA AND LATERAL CHEST X-RAYS

Coronary artery bypass graft changes are noted. The heart is mildly enlarged in size. The lung fields are clear, without infiltrate or effusion. Moderate spondylitic changes are noted in the thoracic spine.

_____

(Continued on next page)

Chapter 5 Review   (Continued)

25. CT SCAN OF THE HEAD WITHOUT INTRAVENOUS CONTRAST

Reveals a diffuse, moderately large area of localized atrophy involving the superiormost portion of the left parietal region. This is seen on images #14, 15, and 16. There is no extra-axial fluid collection, acute intracranial bleeding, midline shift, mass effect, or other significant abnormality.

IMPRESSION: Localized atrophy involving the superiormost portion of the left parietal lobe as described above. This could be old or recent. Short-term interval follow-up CT scan is suggested for further evaluation.

_____

26. Radiologist performed ultrasound guidance intraoperatively

_____

27. Patient has an acute gastrointestinal blood loss imaging study to help determine the source of the blood loss.

_____

28. Due to the possibility of a pulmonary embolus, the patient undergoes a ventilation and perfusion study in the Nuclear Medicine Department.

_____

Pathology and Laboratory Services

6

Learning Objectives

- Describe the use of a chargemaster file for billing pathology/laboratory services.

- Describe the format of an organ- or disease-oriented panel.
- Explain the use of U codes.

The pathology and laboratory section of the *Current Procedural Terminology* (CPT) code book includes services provided by physicians, including pathologists and technologists under the supervision of a pathologist or other physician. It includes codes for services and procedures such as organ or disease panel tests, automated multichannel tests, urinalysis, hematologic and immunologic studies, and surgical and anatomic pathologic examinations. This chapter discusses specific subsections of the pathology and laboratory section, such as urinalysis, chemistry, hematology, and surgical pathology.

> This specialty area of coding requires involvement of laboratory professionals to differentiate between the codes.

Alphabetic Index

Laboratory and pathology procedures and services are listed in the alphabetic index of the CPT code book under the following main terms:

- Specific name of the test, such as urinalysis, evocative/suppression test, and fertility test
- Specific substance/specimen/sample, such as glucose, CPK, cyanide, enterovirus, bone marrow, and nasal smear
- Specific method used, such as culture, fine needle aspiration, and microbiology

Hospital Billing for Laboratory and Pathology Procedures

In the hospital setting, the chargemaster is used to automate the billing of laboratory and pathology services (see table 6.1 for an example excerpt from a laboratory chargemaster). As mentioned in chapter 5, the chargemaster is a computer program containing codes, abbreviated definition descriptions, charges, and possibly other information used by a given hospital. Therefore, when patients visit the outpatient department with a requisition from their physician for laboratory work, the computer automatically assigns the appropriate code and charge for that particular service. Although coding professionals are not really involved in the actual coding of these services, the health information management (HIM) department may be asked to help the laboratory and pathology department update its portion of the chargemaster.

Table 6.1. Excerpt from a laboratory chargemaster in numeric order by department

Charge Seq Number	Revenue Center*		Description	CPT Code
		DEPT	703 CHEMISTRY	
2120053 320	301		HEPATITIS B CORE HBcAb	86704
2120053 910	301		HEPATITIS B CORE IgM antibody	86705
2120103 320	301		ELECTROLYTES PROFILE I	80051
2120111 999	301		BASIC METABOLIC PANEL	80048
2120129 320	301		GLUCOSE FASTING	82947
2120137 320	301		ACETONE SERUM	82009
2120145 320	301		GLUCOSE 1HR PP	82950
2120152 999	301		HDL CHOLESTEROL	83718
2120186 99ww9	301		UREA NITROGEN	84540

*320 = MDLAB, 999 = INP

Physician Billing

When reporting laboratory services provided by a physician, the coding professional must determine whether the physician performed the complete procedure or only a component of it. Some physician offices and physician-owned clinics have sophisticated laboratory equipment on the premises that enables the physicians to provide complete laboratory testing. A complete test would involve ordering the test, obtaining the sample (for example, blood or urine), handling the specimen, performing the actual test or procedure, and analyzing and interpreting the results. However, most physicians typically send the sample to a freestanding or hospital-based laboratory for testing and analysis. In this instance, the physician may report only the collection and handling of the blood sample or specimen.

Physicians also may send the patient for laboratory testing to a local hospital, where the sample or specimen is taken, the test or procedure is performed, and the results are analyzed and interpreted. The physician may seek reimbursement for these tests from some insurance plans when the tests are purchased from a reference laboratory or a hospital acting as a reference laboratory. Medicare, however, does not allow any provider who does not perform the test to bill for it. The reporting of laboratory tests depends on the organizations involved and the health plan guidelines applicable to the patient.

Example:

Dr. Reynolds performed a bone marrow needle biopsy in an oncology clinic and sent the specimen to a pathologist for review and interpretation. Dr. Reynolds reports 38221 for the actual biopsy of the bone marrow, and the pathologist reports 88305 for the review and interpretation of the specimen. If Dr. Reynolds pays the pathologist for the interpretation, he may report both codes, depending on the guidelines of the health plan involved.

Quantitative and Qualitative Studies

Throughout the laboratory and pathology section of the CPT code book, code descriptions state whether the test performed is quantitative or qualitative in nature. *Qualitative* screening refers to tests that detect the presence of a particular analyte, constituent, or condition. Typically, qualitative studies are performed to determine whether a particular substance is present in the sample being evaluated. In contrast, *quantitative* studies provide results expressing specific numerical amounts of an analyte in a specimen. Usually, these tests are performed after a qualitative study to identify the specific amount of a particular substance in the sample.

Modifiers in the Laboratory Section

Because most of the commonly used modifiers in the pathology and laboratory section have been discussed in earlier chapters, only a brief summary of each is offered here.

22 Increased Procedural Services: This modifier is intended for use by physicians or qualified healthcare professional when the service provided is greater than the one usually required for the listed procedure.

26 Professional Component: In circumstances where a laboratory or pathology procedure includes both a physician or qualified healthcare professional (professional) component and a technical component, modifier 26 can be reported to identify the physician component.

32 Mandated Services: Modifier 32 may be reported when a group such as a third-party payer or a PRO mandates a service.

52 Reduced Services: Modifier 52 may be reported by both hospitals and physicians or qualified healthcare professional to indicate that a laboratory or pathology procedure was partially reduced or eliminated at the discretion of the physician.

53 Discontinued Procedure: Modifier 53 may be reported by physicians or qualified healthcare professional only to indicate that the physician elected to terminate a procedure due to circumstances that put the patient's well-being at risk.

59 **Distinct Procedural Service**: Modifier 59 may be used by both hospitals and physicians to identify that a procedure or service was distinct or independent from other services provided on the same day. This modifier may be used when procedures are performed together because of specific circumstances, even though they usually are not.

90 **Reference (Outside) Laboratory**: Modifier 90 may be reported by physicians or qualified healthcare professional to indicate performance of the test by a party other than the treating or reporting physician.

Example:

Dr. Reynolds performed a venipuncture to obtain a blood sample for a lipid panel. He prepared the sample for transport and had it sent to an outside laboratory for testing, analysis, and interpretation. Dr. Reynolds should report 80061–90 to describe the laboratory test with the interpretation and analysis being performed at an off-site laboratory, along with code 36415 for the venipuncture.

91 **Repeat Clinical Diagnostic Laboratory Test**: Modifier 91 shows the need to repeat the same laboratory test on the same day to obtain multiple test results. It may be used by both hospitals and physicians. It is not to be used to confirm initial results due to testing problems with specimens or equipment or for any reason when a normal one-time reportable result is all that is required. In addition, it is inappropriate for tests where codes describe a series of test results, such as with glucose tolerance or evocative suppression testing.

92 **Alternative Laboratory Platform Testing**: This modifier describes when laboratory testing is being performed using a kit or transportable instrument that wholly or in part consists of a single use, disposable analytical chamber.

Organ or Disease-Oriented Panels

The organ- or disease-oriented panels describe the laboratory procedures performed most commonly for specific diseases, such as hepatitis and arthritis, or for specific organs, such as thyroid and hepatic function. All the tests listed in a panel must be performed for that code to be reported. When additional tests are performed that are not part of that particular panel, the codes describing those tests also must be reported. When some, but not all, of the tests in the panel are performed, the individual CPT codes should be reported, rather than the panel code. The introductory section of the Organ or Disease-Oriented Panels subsection states that coders should not report multiple panel codes that include any of the same constituent tests performed from the same patient collection. In the index, reference the main term Organ for a list of the panels.

Example:

Code 80051 describes an electrolyte panel and includes the following tests: carbon dioxide, chloride, potassium, and sodium. For code 80051 to be reported, all four tests must be performed. If the carbon dioxide test is omitted, separate codes must be assigned for the remaining tests: chloride (82435), potassium (84132), and sodium (84295). Code 80051 should not be reported.

If a glucose test is performed in addition to the electrolyte panel, a separate code is reported for the glucose test (82947), along with the electrolyte panel (80051).

Drug Assay

Beginning with code 88305, CPT divides this section into the following subsections: Therapeutic Drug Assay, Drug Assay, and Chemistry. The codes are assigned based on the purpose and type of patient results obtained. The Drug Assay is further divided into Presumptive and Definitive Drug Class.

Evocative/Suppression Testing

The codes used for evocative/suppression testing (80400–80439) allow the physician to determine a baseline and the effects on the body after evocative or suppressive agents are administered. In reviewing the codes in this series, it should be noted that the description for each panel identifies the type of test(s) included in that panel and the number of times a specific test must be performed.

Example:

Code 80420, Dexamethasone suppression panel, 48-hour. This panel must include:
Free cortisol, urine (82530 × 2)
Cortisol (82533 × 2)
Volume measurement for timed collection (81050 × 2)

Physician attendance and monitoring during the test should be reported with the appropriate E/M services code, as well as the prolonged physician care codes, if they apply.

Overview of Urinalysis and Chemistry Subsections

A variety of tests can be found in the urinalysis and chemistry subsections. Urinalysis tests are performed from a urine sample. Chemistry tests can be performed on several types of specimens, such as urine, blood, sputum, and feces. For this subsection of CPT, accurate coding requires identification of the specific tests performed. In some cases, the codes differentiate between qualitative/ quantitative and automated versus nonautomated.

Molecular Pathology (81105–81479)

The molecular pathology subsection is related to procedures that aid in the discovery of disease-associated genes. Technological advances have permitted the identification of molecular mechanisms of numerous diseases. There are two categories of codes: Tier 1 and Tier 2. The first set of codes in Tier 1 account for a large percentage of molecular pathology procedures performed such as testing for cystic fibrosis and breast cancer. The Tier 2 section is grouped into broad levels, and Tier 1 codes are more specific. This subsection has expanded in past years and has the majority of new codes in CPT 2019.

Multianalyte Assays with Algorithmic Analyses (81490–81599)

The Multianalyte Assays with Algorithmic Analyses (MAAA) section is for MAAA procedures that utilize multiple results derived from assays of various types.

Chemistry

This series of chemistry codes (82009–84999) is used to report individual chemistry tests that are not performed as part of the automated organ- or disease-oriented panels (80047–80076). Unless otherwise noted in the code description, these tests are quantitative in nature.

Example:

Patient was seen in the laboratory department and the calcium level test was performed. Results: total calcium: 82310

Hematology and Coagulation

The codes in the hematology and coagulation subsection (85002–85999) are used to report hematological procedures, such as complete blood count (CBC), and coagulation procedures, such as clotting factor and prothrombin time.

To assign the appropriate code, careful attention must be paid to the specific type of procedure performed. Collaboration with the medical laboratory director or technician is helpful in ensuring that CPT codes are correct and consistent with the equipment available and the actual test performed.

Immunology

Beginning with 86000, these sections of CPT codes introduce tests to evaluate aspects of the immune system. For example, CPT code 86038, Antinuclear antibodies (ANA) is a test to help evaluate a patient for autoimmune disorders such as systemic lupus erythematous (SLE).

Microbiology

This section of codes (beginning with 87003) includes bacteriology, mycology, parasitology, and virology. For example, CPT code 87110 tests for chlamydia and CPT code 87230 can identify Clostridium difficile toxin. Clostridium difficile (called C. difficile) is a bacterium that causes diarrhea which can easily spread.

Surgical Pathology

In surgical pathology coding (88300–88399), the unit of service is known as the specimen. The CPT code book defines a specimen as tissue or tissues submitted for individual and separate attention, requiring individual examination and pathologic diagnosis. Codes are differentiated by six levels. Level I (88300) identifies the gross examination of tissue only. Levels II through VI (88302–88309) refer to the gross and microscopic examination of tissue. Selection of a level between II and VI is made based on the type of specimen submitted. When two or more specimens are obtained from one patient, separate codes identifying the appropriate level for each should be reported.

Example 1:
Gross examination of a gallstone. The pathologist reports code 88300.

Example 2:
Gross and microscopic examination of a pituitary adenoma. The pathologist reports code 88305.

Example 3:
Gross and microscopic examination of two separate colon polyps. The pathologist reports codes 88305 and 88305 to identify examination of two separate specimens.

It should be noted that codes 88300 through 88309 include the accession or acquisition, examination, and reporting of a specimen.

Proprietary Laboratory Analyses (U Codes)

The 2018 edition of CPT introduced new alphanumeric codes after 89398. This new section, Proprietary Laboratory Analyses, identifies advanced diagnostic laboratory tests and clinical tests that are cleared or approved by the Food and Drug Administration (called Clinical Diagnostic Laboratory Tests).

Chapter 6 Review

Answers to odd-numbered questions can be found in appendix C of this book. The answers to even-numbered questions are located in the instructor materials and are available to approved instructors.

Assign the appropriate codes for the following pathology and laboratory procedures.

1. Gross and pathologic examination for a fallopian tube biopsy

   _____

2. Therapeutic drug testing for Haloperidol

   _____

3. Evaluation of blood gases—pH, pCO_2, pO_2, CO_2, and HCO_3

   _____

4. Confirmatory test for HTLV-II antibody

_____

5. Reticulated platelet assay

_____

6. Blood chemistry test for cyanide

_____

7. Histoplasmosis skin test

_____

8. HAI test

_____

9. The following tests were performed as a group from one blood sample: (lipid panel) total serum cholesterol, high-density lipoprotein and triglycerides; (electrolyte panel) carbon dioxide, chloride, potassium, and sodium.

_____

10. Serum nickel testing to detect potential toxic exposure

_____

11. ACTH stimulation panel for 21-hydroxylase deficiency

_____

12. Antibody test for herpes virus -6 detection (direct probe technique)

_____

13. Partial thromboplastin time (PTT) of whole blood and prothrombin time (PT)

_____

14. Automated urinalysis (dip stick), without microscopy

_____

15. Pathology consultation provided during surgery with frozen section of single specimen

_____

16. Physician orders ferritin blood level to determine how much iron the body is storing

_____

17. Pediatric specialist orders a vanillylmandelic acid urine test to rule out a neuroblastoma

_____

18. Epstein-Barr virus nuclear antigen (EBNA)

_____

19. Physician orders Bordetella antibody blood test to rule out whooping cough

_____

20. Patient presents to the outpatient laboratory department with an order for Giardia lamblia to rule out the parasite as a source for severe diarrhea

_____

Evaluation and Management Services

7

Learning Objectives

- Describe the format and organization of E/M services.
- Differentiate between a new and established patient.
- List the three key components for levels of E/M services.
- Given a scenario, assign the correct E/M code.

The section dedicated to evaluation and management (E/M) services was added to the *Current Procedural Terminology* (CPT) code book in 1992. For billing, E/M services require the selection of a CPT code that best represents:

- Patient type (new or established patient)
- Setting of service (office or outpatient setting, inpatient)
- Level of E/M service performed (various categories and levels)

The E/M codes are designed to classify the cognitive services provided by physicians during hospital and office visits, skilled nursing facility (SNF) visits, and consultations. The various levels of the E/M codes describe the wide variety of skills and the amount of effort, time, responsibility, and medical knowledge that physicians dedicate to the prevention, diagnosis, and treatment of illnesses and injuries as well as the promotion of optimal health. Healthcare facilities such as hospitals also report E/M codes to designate encounters or visits for outpatient services.

In claims processing for physicians, E/M codes are reported to document the professional services provided to patients. The level of medical decision-making is a key factor in the selection of appropriate E/M codes, but the level of decision-making is sometimes difficult to quantify in documentation. Generally, it is preferable that physicians select E/M codes. Coding professionals can then validate and verify the physicians' code selections according to the documentation guidelines developed jointly by the American Medical Association (AMA) and the Centers for Medicare and Medicaid Services (CMS). Documentation guidelines will be described in chapter 8 of this textbook.

In the hospital setting, E/M codes are assigned for Emergency Department Visits (99281–99285). E/M code assignment helps distinguish medical services from surgical services when assigning patients to a particular payment group. It also facilitates data collection by counting patients rather than services for outpatient reporting because one patient may have a number of outpatient services during a single visit. Under the prospective payment system, CMS instructed hospitals to develop their own method for assignment of the facility E/M codes.

CMS and the American Academy of Family Physicians websites provide additional information pertinent to E/M coding (see the online resources of this book for a list of relevant websites).

Classification of the Evaluation and Management Services

The E/M services section of CPT is divided into broad subsections that are further divided into subcategories. The first subsection is called Office or Other Outpatient Services. This group is further divided to New Patient vs. Established Patient. The following exercise will delve into the various subsections in Evaluation and Management

Exercise 7.1 Exploring Evaluation and Management

Answers to odd-numbered questions can be found in appendix C of this book. The answers to even-numbered questions are located in the instructor materials and are available to approved instructors.

Locate the subsection for each of the following CPT codes.

1. 99381
2. 99490
3. 99492
4. 99341
5. 99304
6. 99221

Format of Evaluation and Management Codes

The basic format of the E/M service codes followed in most of the categories in the section consists of five elements:

1. A unique code number beginning with 99
2. The place or type of service (for example, physician office or other outpatient service; initial or subsequent hospital care)

3. The extent or level of service (for example, detailed history and detailed examination)

4. The nature of the presenting problem (for example, moderate severity)

5. The amount of time typically required to provide a service

Peruse the E/M chapter beginning with code 99201 to discover the organization and format. Each level of service requires documentation to support the code selection for physician (or other healthcare professional) reporting. For example, note the excerpt for code 99204. This is a code for an office/outpatient visit for a **new** patient.

> 99204 Office or other outpatient visit for evaluation and management of a new patient, which requires these 3 key components:
>
> - A comprehensive history;
> - A comprehensive examination; and
> - Medical decision making of moderate complexity

Note that documentation requires that all three key components be met or exceeded.

In addition to the three key components, the CPT code descriptions provide guidance pertaining to the presenting problem and time. For example, code 99204 states that the presenting problem(s) are moderate to high severity and the typical face-to-face time with the physician is approximately 45 minutes. Compare this description to a lower-level E/M code, 99203, which states that the presenting problem is moderate and time is 30 minutes.

Time is not a key component for determining an E/M code assignment unless counseling and coordination of care dominates the encounter (more than 50 percent of total time of visit).

Compare the key components requirements to 99215 below.

> 99215 Office or other outpatient visit for the evaluation and management of an established patient, which requires 2 of these key components:
>
> - A comprehensive history
> - A comprehensive examination
> - Medical decision-making of high complexity

Note the change to two instead of three for key component documentation.

The Role of Coding Professionals

Due to the complexity of E/M coding, typically physicians select the E/M code or have software decision-making tools to help determine the code. Experienced coding professionals may transition to the role of auditor that reviews documentation to support the E/M code. This process is presented in chapter 8 of this textbook.

Qualified Healthcare Professional

Several years ago, CPT revised codes to include reference to "qualified healthcare professional" for codes that have been focused on physician services.

Example:

99201 Office or other outpatient visit
Counseling and/or coordination of care with other physicians, *other qualified healthcare professionals*, or agencies are provided consistent with the nature of the problem(s) and the patient's and/or family's needs.

A "physician or other qualified healthcare professional" is an individual who is qualified by education, training, licensure/regulation (when applicable), and facility privileging (when applicable) who performs a professional service within his/her scope of practice and independently reports that professional service. In addition, any procedure or service in any section of the book may be used to designate the services rendered by any qualified physician or other qualified healthcare professional or entity (such as, hospital, clinical laboratory, or home health agency).

The qualified healthcare professionals are distinct from "clinical staff." A clinical staff member is a person who works under the supervision of a physician or other qualified healthcare professional and who is allowed by law, regulation, and facility policy to perform or assist in the performance of a specified professional service, but who does not individually report that professional service.

New or Established Patient

Some of the E/M categories provide separate code ranges to identify new and established patients:

Office or Other Outpatient Services	99201–99215
New patient range is 99201–99205	
Domiciliary, Rest Home, or Custodial Care Services	99324–99337
New patient range is 99324–99328	
Home Services	99341–99350
New patient range is 99341–99345	
Preventive Medicine Services	99381–99397
New patient range is 99381–99387	

> Not all E/M codes use *new* versus *established* in the coding selection.

In this context, a patient who has not received any professional services from the physician or qualified healthcare professional (or another physician [or qualified healthcare professional] of the exact same specialty and subspecialty who belongs to the same group practice) within the past three years is considered a *new patient*. Professional services are those face-to-face services rendered by a physician or qualified healthcare professional and reported by a specific CPT code or codes. An *established patient* is a patient who has received professional services from the physician or qualified healthcare professional (or another physician or qualified healthcare professional of the exact same specialty and subspecialty who belongs to the same group practice) within the past three years. In the E/M Services Guidelines, a decision tree is provided to aid in distinguishing between a new or established patient encounter.

Exercise 7.2 New or Established Patient

Answers to odd-numbered questions can be found in appendix C of this book. The answers to even-numbered questions are located in the instructor materials and are available to approved instructors.

Identify if the patient is new or established.

1. A patient is seen by his primary care physician on January 9, 20XX for flu symptoms. The following summer (July 5), the patient is seen for a skin rash. Would the July 5th visit be classified as new or established?

2. A patient is seen by his primary care physician (Dr. Welling) on July 17, 20XX complaining of headaches. The patient returns two months later and sees a partner of Dr. Welling (Dr. Thomas), who is also a primary care physician, with the chief complaint of dizziness. Would the visit for Dr. Thomas be considered new or established?

3. A patient is seen by Dr. Parsons on July 12, 2014 for back pain. The patient returns to see Dr. Parsons on June 9, 2017 for allergies. Would the visit on June 9th be new or established?

4. An established patient is seen by a primary care physician (Dr. Fowler) after falling and hurting her ankle. After x-rays, Dr. Fowler refers the patient to an orthopedic surgeon (Dr. Florez). Would the visit for Dr. Florez be considered new or established?

5. An established patient is seen by his primary care physician (a member of University Associates) on January 23, 2018 for chest pains and shortness of breath. The primary care physician refers the patient to another member of University Associates who is a cardiologist. Would the visit to the cardiologist be considered new or established?

Concurrent Care and Transfer of Care

The CPT code book defines *concurrent care* as the circumstance in which more than one physician or qualified healthcare professional provides similar services (for example, hospital visits or consultations) to the same patient on the same day. Health plans often limit reimbursement to one physician per day unless the physicians have different specialties and the services of more than one physician are medically necessary. CMS assigns a specialty number that is used for this purpose.

Correct assignment of ICD-10-CM diagnosis codes also plays an important role in billing and receiving payment for concurrent care services. The physicians (or qualified healthcare professionals) involved in the concurrent care episode must identify the appropriate ICD-10-CM code for each service provided. Assigning the same ICD-10-CM code could result in one of the physicians (or qualified healthcare professional) being denied payment, usually the one who submitted the claim last.

Example:

Patient is admitted to the hospital complaining of unstable angina and uncontrolled type 2 diabetes mellitus. Dr. Smith treats the patient's angina, and Dr. Reynolds follows the patient's diabetes. The following codes should be reported:

Dr. Smith: I20.0, Intermediate coronary syndrome, and the appropriate E/M level of service code from the hospital inpatient services category

Dr. Reynolds: E11.65, Diabetes mellitus, uncontrolled, and the appropriate E/M level of service code from the hospital inpatient services category

Transfer of care is the process whereby a physician or qualified healthcare professional who is providing management for some or all of a patient's problems relinquishes this responsibility to another physician or qualified healthcare professional who explicitly agrees to accept this responsibility and who, from the initial encounter, is not providing consultative services. An extended definition is found in the guidelines at the beginning of the E/M Section. In addition, all of the sections of CPT have "Coding Tip" elements disseminated throughout the book that provide guidance.

Selection of Modifiers

Under certain circumstances, a listed service may be modified slightly without changing its basic definition. In these situations, several modifiers are available for use with E/M services codes. Modifiers are reported as two-digit numbers attached to the main code.

The following modifiers are available for use with E/M codes:

24 Unrelated Evaluation and Management Service by the Same Physician or Other Qualified Healthcare Professional during a Postoperative Period: Modifier 24 can be reported by physicians with an E/M service provided during the postoperative period by the same physician/other qualified healthcare professional who performed the original procedure. The E/M service must be unrelated to the condition for which the original procedure was performed.

Example:

Office visit provided to a patient who is in the postoperative period for a cholecystectomy performed three weeks earlier. The patient's current complaint is a possible infection of a finger that was lacerated four days ago. The physician may report the appropriate office visit code and attach modifier 24 to identify this activity as an unrelated service provided during the postoperative period of the cholecystectomy.

25 Significant, Separately Identifiable Evaluation and Management Service by the Same Physician or Other Qualified Healthcare Professional on the Same Day of the Procedure or Other Service: Modifier 25 may be reported by hospitals and physicians (or other qualified healthcare professional) to indicate that the patient's condition required a separate E/M service on the day a procedure or other service was performed because the care provided went beyond the usual procedures associated with the activity. By definition, CPT guidelines state that this modifier is not to be reported with an E/M service that resulted in a decision to perform surgery.

Example:

Office visit is provided to a patient for evaluation of diabetes and associated chronic renal failure, as well as a mole on the arm that has increased in size. Suspecting the mole is malignant, the physician excises it. The pathology report confirms a 1.1-cm malignant lesion. The physician can bill for the malignant lesion removal and use the office visit code accompanied by modifier 25 to identify that, during the visit, a separate condition was addressed (in this example, the diabetes and the renal failure). Generally, two diagnosis codes are required to explain the reporting of two separate services during the same encounter, although CPT guidelines do not require it.

It is important to note that CMS and other payers may have guidelines for use of this modifier.

Example:

A patient is seen in the emergency department for chest pains. An EKG is performed. The hospital would report the emergency department E/M code of 99283–25 with 93005 (EKG).

27 Multiple Outpatient Hospital E/M Encounters on the Same Date: Modifier 27 was developed to allow hospitals to report multiple outpatient hospital E/M encounters on the same date. The modifier is appended to the second encounter and each subsequent E/M code.

Example:

Patient is seen in the dermatology clinic in the morning and the orthopedic clinic in the afternoon. A level III clinic visit is performed at both visits. The hospital would report 99213 with 99213–27.

CMS has instructed hospitals to assign E/M codes for facility billing based on their own system, which reflects the facility's resources to give care to the patient. The hospital must have a policy for determining the level of care.

32 Mandated Services: Modifier 32 can be reported by physicians when an entity such as a third-party payer or a quality improvement organization mandates a service. Most often, this modifier is reported with the consultation codes.

57 Decision for Surgery: Modifier 57 can be reported by physicians along with the appropriate E/M services code when an E/M service was the result of an initial decision to perform surgery on a patient. Modifier 57 is appropriate with procedures that Medicare designates as major, which typically are those with a 90-day global fee period assigned. Generally, it is not required when the decision for surgery occurs at a time earlier than the day of or before surgery. Some insurance plans include consultation and/or visit codes where the decision is made in the global fee for surgery and do not provide separate payment.

Example:

An office visit is provided to a Medicare patient complaining of acute right, upper-quadrant pain and tenderness referred to the right scapula, nausea and vomiting, and anorexia. A low-grade fever and an elevated white blood cell count are noted. An ultrasound confirms the diagnosis of acute cholecystitis with cholelithiasis. The physician recommends that surgery be performed later that day. The physician can report the appropriate office visit code along with modifier 57 to identify that, during this office visit, it was decided to perform a cholecystectomy.

Categories of E/M Services

E/M services are divided into many different types of services as listed previously. CPT guidelines are provided within each section. A summary of the services is provided below.

Office or Other Outpatient Services (99201–99215)

The most commonly reported E/M codes are from the Office/Outpatient Services. The office or other outpatient services category may be used to describe services provided in the physician's office, the outpatient clinic, or some other ambulatory facility. This category is divided into two subcategories: new patient and established patient. It is important to remember that the basic difference between a new and established patient is whether the patient received professional services within the past three years from the same physician or healthcare professional or another physician within the same group practice. Whereas the new patient level of services requires meeting all three of the key components prior to assigning a code, the established patient level of services requires meeting only two of the three key components.

Reporting an office visit code is inappropriate if, during the course of events within a specific encounter, the physician admits the patient to the hospital as an inpatient or observation patient or to a nursing care facility. Only the resulting admission service should be reported in such a situation, which should incorporate the level of care provided in the office. There may be a rare circumstance where the patient receives office services early in the day and then returns later and must be admitted to the hospital from the office. Such a situation would merit use of modifier 25 to show that the services were separately identifiable.

Hospital Observation Services (99217–99220, 99224–99226) and Hospital Observation or Inpatient Care Services (Including Admission and Discharge Services (99234–99236)

The hospital observation services category identifies patients who are admitted to a hospital or are placed in observation status in a hospital and the services span more than one calendar date. For observation and inpatient care where admission and discharge occur on the same date, codes 99234 through 99236 would be used.

Consulting physicians providing services while patients are in observation status would use either outpatient consultation (99241–99245) or inpatient consultation codes (99251–99255), depending on the patient's status at the time of service. When a patient is admitted to the hospital (and not discharged on the same date), the initial hospital or inpatient consultation codes will be used, as appropriate.

The initial encounter with a patient in observation status is reported with a code from 99218 to 99220. Coding professionals should note that all three key components must be met to assign a particular level of service. In the rare circumstance that a patient remains in observation status after the date of admission, but is removed before the date of discharge, codes 99211–99215 may be used to report a physician visit on the intervening dates between removal from observation status and discharge.

Code 99217 (Observation care discharge services) is used to describe the services provided to a patient on discharge from outpatient hospital "observation status," but only if the discharge was not on the same date as the initial care. These services include a final examination of the patient, discussion of the hospital stay, instructions for continuing care, and completion of the health record.

Hospital Inpatient Services (99221–99239)

The hospital inpatient services category includes codes for initial hospital care (99221–99223), subsequent hospital care (99231–99233), and hospital discharge services (99238–99239). These codes also may be used to describe services provided to patients in a so-called partial hospital setting. Partial hospitalization is used for crisis stabilization, intensive short-term daily treatment, or intermediate-term treatment of psychiatric disorders.

The initial hospital care codes (99221–99223) are used to report the physician's first inpatient hospital visit with a new or established patient. Coding professionals should note that all three of the key components must be met to assign a particular level of service.

Codes 99231–99233 are reported for subsequent hospital services provided by the physician. Changes in the patient's medical status and the related documentation in the health record allow the physician to report various levels of service for the subsequent hospital care. It should be noted that only two of the three key components must be met to assign a specific level of service for subsequent hospital care services.

Codes 99238–99239 are used to report the services related to discharging a patient from the hospital. This reflects the added work the physician must perform, such as final examination of patient, discussion of hospital stay, instructions for home care, and completion of the health record. Code selection is based on time. For example, code 99238 describes discharge services requiring 30 minutes or less, and code 99239 identifies those services requiring more than 30 minutes.

Patients receiving inpatient or observation services when admission and discharge occur on the same date are reported using codes 99234 through 99236.

Consultations (99241–99255)

The CPT code book defines a consultation as a type of service provided by a physician at the request of another physician or appropriate source to either recommend care for a specific condition or problem or to determine whether to accept responsibility for ongoing management of the patient's entire care or for the care of a specific condition or problem. Although consulting physicians may

Medicare does not accept consultations codes; instead, providers must report E/M office codes. Other payers may or may not accept the codes.

initiate diagnostic and/or therapeutic services, they cannot assume responsibility for any portion of that patient's care. If responsibility is assumed, the service is no longer considered a consultation and the appropriate code should be assigned for hospital care or office or other outpatient services.

Documentation to support a consultation is essential and should include the request and need for a consultation, the opinion of the consultant, and any services ordered and/or performed. All this information should be documented in the health record and communicated by written report to the requesting physician or other appropriate source.

When a consultation is requested by the patient and/or his or her family, but not by another physician or other appropriate source (for example, physician assistant, nurse practitioner), the physician should report the service using the office visit, home services, or domiciliary or rest home care codes.

Introductory language for consultation codes in CPT is provided preceding code 99241.

Office or Other Outpatient Consultations (99241–99245)

Codes 99241–99245 describe office or other outpatient consultation services provided to new or established patients. These services may be provided in an office, outpatient or other ambulatory facility, hospital observation services program, home services program, domiciliary, rest home, custodial care program, or emergency department. Subsequent visits to the consulting physician's office are reported using the office visit codes for established patient (99211–99215). All three key components must be met in the selection of a level of service code from 99241 to 99245.

Inpatient Consultations (99251–99255)

Inpatient consultation codes (99251–99255) are used to report consulting services provided to hospital inpatients, residents of nursing facilities, or patients in a partial hospital setting. All three key components must be met in the selection of a level of service code from 99251 to 99255. In addition, a consultant can report only one consultation code per admission.

Emergency Department Services (99281–99288)

Emergency department services category codes are used to report E/M services that a physician provides when treating a patient in the emergency department. The CPT code book defines the emergency department as an organized hospital-based facility for the provision of unscheduled episodic services to patients who present for immediate medical attention. Moreover, the facility must be available 24 hours a day. All three of the key components, as stated within each level, must be met prior to selection of an emergency services code.

Special attention should be given to the description of code 99285, "which requires these three key components within the constraints imposed by the urgency of the patient's clinical condition and mental status." This description allows the code to be assigned, even when not all the documentation meets the criteria so stated. For example, when the patient is unconscious, it may be impossible to document a comprehensive history.

Again, code selection by physicians rather than coding or billing professionals is important because a physician is the only one in a position to determine clinical condition and mental status. Nonphysicians may verify compliance of the code selection to the current guidelines, but the provider of service best determines the level of code selection.

When a patient receives critical care services in the emergency department, codes 99291 and 99292 may be reported for these services, provided the requirements for critical care are met.

Critical Care Services (99291–99292)

The critical care services category involves the care of critically ill patients in a medical emergency that requires the constant attention of the physician. However, the physician's constant attendance or monitoring does not have to be continuous on a given date. Types of medical emergencies can include cardiac arrest, shock, bleeding, respiratory failure, and postoperative complications. Although usually provided in critical care areas such as a coronary care unit, intensive care unit (ICU), or emergency department, this type of care may be offered in other settings as well.

Critical care provided to neonatal and pediatric inpatients is reported with codes 99468 through 99480. CPT provides a Coding Tip that outlines which services are included in Critical Care Service codes, such as pulse oximetry.

Time is a key factor when selecting a critical care code. Code 99291 is reported for the first 30 to 74 minutes of critical care on a given date and may be reported only once per date. Code 99292 is reported for each additional 30 minutes of care beyond the first 74 minutes. As mentioned previously, coding professionals should note that the constant attention the physician provides need not be continuous on a given date. Critical care of less than 30 minutes on a given date should be reported with an appropriate E/M services code, such as subsequent hospital inpatient services, rather than a critical care code. A comprehensive explanation of time as an element in code selection can be found in the note under the critical care services subcategory.

Nursing Facility Services (99304–99310)

The codes in the nursing facility services category are used to report services in the following facilities:

- Skilled nursing facilities (SNFs), including hospital-based skilled care or swing beds in rural hospitals
- Intermediate care facilities
- Long-term care facilities

Nursing facilities (NFs) are required by law to perform a comprehensive assessment of each resident's functional capacity upon admission. Additional assessments must be conducted immediately after significant changes in a resident's condition, or at least every 12 months. The assessments are documented in a form called the resident assessment instrument (RAI), which is composed of a uniform Minimum Data Set (MDS) and resident assessment protocols (RAPs). The MDS includes a minimum set of assessment elements to evaluate SNF and NF residents. SNFs and NFs are responsible for completing the RAI, although specific portions of the form must be completed by a physician only.

CPT recognizes two types of NF services: initial nursing facility care and subsequent nursing facility care. Both subcategories apply to new or established patients. All three of the key components must be met in initial visits before code selection. The CPT descriptions include time to assist physicians in selecting the most appropriate level of service. The Coding Tip (before code 99304) outlines the guidelines for specific application of "time" in the coding selections.

Subsequent NF care (99307–99310) includes reviewing the health record, noting changes in the resident's status since the last visit, and reviewing and signing orders. Subsequent NF care requires that only two of the three key components be met before assigning a specific level of service code. The time designation for these codes specifies that the physician must be at the bedside and on the patient's facility floor or unit.

NF discharge day management codes are used to report the total duration of time spent by a physician for the final NF discharge of a patient. These include final examination of the patient and discussion of the NF stay, even when the time spent on that date is not continuous. Instructions are given for continuing care to all relevant caregivers and for preparation of discharge records, prescriptions, and referral forms. These codes are 99315 for services of 30 minutes or less and 99316 for services of more than 30 minutes.

Domiciliary, Rest Home, or Custodial Care Services (99324–99337)

Physician visits to patients being provided room, board, and other personal assistance services (usually on a long-term basis) are reported using codes 99324–99337. A medical component is not part of the facility's services. Such facilities may include group homes, assisted-living, or correctional facilities. All three key components, as defined in the levels of service, must be met before code assignment in the new patient subcategory (99324–99328). However, only two of the three key components must be met in the established patient subcategory (99334–99337).

Domiciliary, Rest Home (e.g., Assisted Living Facility), or Home Care Plan Oversight Services (99339–99340)

These codes identify physician's time in care-plan development and oversight for patients cared for in assisted living. Physicians report 15 minutes or more within a calendar month of care-plan oversight for patients not enrolled in a home healthcare agency or a hospital and not in a nursing facility. Codes 99339 and 99340 report development of complex and multidisciplinary care modalities and/or revision of care plans, review of subsequent reports of patient status, review of related laboratory and other studies, communication (including telephone calls) for purposes of assessment or care decisions with healthcare professional(s), family member(s), surrogate decision-maker(s) (such as a legal guardian), and/or key caregiver(s) involved in the patient's care, integration of new information into the medical treatment plan, and/or adjustment of medical therapy.

Home Services (99341–99350)

Home services codes 99341–99350 are used to report E/M services provided in a private residence. As stated in the levels of service, all three key components are required prior to code assignment in the new patient subcategory (99341–99345). However, only two of the three key components must be met in the established patient subcategory (99347–99350).

Prolonged Services (99354–99416) and Physician Standby Services (99360)

The series of codes capture prolonged service with the patient that is beyond the usual service in either the inpatient or outpatient setting. The time the physician spends providing prolonged service on a given date need not be continuous. Coding professionals should note that these codes may be reported in addition to other services, including E/M services at any level. Moreover, other procedures or supplies provided during the same encounter should be reported according to payer directions or guidelines. Coders should review the complete set of instructions with a reference table (before code 99354) before attempting to assign codes in this area.

The codes are further subdivided to identify prolonged services provided in the outpatient setting (99354–99355) and the inpatient or observation setting (99356–99357). Codes 99354 and 99356 describe the first hour of prolonged service and should be reported only once per any given date. Codes 99355 and 99357 describe each additional 30 minutes of prolonged service. Coding professionals should note that prolonged service of less than 30 minutes should not be reported separately.

Codes 99358–99359 describe prolonged physician service without direct or face-to-face contact with the patient that is beyond the usual non-face-to-face component of physician service time. These codes may be reported along with other services, including E/M services at any level. Code 99358 is used to report the first hour of prolonged service (reported only once per date) regardless of the place of service, and code 99359 describes each additional 30 minutes of service. Prolonged service of less than 30 minutes should not be reported separately.

Another subcategory allows for reporting of prolonged clinical staff services with physician or other qualified healthcare professional supervision. These codes (99415–99416) focus on prolonged services in the office or outpatient setting. Guidance for use of these codes is provided within the CPT code book, before code 99415.

Code 99360 is used to report physician or other qualified healthcare professional standby services requested by another individual that requires prolonged attendance without direct or face-to-face contact. This type of service may involve a physician who stands by for assistance in surgery or high-risk delivery for care of a newborn. Code 99360 may be reported for each full 30-minute period for stand-by services. Less than 30 minutes of standby service may not be reported separately.

Coding professionals should reference the detailed instructions and illustration provided before code 99354 for additional guidance.

Case Management Services (99366–99380)

The case management services category includes services when a physician (or another qualified healthcare professional) is responsible for providing direct care for a patient, as well as coordinating and controlling access to other healthcare services or initiating and/or supervising them.

Medical Team Conferences

Codes 99366 through 99368 describe a team conference that includes a physician, an interdisciplinary health team, or representatives of community agencies for the purpose of coordinating the activities of the patient. The two codes differentiate between direct (face-to-face) contact or without direct contact with patient and/or family.

Care Plan Oversight Services (99374–99380)

The care plan oversight services category describes the services required when supervising and coordinating the patient's care within a 30-day period, but not actually seeing the patient face-to-face. These codes are appropriate for recurrent supervision of therapy for patients in NFs, home health agencies, or hospice beds. Care plan oversight services for patients in home, domiciliary, or rest home (for example, assisted living facility) are assigned codes in the 99339–99340 range.

Code 99374 (home health), code 99377 (hospice), or code 99379 (NF) is reported for services lasting between 15 and 29 minutes, whereas codes 99375, 99378, and 99380 cover services lasting longer than 30 minutes. Only one individual may report this type of service within a 30-day period. Work involved in providing very low-intensity services or infrequent supervision is included in the pre-encounter and post-encounter work for the home, office or outpatient, and NF or domiciliary visit codes and should not be reported with care plan oversight codes.

Preventive Medicine Services (99381–99429)

The preventive medicine services category codes are used to report the preventive medicine evaluation and management of infants, children, adolescents, and adults. When an abnormality is discovered or a preexisting condition is addressed during this service, the appropriate office visit code also should be reported if the condition or abnormality proves significant enough to require additional workup. Moreover, modifier 25 should be added to the office visit code to indicate that the same physician or other qualified healthcare professional provided a significant and separate E/M service on the same date as the preventive medicine service. Any insignificant conditions or abnormalities discovered during the preventive medicine services that do not require additional workup should not be reported separately.

Ancillary procedures (such as laboratory or radiologic procedures), screening tests identified with a specific CPT code, and immunizations provided during the preventive medicine encounter should be coded and reported separately.

The subcategories of preventive medicine services distinguish between new and established patients, with the individual codes identifying specified age ranges. Codes 99401 through 99412 are used to report services provided to individuals at a separate encounter for the purpose of promoting health and preventing illness or injury. Counseling and/or risk factor reduction intervention vary with age and should address issues such as family problems, diet and exercise, substance abuse, sexual practices, injury prevention, dental health, and diagnostic and laboratory test results available at the time of visit.

A separate code is not needed for counseling (99401–99412) when provided as part of preventive medicine services (99381–99397) or during an E/M service. The preventive medicine codes (99381–99397) include counseling, anticipatory guidance, and risk factor reductions in the service provided. An additional code is not required to identify them. The E/M services codes also include counseling in the care provided.

Non-Face-to-Face Physician Services (99441–99444)

Certain services provided by physicians/other qualified healthcare professional, such as telephone services and online medical evaluations, do not require face-to-face contact with the patient. CPT guidelines are provided to direct the coding of these services.

Telephone Services

Codes 99441 through 99443 describe E/M services provided by the physician or other qualified healthcare professional via the telephone. The codes are differentiated by time (for example, 5 to 10 minutes for code 99441). The detailed guidelines outline the use of these codes, such as:

- Care initiated by established patient (or guardian of patient)
- If the telephone call ends with a decision to see the patient within 24 hours (or soonest available appointment), then this code is not reported.
- If the call refers to an E/M service performed and reported by the individual within the previous seven days (for example, postoperative follow-up) then these telephone services are considered part of that previous E/M service or procedure.

Online Medical Evaluations

Guidelines for online medical evaluations (99444) are similar to those for telephone services, but these services are provided via the internet. Documentation guidelines state that the patient's inquiry and physician's response must be maintained in permanent storage (electronic or hard copy).

Interprofessional Telephone/Internet Consultants (99446–99454)

These series of codes are used to report telephone or internet consultations or electronic health record assessment and management services based on the number of minutes. Guidance for use of the codes is provided before code 99446.

Special E/M Services (99450–99456)

The special E/M services category codes were developed to report services that can be performed in the office setting or other setting to establish baseline information before life or disability insurance certificates are issued. Coding professionals should note that no active management of the patient's problem is performed during this visit. If other E/M services and/or procedures are performed on the same date, the appropriate E/M services codes also should be reported, with modifier 25 appending them.

Newborn Care (99460–99463)

The newborn care codes are used to report services provided to normal newborns in different settings. Codes are applicable from the initial first days after birth (per day) until home discharge. Codes differentiate between initial and subsequent days of service. Reporting of these codes reflect services such as newborn history, physician exam, ordering tests, treatments, meeting with family, and preparation of hospital records.

Delivery or Birthing Room Attendance (99464–99465)

Code 99464 is used to report attendance at a delivery at the request of the delivering physician or qualified healthcare professional for initial stabilization of the newborn. Newborn resuscitative services are reported with code 99465, which includes the provision of positive pressure ventilation and/or chest compressions in the presence of acute inadequate ventilation and/or cardiac output. Code 99464 cannot be reported with 99465. When other procedures are performed in addition to the resuscitative services, additional codes should be reported.

Inpatient Neonatal Intensive Care Services and Pediatric and Neonatal Critical Care Services (99466–99482)

Pediatric Critical Care Patient Transport (99466, 99467, 99485, 99486)

The first two codes in this subsection (99466–99467) are used to report face-to-face critical care services delivered by a physician during the interfacility transport of a critically ill or injured pediatric patient, 24 months of age or younger.

Code 99466 is used to report the first 30 to 74 minutes, and code 99467 is an add-on code for each additional 30 minutes. Transport time less than 30 minutes should be reported with the appropriate E/M code.

Code 99485 and 99486 are used to report control physician's non-face-to-face supervision of interfacility pediatric critical care transport.

Inpatient Neonatal and Pediatric Critical Care (99468–99476)

These codes are used to report services performed by a physician to direct the care of a critically ill neonate or infant. Code 99468 should be assigned for the initial critical care services provided to a neonatal patient (birth through 28 days of age), and code 99469 should be assigned for subsequent critical care. Code 99471 should be assigned for the initial critical care services provided to a pediatric patient (29 days to 24 months of age), and code 99472 should be assigned for subsequent critical care. The last set of codes (initial and subsequent) identifies patients that are two years of age through five years of age.

Coding guidelines dictate that these codes may be reported only once by a single individual per patient per day. It is important to note that the CPT book provides detailed coding guidelines before code 99468.

Initial and Continuing Intensive Care Services (99477–99480)

CPT code 99477 is provided to report initial services for the neonate requiring intensive observation, frequent interventions, and other intensive care services.

Codes (99478–99480) are used by physicians to report intensive (noncritical) care given to infants with low birth weights. Subsequent intensive care visits (per day) can be distinguished by body weight: 99478 (body weight of less than 1,500 grams), 99479 (body weight of 1,500–2,500 grams), and 99480 (body weight of 2,501–5,000 grams).

Care Management Services

CPT provides for two categories of care management codes: chronic care management services (99490) and complex chronic care management services (99487–99489). These codes are used to identify the complexity of coordination by multiple disciplines and community service agencies for patients with chronic conditions. Specific criteria for the use of these "time-based" codes are stated in CPT before code 99490.

Psychiatric Collaborative Care Management Services (99492–99494)

This section of codes was developed under the collaborative care model managed in the primary care setting by a team. The time-based codes are provided for initial or subsequent care over a calendar month. The Professional Edition of CPT has a table in the Notes section that helps guide the selection of codes.

Transitional Care Management Services (99495–99496)

Service codes 99495–99496 are for an established patient whose medical and/or psychosocial problems require *moderate or high complexity medical decision-making* during transitions in care from an inpatient hospital setting (hospital, long-term care, or skilled care) to patient's community setting (home, domiciliary, rest home, or assisted living). These services start on the date of discharge and continue for the next 29 days. Reporting and documentation requirements are stated in the CPT note before code 99495.

Advance Care Planning Services (99497–99498)

These codes are for reporting face-to-face services to the patient and/or family associated with advance care planning, such as writing advance directives, durable power of attorney, or living will.

General Behavioral Health Integration Care Management

One CPT code (99484) uses a 20-minute threshold to report clinical staff time, directed by a physician or other qualified health care professional, for management and oversight of behavioral health issues.

Other E/M Services (99499)

The other E/M services category code is used to report an unlisted E/M service that does not fit into the previous categories.

Step-by-Step Instructions for Selection of E/M Codes

1. Identify the correct category of service (such as Office Visit, Critical Care Services).
2. Review specific notes and instructions for the selected category and subcategory.
3. Review narrative descriptors and apply definitions and supportive documentation for key components.

Example:

Office Visit: The established patient is seen for a rash on the arms and legs. The physician's documentation supports an expanded problem focused history and expanded problem focused examination with moderate decision-making.

> 99214 would not be selected unless the history or examination was documented as detailed.

Step 1: The category of service is Office/Outpatient Visit codes (99201–99215)

Step 2: The services are differentiated by New vs. Established patient status. The scenario identified that the patient was established (applicable codes 99211–99215).

Step 3: Documentation of key components revealed 2 of the 3 from code 99213. The correct code is 99213.

Chapter 7 Review

Answers to odd-numbered questions can be found in appendix C of this book. The answers to even-numbered questions are located in the instructor materials and are available to approved instructors.

Assign only the appropriate E/M services code(s) for the following cases.

1. An established patient with hypertension visits a physician's office for a blood pressure check. The nurse performs the service under the physician's supervision.

_____

2. A new patient was seen in the physician's office for abdominal pain. The physician performs a comprehensive history and examination. Medical decision-making is of moderate complexity.

_____

3. A patient with rectal bleeding was seen in the office of a gastroenterologist. The patient's primary care physician requested that the gastroenterologist provide advice about this case. The specialist conducted a comprehensive history and examination, and medical decision-making was of high complexity. The consultant documented his findings and communicated them via written report to the primary care physician.

_____

4. A new patient is seen in the physician's office for a cough, sore throat, and fever. The physician performs an expanded problem-focused history and a detailed examination, and medical decision-making was of low complexity.

_____

5. Dr. Ramirez provides critical care services in the emergency department for a patient in respiratory failure and with congestive heart failure. Ventilator management is initiated. Dr. Ramirez spends 1 hour and 50 minutes providing critical care for this patient.

_____

6. A physician provides E/M services for a patient in acute hysteria who has been admitted to the emergency department. After performing a problem-focused history and examination with straightforward medical decision-making, he determines that the patient is suffering from acute grief reaction secondary to the death of her granddaughter due to sudden infant death syndrome (SIDS). At discharge, the patient is in complete control of her actions and is referred to a SIDS organization.

_____

7. Dr. Gerald provides preventive medicine services to an established 45-year-old patient who is in good health and has no complaints. Dr. Gerald obtains a comprehensive history, performs a comprehensive examination, and counsels the patient on proper diet and exercise.

_____

8. A physician sees an established patient in his office for evaluation of Type I diabetes mellitus with nephropathy. In addition to a problem-focused history, he performs an expanded problem-focused examination that includes a limited examination of the genitourinary, immunologic, skin, and musculoskeletal systems, and documents all positive and negative findings. The patient's status does not seem to have changed, and medical decision-making is of low complexity. The doctor discusses the patient's insulin dosage, diet, and exercise, and plans to see the patient in six months.

_____

9. In her office, Dr. Rossi sees an established patient who complains of abdominal pain. She provides a problem-focused history and examination, which reveals the onset of abdominal pain beginning early that morning and characterized by a sharp, crampy feeling with some radiation to the back. Nausea and dry heaves are present, but no vomiting. The patient had a normal bowel movement in the morning. No fever or chills are noted, and bowel sounds are active. A rectal examination reveals hard stool in the rectal vault, guaiac negative. An x-ray of the abdomen is negative except for extensive gas. Dr. Rossi tells the patient to take an enema and return if the pain is not relieved. A change in diet would involve increasing the intake of fiber. The impression is that the patient's pain is the result of impacted feces.

_____

10. A new patient sees Dr. Reynolds in his office complaining of diarrhea and watery stool the previous night, as well as nausea, vomiting, and crampy, lower abdominal pain. Dr. Reynolds provides a detailed history and examination, and medical decision-making of moderate complexity.

_____

(Continued on next page)

11. An established patient sees Dr. Rao in his office with complaints of chest pain. Dr. Rao decides to admit the patient to Central Hospital on March 2 under observation status. He obtains a comprehensive history that includes a complete review of body systems and complete past, family, and social histories. The patient reveals that he has been under emotional stress the past month due to his recent divorce and that this is the first time he has experienced chest pain. Dr. Rao performs a comprehensive examination that includes a complete evaluation of the respiratory and cardiovascular systems. Pertinent diagnostic tests reveal no coronary artery disease. Dr. Rao performs medical decision-making of moderate complexity and determines the origin of the pain to be musculoskeletal secondary to stress. He discharges the patient on March 2 and recommends that he join a stress management group.

12. An established patient is seen in the primary care physician's office complaining of a cough, generalized weakness, joint aches, and a sore throat. She states that the sore throat started a week ago and there has been some green productive sputum with her cough. Patient added that a number of her co-workers have the flu. Examination reveals the following: T: 100.5, B/P 125/68, P 76, appears tired. HEENT: normal. PERLA: No bruits. TMs clear, nares are erythematous. Oropharynx mildly inflamed. Lungs: bronchial breath sounds, some coarseness in upper airways. Heart: regular rate and rhythm. Abdomen: Soft, no obvious masses; bowel sounds normal. Assessment: #1 Influenza, #2 Bronchitis. Prescribed Tamiflu and Z-pack.

The documentation supports a detailed history, expanded problem-focused examination, and moderate-complexity decision-making.

Evaluation and Management Documentation Requirements

8

Learning Objectives

- Describe the documentation requirements for E/M coding.
- Identify the documentation elements for history, examination, and medical decision-making.
- Translate elements of documentation to auditing format.
- Given a scenario, identify documentation requirements to support E/M coding selection.

Documentation Guidelines for Evaluation and Management (E/M) Services

Documentation is the basis for all coding, including E/M services. In 1994, the AMA and CMS developed documentation guidelines for E/M reporting in an effort to clarify code assignment for both physicians and claims reviewers. These guidelines were implemented in 1995.

In 1997, CMS and the AMA collaborated again on a revised edition of the guidelines that includes specific elements that should be performed and documented for general multisystem and selected single-specialty examinations. However, the 1997 revised version did not replace the 1995 documentation guidelines. Physicians may use either set of guidelines, whichever is more advantageous to the individual physician (see the online appendix for this book, which includes an excerpt from the 1997 documentation guidelines for E/M). A complete set of the 1995 and 1997 documentation guidelines is available on the CMS website.

Role of Auditing E/M Codes

As mentioned in chapter 7 of this textbook, many physicians assign their own E/M visit codes with the help worksheets or software tools. The role of the coding professional in this process varies. Auditing of documentation requires advanced study and mentoring. This chapter provides the foundation for reviewing documentation to support E/M coding.

Instructions for Validation of E/M Service Levels

The following steps should be followed in validating a level of E/M services:

1. Identify setting for service (such as outpatient or inpatient).
2. If applicable, distinguish between new and established patient.
3. Review specific notes and instructions for the selected category and subcategory.
4. Verify the level of E/M service provided based on the documentation and identification of documentation requirements (1995 or 1997 guidelines).

For consistency and simplicity, this textbook will use the 1995 documentation guidelines.

Seven Factors in Evaluation and Management Services

Validating physician documentation for E/M coding is an advanced skill that requires knowledge of documentation in the health record.

The documentation for three key factors and four contributing factors determines appropriate E/M code assignment. The key factors are *history, examination,* and *medical decision-making.* The contributing factors include *counseling, coordination of care, presenting problem,* and *time.* Information about the three key factors should be documented in the patient's health record as should information pertaining to any or all of the other four factors when they apply to a case. All applicable factors must be considered in code assignment.

History, examination, and medical decision-making are essential factors because they represent the amount of resources expended by a provider in rendering a service to a patient. For example, when counseling and coordination comprise more than 50 percent of a physician-patient or physician-family encounter, time is considered the controlling factor for determining the correct code.

Example:

Established patient seen in the physician's office for disease management. The physician documents that 40 minutes of the 60-minute visit were devoted to counseling and coordination. With time as the controlling factor, the appropriate code assignment would be 99215.

Documentation in the health record must support code-level selection by describing the key components and the pertinent contributing factors. Physician selection of E/M codes is recommended to ensure clinical validity for service levels. Coding professionals may validate code selection with documentation and assist physicians in meeting the current guidelines for code selection. Facility use of E/M coding is usually assigned via a chargemaster, which is a computerized program that contains codes, abbreviated definition descriptions, and charges (chargemaster programs are discussed further in chapters 5 and 6).

Appendix C of the CPT code book includes a supplement of clinical examples illustrating the appropriate selection of E/M services codes for specific medical specialties. However, these examples are only guidelines, and the documentation in the health record remains the most authoritative and final source when assigning a code for a particular level of service.

The CPT code book defines each level of E/M services by basing it on a unique combination of the three essential factors. The key elements that define E/M services, and the variation within these elements, are reflected in table 8.1.

Table 8.1. Key elements that define E/M services

History	Examination	Medical Decision-Making
Problem-focused	Problem-focused	Straightforward
Expanded problem-focused	Expanded problem-focused	Low complexity
Detailed	Detailed	Moderate complexity
Comprehensive	Comprehensive	High complexity

The following section of this chapter will reveal the criteria for history, examination and medical decision-making that supports the coding selection.

History

According to the documentation guidelines, the following types of histories are recognized. The level of complexity is based on the amount of information (number of elements) obtained by the physician:

- *Problem-focused:* Limited to a chief complaint and a brief history of the present illness or condition.
- *Expanded problem-focused:* A chief complaint, brief history, and a problem-pertinent system review.
- *Detailed:* A chief complaint, expanded history of the present illness, a problem pertinent system review extended to include a review of a limited number of additional systems; pertinent past, family, and/or social history directly related to the patient's problem.
- *Comprehensive:* A chief complaint, extended history of present illness, review of systems that is directly related to the problem(s) identified in the history of the present illness plus a review of all additional body systems; complete past, family and social history.

Each type of history includes some or all of the following elements:

- Chief complaint
- History of present illness
- Review of systems
- Past, family, and/or social history

Chief Complaint

The chief complaint (CC) is a concise statement describing the symptom, problem, condition, diagnosis, a return visit recommended by the physician, or other factor as the reason for the visit.

History of Present Illness

The history of present illness (HPI) describes the patient's developing condition or problem from the first sign and/or symptom in chronological order, starting from the initial visit to the present. Table 8.2 reflects the elements included in the HPI. Remember the HPI is only one portion of the element History. The future exercises contain a worksheet to abstraction documentation for all of the portions of the History.

Table 8.2. Elements included in the HPI

HPI Element	Examples
Location	Abdomen, chest, leg, head
Severity	Bad, intolerable, minimal, slight
Timing	Two hours after eating, 1 hour after waking, comes and goes
Quality	Burning, dull, puffy, pus-filled, red
Duration	For two months, since prescription began
Associated signs/manifestations	Rash with blistering, nausea and vomiting, abdominal pain
Context	When walking in company of smokers
Modifying factors	Improves when lying down, worse after eating

There are two types of HPI: a *brief HPI* and an *extended HPI*. A *brief HPI* refers to the documentation of no more than one to three HPI elements. It may involve a single problem without any complicating factors or symptoms. An *extended HPI* refers to the documentation of four or more HPI elements. It may be appropriate when multiple, confusing, or complex symptoms are present; when the symptoms are prolonged in development; when the history is obtained from an individual other than the patient; and when other complicating factors are present. Consider the following documentation in figure 8.1 with the elements outlined.

Figure 8.1. History of present illness elements

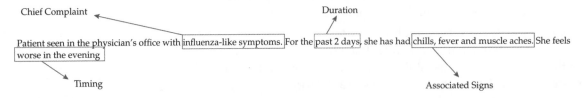

In the example in figure 8.1, *three* HPI elements are documented (duration, associated signs, and timing). Therefore, this would be considered a brief HPI. In the table 8.3, brief is a component of both problem-focused and expanded-problem focus. The history element is not computed on this portion of the history documentation requirements, it is factored with review of systems (ROS) and past, family and social history (PFSH).

Documentation requirements differ slightly for *new* versus *established* patients.

Table 8.3. History of present illness worksheet

History Component (equal to lowest category documented)	Problem-Focused	Expanded Problem-Focused	Detailed	Comprehensive
Chief Complaint _____ HPI—History of Present Illness __ Location __ Duration __ Severity __ Quality __ Context __ Timing __ Modifying factors __ Associated signs and symptoms	Brief: one to three HPI elements documented	Brief: one to three HPI elements documented	Extended: four or more HPI or status of three or more chronic conditions documented	Extended: four or more HPI or status of three or more chronic conditions documented

Exercise 8.1 History of Present Illness Component

Answers to odd-numbered questions can be found in appendix C of this book. The answers to even-numbered questions are located in the instructor materials and are available to approved instructors.

Remember that the HPI is just one component of the entire History section for key components. For this exercise, identify the documentation elements (location, duration, etc.) and if the result was *brief* or *extended*. Use table 8.3 as a guide.

1. The patient is seen with a sore throat that started three days ago and is getting worse.

   _____

2. Mother presents with an 11-month-old child after the child fell and injured her forehead this morning. The child is just beginning to walk but lost her balance and fell into the coffee table. Reports no loss of consciousness.

   _____

3. Patient presents with constant pain the left knee that has been getting worse over the course of the last two months. He states that the pain is not relieved by ibuprofen.

   _____

4. Mother presents with a 5-year-old who has had red eyes for the past two days, with itching and watery discharge. Mother reports that several children in his class have pink eye.

   _____

Review of Systems

Another section of the History component is the review of systems (ROS). ROS is an inventory of body systems obtained by the physician through a series of questions seeking to identify signs and symptoms the patient may be experiencing or has experienced. An ROS includes the following 14 systems:

- Constitutional symptoms (for example, fever or weight loss)
- Eyes
- Ears, nose, mouth, throat
- Cardiovascular
- Respiratory
- Gastrointestinal
- Genitourinary
- Musculoskeletal
- Integumentary (skin and/or breast)
- Neurologic
- Psychiatric
- Endocrine
- Hematologic/lymphatic
- Allergic/immunologic

Three types of ROS are recognized:

- A *problem-pertinent ROS* is directly related to the problem(s) identified in the HPI. The patient's positive responses and pertinent negatives for the system related to the problem should be documented.
- An *extended ROS* is directly related to the problem(s) identified in the HPI and a limited number of additional systems. The patient's positive responses and pertinent negatives for two to nine systems should be documented.
- A *complete ROS* is directly related to the problem(s) identified in the HPI and all additional body systems. At least 10 organ systems must be reviewed. Those systems with positive or pertinent negative responses should be documented individually. For the remaining systems, a notation indicating that all other systems are negative is permissible. In the absence of such a notation, at least 10 systems must be documented individually.

Example:

A patient presents with nausea (chief complaint). She has lost seven pounds in the past month (constitutional). She denies abdominal pain, diarrhea, and vomiting (gastrointestinal).

According to documentation guidelines, the preceding example would demonstrate an *extended* ROS because two systems are documented. Again, this is only one part of the History component along with HPI and PFSH.

Note the ROS portion of the worksheet in table 8.4 below

Table 8.4. Review of systems worksheet

ROS—Review of System(s)	None	Problem Specific: one system	Extended: two to nine systems	Complete: more than 10 systems or some with all others negative
__ Constitutional __ Integumentary (wt loss, etc.) __ Endocrine __ Eyes __ GI __ Hem/lymph __ ENT, mouth __ GU __ Allergy/Immune __ Respiratory __ MS __ Cardiovascular __ Neuro __ Psychiatric				

Exercise 8.2 Review of Systems Component

Answers to odd-numbered questions can be found in appendix C of this book. The answers to even-numbered questions are located in the instructor materials and are available to approved instructors.

For this exercise, identify the ROS elements and if the result was *problem-specific*, *extended*, or *complete*. Use table 8.4 as a guide.

1. Patient reports no fever. No shortness of breath or cough. No chest pain. Periumbilical abdominal pain.

   _____

2. Patient states loss of appetite, no blurred vision, no arm or leg weakness. She has a cough and mild congestion.

   _____

3. Patient reports splinter embedded deep in skin.

   _____

Past, Family, and/or Social History

The last section of the History component is the past, family, and/or social history (PFSH) element, which is broken down as follows:

- A *past history* consists of the patient's past experiences with illnesses, operations, injuries, and treatments (including medications). For pediatric populations, the past history also should include prenatal and birth history, feedings, food intolerance, and immunization history.

- A *family history* consists of a review of medical events in the patient's family, including diseases that may be hereditary or may place the patient at risk, as well as the age and status (alive or dead) of blood relatives.

- A *social history* consists of an age-appropriate review of past and current social activities. It also may include the patient's marital status and number of children, present and past employment, exposure to environmental agents, religion, hobbies, living conditions, water supply, and daily habits such as alcohol, tobacco, drug, and caffeine use. For veterans, it includes military service history. For pediatric populations, it may include school grades and sleep or play habits.

There are two types of PFSH:

- A *pertinent PFSH* includes the documentation of at least one specific item from any of the three history areas.
- A *complete PFSH* refers to the documentation of at least one specific item from two of the three history areas for the following E/M categories: office or other outpatient services, established patient; emergency department; subsequent nursing facility care; domiciliary care, established patient; and home care, established patient.

At least one specific item from each of the three history areas must be documented for a complete PFSH for the following E/M categories: office or other outpatient services, new patient; hospital observation services; hospital inpatient services, initial care; consultations; comprehensive nursing facility assessments; domiciliary care, new patient; and home care, new patient. The worksheet snapshot in table 8.5 highlights the PFSH of the History component.

Table 8.5. Past, family, and social history worksheet

PFSH (past medical, family, and social histories)	None	None	Pertinent: at least one item from at least one history area	Complete: specifics of at least two history areas documented
__ Previous medical (past experience with illness, injury, surgery, medical treatments, etc.) __ Family medical history (diseases, which may be hereditary or with increased risk of occurrence) __ Social (relationships, diet, exercise, occupation, and so on)				
Note: A chief complaint (CC) is required for all history types.				

Exercise 8.3 Past, Family and Social History Component

Answers to odd-numbered questions can be found in appendix C of this book. The answers to even-numbered questions are located in the instructor materials and are available to approved instructors.

For this exercise, identify the PFSH documentation elements and if the result was *pertinent* or *complete*. Use table 8.5 as a guide.

1. Patient is single and lives alone. He has a history of a total right knee replacement five years ago.

   _____

2. Patient has no known drug allergies. He is employed by the postal service. Father died of lung cancer 10 years ago.

   _____

Putting It All Together: History Component

In the previous discussion for evaluating documentation of HPI, ROS, and PFSH, elements were counted to determine the level for each. According to documentation guidelines, *all three levels* must be met to qualify for the specific level. The chief complaint is required for all levels.

Table 8.6 incorporates all the elements of a history.

The following examples illustrate how the worksheet is used to support the documentation required for History. Assume the chief complaint was documented in each case. Remember that the History component is equal to the *lowest category* documented.

> The criteria for Detailed and Comprehensive are the same; the difference is in the amount of detail in the documentation element.

Table 8.6. Elements of a history

History Component (equal to lowest category documented)	Problem-Focused	Expanded Problem-Focused	Detailed	Comprehensive
Chief Complaint _____ HPI—History of Present Illness __ Location __ Duration __ Severity __ Quality __ Context __ Timing __ Modifying __ Associated signs and factors factors symptoms	Brief: one to three HPI elements documented	Brief: one to three HPI elements documented	Extended: four or more HPI or status of three or more chronic conditions documented	Extended: four or more HPI or status of three or more chronic conditions documented
ROS—Review of System(s) __ Constitutional __ Integumentary (wt loss, etc.) __ Endocrine __ Eyes __ GI __ Hem/lymph __ ENT, mouth __ GU __ Allergy/ Immune __ Respiratory __ MS __ Cardiovascular __ Neuro __ Psychiatric	None	Problem specific: one system	Extended: two to nine systems	Complete: more than 10 systems or some with all others negative

PFSH (past medical, family, and social histories)
 __Previous medical (past experience with
   illness, injury, surgery, medical treatments,
   and so on)
 __Family medical history (diseases, which
   may be hereditary or with increased
   risk of occurrence)
 __Social (relationships, diet, exercise,
   occupation, and so on)
	None	None	Pertinent: at least one item from at least one history area	Complete: specifics of at least two history areas documented

Note: A chief complaint (CC) is required for all history types.

Example 1:

The physician documented 4 HPI elements and 4 ROS with no PFSH. The History component for this case would be expanded problem-focused. Because the PFSH was not documented, the History level could not be above expanded problem-focused.

Example 2:

The physician documents an extended HPI and complete ROS and the PFSH is pertinent. The History component for this case would be Detailed. In order for this case to be comprehensive, the PFSH would have to be complete.

In addition, the following are some general history documentation guidelines:

- The CC, ROS, and PFSH may be listed as separate elements of the history or included in the description of the HPI.

- An ROS and/or PFSH obtained during an earlier encounter do not need to be re-documented if there is evidence that the physician has reviewed and updated the previous information. The review and update may be documented by:

    ○ Describing any new ROS and/or PFSH information or noting that no change in the previous information has occurred

    ○ Noting the date and location of the earlier ROS and/or PFSH

- The ROS and/or PFSH may be recorded by ancillary staff or the patient on a completed form. To indicate that the physician has reviewed the information, a notation must supplement or confirm the documentation recorded by the other parties.

- If the physician is unable to obtain a history from the patient or other source, the documentation in the record should describe the patient's condition or other circumstance that precludes obtaining a history.

Exercise 8.4 Evaluation and Management (History)

Answers to odd-numbered questions can be found in appendix C of this book. The answers to even-numbered questions are located in the instructor materials and are available to approved instructors.

Using the template (table 8.6) as a guide and applying the documentation guidelines, assign only the <u>history</u> level (problem-focused, expanded problem-focused, detailed, comprehensive) to the following scenarios.

1. Patient seen in the physician's office complaining of a right eye that is itchy, watery, and red. Symptoms began on Saturday. Patient denies any loss of vision.

History Component (equal to lowest category documented)	Problem-Focused	Expanded Problem-Focused	Detailed	Comprehensive
Chief Complaint _____ HPI—History of Present Illness __ Location __ Duration __ Severity __ Quality __ Context __ Timing __ Modifying __ Associated signs and factors factors symptoms	Brief: one to three HPI elements documented	Brief: one to three HPI elements documented	Extended: four or more HPI or status of three or more chronic conditions documented	Extended: four or more HPI or status of three or more chronic conditions documented
ROS—Review of System(s) __ Constitutional __ Integumentary (wt loss, etc.) __ Endocrine __ Eyes __ GI __ Hem/lymph __ ENT, mouth __ GU __ Allergy/ Immune __ Respiratory __ MS __ Cardiovascular __ Neuro __ Psychiatric	None	Problem specific: one system	Extended: two to nine systems	Complete: more than 10 systems or some with all others negative

PFSH (past medical, family, and social histories)	None	None	Pertinent: at least one item from at least one history area	Complete: specifics of at least two history areas documented
__ Previous medical (past experience with illness, injury, surgery, medical treatments, and so on) __ Family medical history (diseases, which may be hereditary or with increased risk of occurrence) __ Social (relationships, diet, exercise, occupation, and so on)				

Note: A chief complaint (CC) is required for all history types.

2. Established patient seen in the urgent care center for back pain extending down in both legs and feeling numb at times. This has been ongoing for about five months but has become intolerable. She notices it more when she is driving the car. The patient denies any trauma. She recently started a new job. She denies any sense of weakness. No bowel or bladder habit changes. She is not allergic to any medications. Has a history of diabetes and takes glucose tablets. She smokes two packs of cigarettes a day and drinks alcohol occasionally.

History Component (equal to lowest category documented)	Problem-Focused	Expanded Problem-Focused	Detailed	Comprehensive
Chief Complaint _____ HPI—History of Present Illness __ Location __ Duration __ Severity __ Quality __ Context __ Timing __ Modifying __ Associated signs and factors factors symptoms	Brief: one to three HPI elements documented	Brief: one to three HPI elements documented	Extended: four or more HPI or status of three or more chronic conditions documented	Extended: four or more HPI or status of three or more chronic conditions documented
ROS—Review of System(s) __ Constitutional (wt loss, etc.) __ Eyes __ GI __ ENT, mouth __ GU __ Respiratory __ MS __ Cardiovascular __ Neuro __ Psychiatric __ Integumentary __ Endocrine __ Hem/lymph __ Allergy/ Immune	None	Problem specific: one system	Extended: two to nine systems	Complete: more than 10 systems or some with all others negative
PFSH (past medical, family, and social histories) __ Previous medical (past experience with illness, injury, surgery, medical treatments, and so on) __ Family medical history (diseases, which may be hereditary or with increased risk of occurrence) __ Social (relationships, diet, exercise, occupation, and so on)	None	None	Pertinent: at least one item from at least one history area	Complete: specifics of at least two history areas documented

Note: A chief complaint (CC) is required for all history types.

3. Patient seen in the clinic complaining of irritated throat, runny nose, and pressure in the cheek area for the past three days. Pressure seems to be worse today. Patient reports some coughing but denies headaches, just pressure in cheeks. Temperature has been normal. No daily meds. Takes Claritin 10 mg as needed.

(Continued on next page)

Exercise 8.4 (Continued)

History Component (equal to lowest category documented)	Problem-Focused	Expanded Problem-Focused	Detailed	Comprehensive
Chief Complaint _____ HPI—History of Present Illness __ Location __ Duration __ Severity __ Quality __ Context __ Timing __ Modifying __ Associated signs and factors factors symptoms	Brief: one to three HPI elements documented	Brief: one to three HPI elements documented	Extended: four or more HPI or status of three or more chronic conditions documented	Extended: four or more HPI or status of three or more chronic conditions documented
ROS—Review of System(s) __ Constitutional __ Integumentary (wt loss, etc.) __ Endocrine __ Eyes __ GI __ Hem/lymph __ ENT, mouth __ GU __ Allergy/ Immune __ Respiratory __ MS __ Cardiovascular __ Neuro __ Psychiatric	None	Problem specific: one system	Extended: two to nine systems	Complete: more than 10 systems or some with all others negative
PFSH (past medical, family, and social histories) __ Previous medical (past experience with illness, injury, surgery, medical treatments, and so on) __ Family medical history (diseases, which may be hereditary or with increased risk of occurrence) __ Social (relationships, diet, exercise, occupation, and so on)	None	None	Pertinent: at least one item from at least one history area	Complete: specifics of at least two history areas documented

Note: A chief complaint (CC) is required for all history types.

Examination

The physical examination is the objective description of the patient's chief complaint, illness, or injury. Four types of examinations are recognized:

- *Problem-focused:* Examination limited to the affected body area or organ system
- *Expanded problem-focused:* Examination of affected body area or organ system, as well as symptomatic or related organ systems
- *Detailed:* Extended examination of affected body area(s) and other symptomatic or related organ system(s)
- *Comprehensive:* A general multisystem examination or complete examination of a single-organ system and other symptomatic or related body area(s) or organ system(s)

The types of examination have been defined by the revised guidelines for general multisystems as well as the following single-organ systems:

- Cardiovascular
- Ears, nose, mouth, and throat
- Eyes
- Genitourinary (female)
- Genitourinary (male)

- Hematologic/lymphatic/immunologic
- Musculoskeletal
- Neurological
- Psychiatric
- Respiratory
- Skin

The following areas of the body are examined:

- Head, including the face
- Genitalia, groin, buttocks
- Neck
- Back, including spine
- Chest, including breasts and axillae
- Each extremity
- Abdomen

The following systems are examined:

- Constitutional (vital signs, general appearance)
- Genitourinary
- Eyes
- Musculoskeletal
- Ears, nose, mouth, and throat
- Skin
- Cardiovascular
- Neurologic
- Respiratory
- Psychiatric
- Hematologic/lymphatic/immunologic
- Gastrointestinal

Table 8.7 lists all the components of an examination.

Table 8.7. Components of an examination

Examination Component			Problem-Focused	Expanded Problem-Focused*	Detailed	Comprehensive
Body Areas __ Head, face __ Neck __ Chest, breasts __ Abdomen __ Genit, groin __ Back, spine __ Each extremity	**Organ Systems** __ Const. (vitals, general appearance) __ Eyes __ ENT, mouth __ Respiratory __ Cardiovascular __ Gastrointestinal __ Lymph/hem/immune	__ GU __ Skin __ Integumentary __ MS __ Neurological __ Psychiatric	One body area or system	Two to four body systems or two to seven basic systems, including affected area	Two to seven detailed systems, including affected area	Eight or more systems

Some texts use two to four body systems for expanded problem-focused and five to seven body systems for detailed. Both methods have been published in CMS publications. This is a controversy in the industry, and CMS will not give an opinion on whether one method is more acceptable than the other. Physicians frequently find that the two–four and five–seven distinction is easier to understand and follow.

Exercise 8.5 Evaluation and Management (Physical Examination)

Answers to odd-numbered questions can be found in appendix C of this book. The answers to even-numbered questions are located in the instructor materials and are available to approved instructors.

Using the template provided, assign the level of examination based on the documentation in the following scenarios.

1. Vital signs: temperature is 98.4° F, respirations 16, and blood pressure is 119/81. General: well-nourished, well-developed female in no apparent distress. HEENT: normocephalic, atraumatic. Mucous membranes appear moist. Lungs: clear. Heart: regular rate and rhythm. Abdomen: positive bowel sounds, soft, nontender, and nondistended. Back: no swelling, bruising, or erythema. Extremities: lower extremities show no muscle wasting. Patient has 2+ patellar and ankle jerks, 5/5 muscle strength bilaterally, and a negative straight leg raise bilaterally.

Examination Component			Problem-Focused	Expanded Problem-Focused*	Detailed	Comprehensive
Body Areas __ Head, face __ Neck __ Chest, breasts __ Abdomen __ Genit, groin __ Back, spine __ Each extremity	**Organ Systems** __ Const. (vitals, general appearance) __ Eyes __ ENT, mouth __ Respiratory __ Cardiovascular __ Gastrointestinal __ Lymph/hem/immune	__ GU __ Skin __ Integumentary __ MS __ Neurological __ Psychiatric	One body area or system	Two to four body systems or two to seven basic systems, including affected area	Two to seven detailed systems, including affected area	Eight or more systems

2. Temperature: 98; pulse 86; respirations 16; blood pressure 150/65. General: Patient is a well-nourished female who is wearing corrective lenses and looks to be somewhat uncomfortable. HEENT: head examination is normocephalic, atraumatic. Eyes: clear. Pupils equally round and reactive to light and accommodation. Discs sharp bilaterally. Ears, tympanic membranes pearly white bilaterally. Negative fluid. Neck: trachea midline, supple, no adenopathy. Cervical spine shows no swelling, bruising, or erythema. She had tenderness in the sternocleidomastoid muscle. C-spine itself was nontender to palpation.

Examination Component			Problem-Focused	Expanded Problem-Focused*	Detailed	Comprehensive
Body Areas __ Head, face __ Neck __ Chest, breasts __ Abdomen __ Genit, groin __ Back, spine __ Each extremity	**Organ Systems** __ Const. (vitals, general appearance) __ Eyes __ ENT, mouth __ Respiratory __ Cardiovascular __ Gastrointestinal __ Lymph/hem/immune	__ GU __ Skin __ Integumentary __ MS __ Neurological __ Psychiatric	One body area or system	Two to four body systems or two to seven basic systems, including affected area	Two to seven detailed systems, including affected area	Eight or more systems

3. Alert 16-year-old boy. Temperature: 98.6° F; pulse: 86; respirations: 14; blood pressure: 126/80. Has 2-cm laceration of chin.

Examination Component		Problem-Focused	Expanded Problem-Focused*	Detailed	Comprehensive
Body Areas __ Head, face __ Neck __ Chest, breasts __ Abdomen __ Genit, groin __ Back, spine __ Each extremity	**Organ Systems** __ Const. (vitals, general appearance) __ Eyes ___ GU __ ENT, mouth ___ Skin __ Respiratory ___ Integumentary __ Cardiovascular ___ MS __ Gastrointestinal ___ Neurological __ Lymph/hem/immune ___ Psychiatric	One body area or system	Two to four body systems or two to seven basic systems, including affected area	Two to seven detailed systems, including affected area	Eight or more systems

Medical Decision-Making

Medical decision-making involves the complexity of establishing a diagnosis and/or selecting a management opinion or treatment plan as measured by the following:

- The number of possible diagnoses and/or management options or treatment plans to be considered
- The amount and/or complexity of the data (health records, diagnostic tests, and/or other information) to be obtained, reviewed, and analyzed
- The risk of significant complications, morbidity, and/or mortality associated with the patient's presenting condition, the diagnostic procedure(s), and/or the possible management options or treatment plans

Number of Possible Diagnoses and/or Management Options

The number of possible diagnoses and/or management options is based on the number and types of problems addressed during the encounter, the complexity of establishing a diagnosis, and the management decisions made by the physician.

The following documentation guidelines apply:

- For each encounter, an assessment, clinical impression, or diagnosis should be documented. It may be stated explicitly or implied in documented decisions regarding management plans and/or further evaluation.
- For a presenting problem with an established diagnosis, the record should reflect whether the problem is improving, well-controlled, resolving, or resolved; or inadequately controlled, worsening, or failing to change as expected.
- For a presenting problem without an established diagnosis, the assessment or clinical impression may be stated in the form of a differential diagnosis, or as a possible, probable, or rule-out diagnosis.
- The initiation of, or changes in, treatment should be documented clearly. Treatment involves a wide range of management options, including patient instructions, nursing instructions, therapies, and medications.

- The record should indicate whether referrals are made and where, whether consultations are requested and with whom, and whether advice is sought and from whom.

Amount and/or Complexity of Data for Review

The amount and/or complexity of data for review is based on the types of diagnostic testing ordered or reviewed. A decision to obtain and review old health records and/or to obtain history from sources other than the patient increases the amount and complexity of data to be reviewed.

The following documentation guidelines apply:

- When a diagnostic service (test or procedure) is ordered, planned, scheduled, or performed at the time of the E/M encounter, the type of diagnostic service should be documented.

- The review of laboratory, radiology, and/or other diagnostic tests should be documented. An entry in a progress note (for example, "WBC elevated" or "chest x-ray unremarkable") is acceptable. Alternatively, the review may be documented by initialing and dating the report containing the test results.

- Relevant findings from any review of old records and/or the receipt of additional history from the family, caretaker, or other sources should be documented. If nothing exists beyond the relevant information that already has been obtained, that fact should be documented. A notation of "old records reviewed" or "additional history obtained from family" without further specification is insufficient.

- Documentation of discussions with the physician(s) who performed or interpreted laboratory, radiology, or other diagnostic tests should be included.

- The direct visualization and independent interpretation of an image, tracing, or specimen previously or subsequently interpreted by another physician should be documented.

Risk of Significant Complications, Morbidity, and/or Mortality

The risk of significant complications, morbidity, and/or mortality is based on the risks associated with the presenting problem(s), the diagnostic procedure(s), and the possible management options. The determination of risk is complex and not readily quantifiable.

The risk assessment of the presenting problem(s) is based on the risk related to the disease process anticipated between the present and the next encounter. The risk assessment of selecting diagnostic procedures and management options is based on the risk during and immediately following any procedures or treatment. The highest level of risk in any one category (presenting problem, diagnostic procedure, or management option) determines the overall risk.

Figure 8.2 outlines the factors that determine medical decision-making. The worksheet in figure 8.1 will be further explained in the following case study.

Figure 8.2. Decision-making process

Number of Diagnosis or Treatment Options

$$A \times B = C$$

Problem Status	Number	Point	Result
Self-limited or minor	(max. two)	1	
Established problem; stable, improving		1	
Established problem; worsening		2	
New problem; no additional workup planned	(max. one)	3	
New problem; additional workup planned		4	

Total _____

Amount and/or Complexity of Data Reviewed

Reviewed Data	Points
Review and/or order clinical lab tests	1
Review and/or order tests in the radiology section of CPT	1
Review and/or order tests in the medicine section of CPT	1
Discussion of test results with performing provider	1
Decision to obtain old records/obtain history from other than patient/discuss case with other provider	2
Independent visualization of image, tracing, or specimen itself (not simply review of report)	2

Total _____

Risk Factors

Level of Risk	Presenting Problem	Dx Procedures Ordered	Management Options
Minimal	One self-limited or minor problem	Lab tests, x-rays, EKG, EEG	Rest, superficial dressings, none required
Low	• Two or more self-limited or minor problems • One stable chronic illness • Acute uncomplicated illness or injury	• Physiologic tests w/o stress • Imaging studies w/contrast • Superficial needle biopsy • Skin biopsy • Arterial blood draw	• Over-the-counter remedy • Minor surgery w/o risk factor • Physical, occupational therapy • IV fluids w/o additive
Moderate	• One or more chronic illness with exacerbation, progression, or treatment side effects • Undiagnosed new problem with uncertain prognosis • Acute complicated injury • Acute illness with systemic symptoms	• Stress tests • Endoscopies w/o risk factor • Cardiovascular imaging study w/o identified risk factors • Deep needle or incisional biopsy • Centesis of body cavity fluid	• Minor surgery with identifiable risk factors • Elective major surgery without identifiable risk factors • Prescription drug management • Therapeutic radiology • IV fluids with additives • Closed treatment of skeletal injury
High	• One or more chronic illness with severe exacerbation, progression, or Tx side effects • Acute or chronic illness or injury that may pose a threat to life or bodily function • An abrupt change to mental status	• Cardiovascular imaging studies with identifiable risk factors • Cardiac electrophysiological tests • Endoscopy with identifiable risk factors	• Elective major surgery with identifiable risk factors • Emergency major surgery • Parenteral-controlled substances • Drug therapy requiring intensive monitoring • DNR status

Final Tabulation of Medical Decision-Making Elements: Highest Two of Three

Diagnosis/Management Options	Minimal (one or none)	Limited (two)	Multiple (three)	Extensive (four or more)
Amount/Complexity of Data	Minimal/Low (one or none)	Limited (two)	Moderate (three)	Extensive (four or more)
Highest Risk (from any category)	Minimal	Low	Moderate	High
Medical Decision Making	*Straightforward*	*Low Complexity*	*Moderate Complexity*	*High Complexity*

Medical Decision-Making Documentation Tabulation Case Study

The three-year-old child is seen by his pediatrician after falling and scraping his knee. Mother is worried that stitches are needed. The wound was cleaned and bandaged, no need for stitches. There is no signs of infection or active bleeding. The physician documented superficial wound.

To determine the medical decision, review the three components:

Final Tabulation of Medical Decision-Making Elements: Highest Two of Three				
Diagnosis/Management Options	Minimal (one or none)	Documentation of self-limiting/minor problem		
Amount/Complexity of Data	Minimal/Low (one or none)	No data to be reviewed		
Highest Risk (from any category)	Minimal	Risk is minimal		
Medical Decision-Making	*Straightforward*			

This case would result in straightforward medical decision-making.

Counseling and Coordination of Care

Both counseling and coordination of care are contributing factors in the selection of an E/M level of service. Counseling involves discussion of the patient's care with the patient and/or his or her family. Examples of counseling or coordination of care activities include discussions about results of diagnostic studies, treatment options, and instructions. An often-overlooked coding guideline states:

> When counseling and coordination of care constitute more than 50% of the physician/patient and/or family encounter (face-to-face time in the office or other outpatient setting or unit/floor time in the hospital or nursing facility), time may be considered the **key or controlling factor** to qualify for a particular level of E/M service.

Time can only be used as a key factor when the E/M codes include typical times, such as 99201–99215. There are no typical times for emergency department services (99281–99285), which eliminates the option of code selection based on time.

There are two important documentation guidelines to support use of counseling and coordination as a key factor for selection of E/M code:

- Physician must include a record of the total time of the visit
- Physician must include the specific time spent in counseling and coordination of care activities

For example, the physician could document, "The established office visit of Mrs. Lee was 25 minutes in duration, and 15 minutes of the visit was spent in discussing her treatment options for cancer treatment."

Analysis of this documentation:

- Did counseling and coordination dominate the visit? Answer: Yes (15 of the 25 minutes)

- Because counseling and coordination dominated the visits, refer to the times stated in the E/M codes for established patients for office visits (99211–99215). Code 99214 would be selected based on the total time of the encounter.

Note that elements of the visit that are not involved in face-to-face time (reviewing lab results, telephone calls) are not reflected in the time stated. Coordination of care with other physicians or healthcare professionals or agencies *without* a patient encounter on that day is reported using the case management codes.

Nature of Presenting Problem

CPT defines presenting problems as diseases, conditions, illnesses, injuries, symptoms, signs, findings, complaints, or other reasons for an encounter, regardless of whether a diagnosis is established at the time of the encounter.

Five types of presenting problems are identified:

- *Minimal:* A problem that does not require the presence of a physician or other qualified healthcare professional, although care is provided under a physician's (or other qualified healthcare professional) supervision (for example, a blood pressure check).

- *Self-limited or minor:* A temporary problem with a definite and prescribed course and good prognosis (for example, an upper respiratory infection). The conditions are typically transient in nature.

- *Low severity:* With no treatment, this problem carries a low risk of morbidity and little or no risk of mortality (for example, a teenager with acne that does not respond to over-the-counter medications). A patient with this type of problem can expect full recovery without impairments.

- *Moderate severity:* With no treatment, this problem carries a moderate risk of morbidity and mortality (for example, Dupuytren's contracture of the hand involving several fingers). The patient's prognosis may be uncertain, or the probability of prolonged functional impairment is increased.

- *High severity:* With no treatment, the risk of morbidity is high and a high probability exists for severe, prolonged functional impairment or moderate to high risk of mortality (for example, Type 1 diabetes mellitus, uncontrolled, with chronic renal failure requiring dialysis).

Exercise 8.6 Evaluation and Management (Medical Decision-Making)

Answers to odd-numbered questions can be found in appendix C of this book. The answers to even-numbered questions are located in the instructor materials and are available to approved instructors.

(Continued on next page)

Exercise 8.6   (Continued)

Using the worksheet provided, assign the level of medical decision-making for the following case studies.

1. Patient seen in the emergency department after an automobile accident. She is complaining of pain in her back and right leg. X-rays, UA, and CBC were normal. Discharge diagnosis: Thoracic/rib cage strain and contusion. Right leg contusion. Discharged on Voltaren 50 mg three times a day for pain and Robaxin 750 mg three times a day for muscle spasms. She is to return to work in a couple of days and follow up with her family doctor as necessary.

Category	Documentation	Tabulation
Number of Diagnosis or Treatment Options		
Amount and/or Complexity of Data Reviewed		
Level of Risk		
Final Tabulation	Note that medical decision-making is determined by the highest two of three	

2. Physician office progress note: Follow-up appointment for bronchitis. Patient reports that she feels tired and weak, and the bronchitis is lingering. Impression: Questionable resolution of her bronchitis. Plan: Refill Tessalon Perles and continue with amoxicillin. Will call if not improved.

Category	Documentation	Tabulation
Number of Diagnosis or Treatment Options		
Amount and/or Complexity of Data Reviewed		
Level of Risk		
Final Tabulation	Note that medical decision-making is determined by the highest two of three	

3. Mother brings 4-year-old child to urgent care after the child sustained a cut on the bottom of the foot. A 2-inch laceration was cleaned and sutured. Tylenol given for pain. Referred to family physician.

Category	Documentation	Tabulation
Number of Diagnosis or Treatment Options		
Amount and/or Complexity of Data Reviewed		
Level of Risk		
Final Tabulation	Note that medical decision-making is determined by the highest two of three	

Software Solutions

Several software companies offer technology solutions for determining the E/M code level. The logic software prompts coding professionals to review the health record documentation and select the elements to calculate the E/M code.

Exercise 8.7   Evaluation and Management Case Study

Answers to odd-numbered questions can be found in appendix C of this book. The answers to even-numbered questions are located in the instructor materials and are available to approved instructors.

Chief Complaint: Cough, fever and chills

This 56-year-old woman has been my patient for two years. She complains of cough, chest congestion, shortness of breath, stuffy nose over the past 3 to 4 days; feels worse today. Denies any fever, chills, but has occasional yellow productive sputum. Denies any chest pain, nausea, vomiting, or diarrhea.

Past Medical History: Cholecystectomy

Medications: None

Allergies: None

Social History: Smoker

Physical Examination:
   General: Alert woman in no apparent distress
   Vital signs: Blood pressure 152/84, temperature 99.2, pulse 84, respirations 18
   HEENT: Pupils equal, round and reactive to light and accommodation. Extraocular movements intact
   Neck: Supple, nontender
   Lungs: Breath sounds are equal. No rales or wheezes.
   Heart: S1, S2, no murmur
   Abdomen: Soft, nontender. Bowel sounds present in all quadrants.
   Extremities: Pulses equal
   Skin: Warm and dry

Studies: Chest x-ray is negative.

Diagnosis: Acute bronchitis

Plan: Zithromax Z-Pak. Follow-up in one week. Call if symptoms worse.

Refer to previous tables and apply the documentation guidelines to assign the E/M code for the preceding case. The following worksheet will help guide your coding decision-making.

(Continued on next page)

Exercise 8.7   (Continued)

Abstracting Documentation Elements Worksheet

Chief Complaint

History Component (equal to lowest category documented)	Problem-Focused	Expanded Problem-Focused	Detailed	Comprehensive
Chief Complaint _____ HPI—History of Present Illness ___ Location ___ Duration ___ Severity ___ Quality ___ Context ___ Timing ___ Modifying ___ Associated signs and factors factors symptoms	Brief: one to three HPI elements documented	Brief: one to three HPI elements documented	Extended: four or more HPI or status of three or more chronic conditions documented	Extended: four or more HPI or status of three or more chronic conditions documented
ROS—Review of System(s) ___ Constitutional ___ Integumentary (wt loss, etc.) ___ Endocrine ___ Eyes ___ GI ___ Hem/lymph ___ ENT, mouth ___ GU ___ Allergy/ Immune ___ Respiratory ___ MS ___ Cardiovascular ___ Neuro ___ Psychiatric	None	Problem specific: one system	Extended: two to nine systems	Complete: more than 10 systems or some with all others negative
PFSH (past medical, family, and social histories) ___ Previous medical (past experience with illness, injury, surgery, medical treatments, and so on) ___ Family medical history (diseases, which may be hereditary or with increased risk of occurrence) ___ Social (relationships, diet, exercise, occupation, and so on)	None	None	Pertinent: at least one item from at least one history area	Complete: specifics of at least two history areas documented

Note: A chief complaint (CC) is required for all history types.

Result of History: _____

Examination Component	Problem-Focused	Expanded Problem-Focused*	Detailed	Comprehensive
Body Areas **Organ Systems** ___ Head, face ___ Const. (vitals, general appearance) ___ Neck ___ Eyes ___ GU ___ Chest, breasts ___ ENT, mouth ___ Skin ___ Abdomen ___ Respiratory ___ Integumentary ___ Genit, groin ___ Cardiovascular ___ MS ___ Back, spine ___ Gastrointestinal ___ Neurological ___ Each extremity ___ Lymph/hem/immune ___ Psychiatric	One body area or system	Two to four body systems or two to seven basic systems, including affected area	Two to seven detailed systems, including affected area	Eight or more systems

Result of Physical Examination: _____

Medical Decision-Making	Supporting Documentation	Category
Dx or Treatment Options		
Complexity		
Risk		
Final Decision-Making		

Result of Medical Decision-Making: _____

Time

The 1992 edition of CPT introduced the notion of time as a separate contributing factor for selecting the appropriate E/M level of service codes. Prior editions had been based on the idea that time was an implicit factor in the definition of each level of service. In the current system, the specific times included in the level of service codes are averages and, as such, may vary according to the actual clinical circumstances. Details about use of time with counseling and coordination of care were discussed previously.

Face-to-Face Time

The criteria for determining "face-to-face" time are defined within CPT. Face-to-face time is the amount of time the physician spends face-to-face with the patient and/or his or her family. This includes the period during which the physician obtains a history, performs an examination, and communicating further with other professionals and the patient through written reports and telephone contact. Face-to-face time applies to several subsections in CPT.

Unit/Floor Time

Unit/floor time is the amount of time the physician is present on the patient's hospital unit and rendering services for the patient at the bedside. This includes the period when the physician establishes and/or reviews the patient's health record, examines the patient, writes notes, and communicates with other professionals and the patient's family regarding the patient's care. Unit/floor time applies to the following four subsections and subcategories: Hospital Observation Services, Inpatient Hospital Care, Initial Inpatient Hospital Consultants, and Nursing Facility Care.

Chapter 8 Review

Answers to odd-numbered questions can be found in appendix C of this book. The answers to even-numbered questions are located in the instructor materials and are available to approved instructors.

Circle the correct answer for each of the following statements.

1. All seven of the following are considered key components in selecting an E/M level of service: history, examination, medical decision-making, coordination of care, counseling, nature of presenting problem, and time.

   True   False

2. The AMA and CMS developed documentation guidelines for use with the CPT code book.

   True   False

3. The review of systems requires the physician to perform a physical examination.

   True   False

(Continued on next page)

Chapter 8 Review   (Continued)

4. A chief complaint (reason for visit) is required for all E/M office visit codes.

True   False

5. The element of time is never considered a factor in selecting an E/M level of service.

True   False

Based on 1995 documentation guidelines, write the answer to each of the following questions in the spaces provided.

6. New patient presents to the office with a CC of nasal congestion and headache. ROS: Denies shortness of breath or fever, stiffness of neck, or visual disturbances. Past history: No drug allergies or other allergies were noted, nor any history of TB, COPD, or asthma. Last physical examination 1 year ago was unremarkable. Based on this information, is this past, family, and/or social history pertinent or complete?

_____

_____

7. The CC is chest pain. The examination determined: respiration quiet and unlabored; skin with good color, warm and dry, and no rashes; mucous membranes moist; ears and throat clear; lungs with good breath sounds in all fields; rare expiratory wheeze, no rales, no rhonchi; heart regular rate and rhythm with normal heart sounds, no murmur; abdomen soft with no liver or spleen enlargement; and bowel sounds active. Based on this information, what is the level of examination?

_____

_____

8. An 86-year-old patient presents with a CC of vomiting and dizziness. Yesterday, she became dizzy while getting ready to go to church. In addition, she vomited bile several times and complained of deafness in her left ear at the start of the dizziness. Based on this information, is this history of present illness (HPI) brief or extended?

_____

_____

9. In the following case, how many key documentation elements are documented for the History of Present Illness (HPI)?
Chief Complaint: Patient is complaining of an earache
The patient complains the he has had a dull ache in his left ear for the past 24 hours. Patient explains that he went swimming two days ago. The symptoms are relieved by warm compresses and taking ibuprofen.

_____

10. In the following excerpt, identify the body system(s) explored in the
Review of Systems (ROS). Chief Complaint: Follow-up visit after cardiac
catheterization. Patient feels good. Patient denies chest pain, syncope,
palpitations, and shortness of breath. Patient states that he has some
asymptomatic edema of the left leg.

_____

Medicine

9

Learning Objectives

- Describe coding guidance for reporting immunization.
- Explain coding principles for coronary therapeutic procedures (angioplasty, cardiac catheterization).
- Describe the hierarchy system for coding injections and infusions.
- Differentiate between coding wound care management and surgical debridement (from Integumentary System).

The medicine section of the *Current Procedural Terminology* (CPT) code book comprises a wide variety of specialty services and procedures such as psychiatric therapy, chemotherapy, rehabilitation, and immunization. The modifiers that apply to medicine codes were discussed extensively in earlier chapters of this workbook.

> As an introduction, scan each page to discover the various types of codes in the section.

Specific subsections are discussed later in this chapter. In some cases, the services listed in the medicine section may be performed in conjunction with services or procedures listed elsewhere in the CPT code book. It may be appropriate to use multiple codes from different sections of the code book to identify the particular circumstances.

Example:

An established 6-year-old patient was seen in the physician's office for DTaP immunization IM injection. In addition to the immunization, the physician provides documentation for a minimal-level office visit. The following codes are reported: 90700, 90471, and 99211–25 (E/M code).

Immunization Injections

Separate codes exist for the administration (immunization procedure) of vaccines and toxoids and for the toxoid products themselves. Codes 90460–90474 are used to report the administration of a toxoid substance, and a code or codes from the 90476–90749 range identify the type of immunization or vaccine (measles, polio, DTP, and so on). The immunization administration codes are selected based on how the immunization was administered (intranasal/oral [codes 90473–90474] or other routes [intramuscular]), number of vaccines (single vs. multiple), age of patient, and whether counseling is performed by the physician or other qualified healthcare professional. Note the following differences between the code selections:

90460	Immunization administration (any route) *through 18 years of age* <u>with counseling</u>; first vaccine/toxoid component
+90461	each additional vaccine or toxoid component (add-on code)
90471	Immunization (no face-to-face counseling) *over age of 18*; 1 vaccine
+90472	each additional vaccine/toxoid
90473	Immunization administration by intranasal or oral route; 1 vaccine
+90474	each additional vaccine/toxoid

When a significant, separately identifiable E/M service (for example, office or other outpatient services or preventive medicine services) is performed, the appropriate E/M services code appended with modifier 25 should be reported in addition to the immunization administration and toxoid substance codes. For some health plans, other types of injections, including immunization administration, are bundled with E/M services and not reported separately.

Exercise 9.1 Immunizations

Answers to odd-numbered questions can be found in appendix C of this book. The answers to even-numbered questions are located in the instructor materials and are available to approved instructors.

Assign the appropriate CPT code(s) for each of the following procedures/services.

1. A 25-year-old patient receives a scheduled, routine IM injection for tetanus and diphtheria toxoids (Td).

2. A 5-year-old patient receives immunization injection for measles, mumps, rubella, and varicella vaccine (MMRV). Pediatrician counsels mother about potential side effects.

_____

3. 50-year-old man traveling abroad requires IM injection for typhoid fever.

_____

4. A 19-year-old female receives IM injection for HPV virus (nonavalent, 9vHPV, 3 dose schedule).

_____

5. IM injection of a combination of hepatitis B and _Haemophilus influenzae_ B vaccine (Hib-HepB).

_____

Psychiatry

The psychiatric services included in codes 90785 through 90899 may be provided in an outpatient or inpatient setting or in a partial hospital setting. The Centers for Medicare and Medicaid Services (CMS) defines psychiatric facility partial hospitalization as a facility for the diagnosis and treatment of mental illness that provides a planned therapeutic program for patients who do not require full-time hospitalization, but who need broader programs than are possible from outpatient visits in a hospital-based or hospital-affiliated facility. Partial hospitalization may be used for crisis stabilization, intensive short-term daily treatment, or intermediate-term treatment of psychiatric disorders.

When E/M services such as hospital or office visits are provided along with services from the psychiatry subsection, a code from the E/M section and a code from the psychiatry subsection are usually reported.

Example:

> A patient in a clinic receives individual psychotherapy for more than 25 minutes. The physician also provides medical E/M services for this established patient that include a problem-focused history, a problem-focused examination, and a straightforward level of medical decision-making. Code 90833 and 99212 should be reported.

The psychiatry subsection is further divided to identify interactive complexity, psychiatric diagnostic procedures, and psychotherapy. Add-on code 90863 is applicable for pharmacologic management, including prescription and review of medication, when performed with psychotherapy services. Note that code 90863 has a star in front of the code to indicate it may be reported for telemedicine services. In addition, another add-on code (90785) identifies interactive complexity that complicates the delivery of psychiatric procedures. Criteria for use of this code are outlined in the notes section of CPT.

Psychiatric Diagnostic Procedures

Codes 90791 and 90792 are used to report the biopsychosocial assessment for patients. The evaluation may include communication with the family and review of laboratory or diagnostic studies. The codes may be reported once per day and not on the same day as an E/M service performed by the same individual for the same patient.

Psychotherapy

The time-based codes (90832–90840) are reported for treatment of mental illness and behavior disturbances. Psychotherapy times are for face-to-face services with the patient and/or family members. In reporting times, coding professionals are instructed to code the closest to the actual time. For example, a 16- to 37-minute session would be assigned to a code for 30 minutes. A 38- to 52-minute session would be assigned to the code for 45 minutes.

Other Psychiatric Services or Procedures

Codes 90863–90899 describe specific psychotherapeutic procedures in the treatment of mental disorders and behavioral disturbances, including narcosynthesis, electroconvulsive therapy, and hypnotherapy. Narcosynthesis (90865) involves the administration of a medication that frees patients of their inhibitions and allows them to reveal information they might otherwise have found difficult to discuss.

Exercise 9.2   Psychiatry

Answers to odd-numbered questions can be found in appendix C of this book. The answers to even-numbered questions are located in the instructor materials and are available to approved instructors.

Assign the appropriate CPT code(s) for each of the following procedures/services.

1. Psychiatric evaluation of patient's health records, psychiatric reports, and tests in order to make a diagnosis

_____

2. Individual behavior modification and insight-oriented psychotherapy in office for 30 minutes

_____

3. Family psychotherapy involving patient and family member

_____

Dialysis

The CPT code selections are divided into four subcategories: Hemodialysis, Miscellaneous Dialysis Procedures, End-Stage Renal Disease (ESRD) Services, and Other Dialysis Procedures. Each subcategory begins with a notes paragraph for coding guidance. Table 9.1 outlines each of the subcategories and differentiates between the codes.

Table 9.1. Dialysis

Subcategory	CPT Code Range	Characteristics
Hemodialysis	90935–90940	• Used for inpatient ESRD and non-ESRD procedures or outpatient non-ESRD dialysis services
Miscellaneous Dialysis Procedures	90945–90947	• Identifies dialysis procedures *other than* hemodialysis
End-Stage Renal Disease Services	90951–90970	Codes differentiate between: • Outpatient setting vs. Home • Age of patient • Number of visits
Other Dialysis Procedures	90989–90999	• Training, Hemoperfusion, and unlisted code

End-Stage Renal Disease (ESRD) Services

Two methods are used to treat patients with end-stage renal disease: hemodialysis and peritoneal dialysis. Hemodialysis can be defined as the process of removing metabolic waste products, toxins, and excess fluid from the blood. Codes 90951–90970 identify services for patients with ESRD. The codes in the first range (90951–90962) are used for services provided in an outpatient setting and are based on the number of face-to-face visits per month. In addition, the levels of services are distinguished by the age of the patient. The codes in the second range (90963–90966) identify services provided in the home setting, per month. Again, age is a determining factor for code selection. If the services provided are less than a full month, codes are selected from the range of 90967–90970. Codes describing development of a shunt, cannula, or fistula for hemodialysis are categorized in the surgery section of the CPT code book.

Peritoneal dialysis involves the insertion of a catheter into the abdominal cavity and infusion of a fluid (dialysate) into the peritoneum that allows for diffusion between the dialyzing fluid and the body fluids containing the waste products. Figure 9.1 illustrates peritoneal dialysis. The fluid containing the waste products then is removed from the peritoneum through the catheter. These services are reported using code 90945 or 90947 based on the physician's (or other qualified healthcare professional) evaluation.

Figure 9.1. Peritoneal dialysis

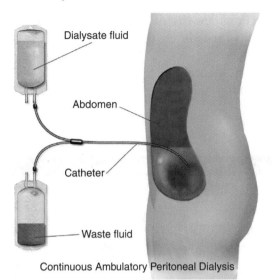

Continuous Ambulatory Peritoneal Dialysis

Source: Blaus, Bruce. "CAPD." Digital Image. Wikimedia Commons. March, 2014. Accessed September, 2018. https://commons.wikimedia.org/wiki/Category:Images_from_Blausen_Medical_Communications# /media/File:Blausen_0160_CAPD.png.

Exercise 9.3   Dialysis

Answers to odd-numbered questions can be found in appendix C of this book. The answers to even-numbered questions are located in the instructor materials and are available to approved instructors.

Assign the appropriate CPT code(s) for each of the following physician procedures/services.

1. A 50-year-old patient with end-stage renal disease treated in the outpatient dialysis unit for the past month. The physician documents one face-to-face visit during that time period.

_____

2. A 19-year-old patient was diagnosed with ESRD. During the first week of service for the month, the patient was treated twice before being transferred to Cleveland Clinic for further treatment.

_____

3. Peritoneal dialysis with a single physician evaluation

_____

Gastroenterology

This subsection contains many types of tests and nonsurgical treatments performed on the esophagus, stomach, and intestine.

Ophthalmology

The ophthalmology subsection includes codes (92002–92499) describing ophthalmologic medical services provided to both new and established patients. The definitions for new and established patient are the same as those mentioned for E/M services:

- A new patient is one who has not received any professional services (face-to-face) within the past three years from the physician or qualified healthcare professional or another physician or qualified healthcare professional of the same specialty who belongs to the same group practice.

- An established patient is one who has received professional services (face-to-face) within the past three years from the physician or qualified healthcare professional or another physician or qualified healthcare professional of the same specialty who belongs to the same group practice.

Complete definitions and examples for intermediate and comprehensive ophthalmologic services are provided in the CPT code book. Briefly, the two types of service can be described as follows:

- *Intermediate services* involve the evaluation of a new or existing condition complicated with a new diagnostic or management problem and include a history, general medical observation, external ocular and adnexal examination, and other diagnostic procedures as indicated.

- *Comprehensive services* involve a general evaluation of the complete visual system and include a history, general medical observation, an external and ophthalmoscopic examination, gross visual fields, and a basic sensorimotor examination. Initiation of diagnostic and treatment programs is always part of a comprehensive service.

An ophthalmologic examination and evaluation performed under general anesthesia is reported with code 92018 or 92019.

The prescription of contact lenses is not part of the general ophthalmologic service and should be reported separately with a code from the series 92310 through 92326. When supplying contact lenses is part of the service of fitting them (92310–92317), a separate code should not be reported.

The prescription of glasses is considered part of a general ophthalmologic service and thus should not be reported separately. Because the actual fitting of the glasses is considered a separate procedure, the fitting should be reported with a code from the series 92340 through 92371.

Exercise 9.4   Ophthalmology

Answers to odd-numbered questions can be found in appendix C of this book. The answers to even-numbered questions are located in the instructor materials and are available to approved instructors.

Assign the appropriate CPT code(s) for each of the following procedures/services.

(Continued on next page)

Exercise 9.4   (Continued)

1. Gonioscopy is performed under general anesthesia.

_____

2. New patient has a comprehensive ophthalmologic examination and evaluation.

_____

Otorhinolaryngologic Services

Special otorhinolaryngologic services include the diagnostic and therapeutic services usually provided by ear, nose, and throat specialists. Vestibular function tests and audiologic function tests are found in this section. No specific coding guidelines apply to these codes other than to use modifier 52, Reduced Services, for audiological function tests when a test is applied to only one ear.

Cardiovascular Services

The cardiovascular subsection includes codes describing diagnostic and therapeutic services such as electrocardiography, cardiac catheterization, atrial septostomy, and percutaneous transluminal coronary atherectomy. The first series of codes in this subsection (92950–92998) describes therapeutic services such as cardiopulmonary resuscitation, cardioversion and percutaneous balloon valvuloplasty.

Coronary Therapeutic Services and Procedures

Coronary therapeutic services and procedures codes are built on progressive hierarchies with more intensive services inclusive of lesser intensive service. This section requires advanced knowledge of anatomy, treatment options, and CPT coding guidance. Codes 92920–92944 describe percutaneous revascularization services for occlusive disease of the coronary vessels typically caused by atherosclerosis. Coronary revascularization is the process of restoring the flow of blood to the heart due to blockages. These procedures are commonly called percutaneous transluminal coronary angioplasty (PTCA). Typically, the surgeon inserts a balloon catheter (thin flexible tube) into the narrowed or blocked artery, inflating a balloon at the tip of the catheter to stretch the narrowed artery. A device called a stent may be placed within the coronary artery to keep the vessel open. Another technique, for removing plaque in the artery, is an atherectomy. The atherectomy procedure is performed with a cutting device (a blade or whirling blade) to remove the plaque buildup. The codes are differentiated by the treatment options such as atherectomy and stenting. A balloon angioplasty is illustrated in figure 9.2 and placement of a stent is depicted in figure 9.3.

Combinations of treatment, including revascularization of _bypass grafts_ are identified in the code range (92937–92944). The coding decision-making process begins with identification of the focus of the percutaneous coronary intervention (PCI). For coding purposes, CPT differentiates between major coronary arteries and coronary artery branches. Refer to table 9.2 and figure 9.4 (Coronary arteries).

Figure 9.2. Balloon angioplasty

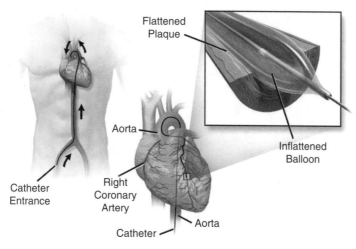

Balloon-tipped Catheter

Source: Blaus, Bruce. "Balloon-tipped Catheter." Digital Image. Wikimedia Commons. February 2016. Accessed September, 2018. https://commons.wikimedia.org/wiki/File:Balloon-Tipped_Catheter.png.

If the operative report revealed that balloon angioplasty (PTCA) was performed for the left anterior descending artery, using the catheter to push the plaque against the wall (figure 9.2), the CPT code assignment would be 92920-LD (PTCA, single major coronary artery).

Figure 9.3. Stent placement

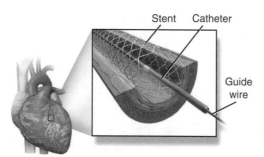

Source: Blaus, Bruce. "Angioplasty Stent." Digital Image. Wikimedia Commons. May, 2014. Accessed September, 2018. https://commons.wikimedia.org/wiki/File:Blausen_0034_Angioplasty_Stent_01.png.

If the operative report said that a PTCA was performed for the left anterior descending artery, pushing back the plaque and inserting a drug-eluting stent (figure 9.3), the CPT code assignment would be 92928-LD (Percutaneous transcatheter placement of intracoronary stent(s), with coronary angioplasty when performed; single major coronary artery or branch).

Table 9.2. Major coronary arteries and coronary artery branches

Major Coronary Arteries	Coronary Artery Branches
Left Main	No recognized branches for reporting purposes
Left Anterior Descending	Diagonals (from left anterior descending branch)
Right Main Coronary Artery	Posterior descending branch & posteriolaterals
Left Circumflex	Marginals (from left circumflex)
Ramus Intermedius Arteries	No recognized branches for reporting purposes

Figure 9.4. Coronary arteries

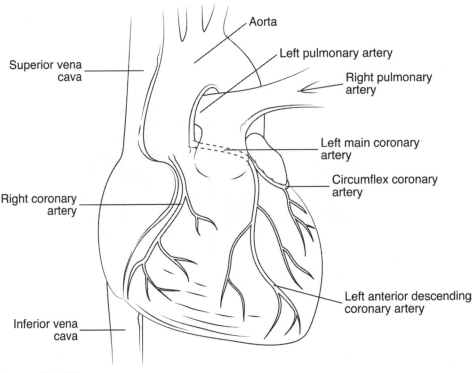

Source: ©AHIMA.

Guidelines for reporting the codes include the following:

- All PCI procedures performed in all segments (proximal, mid, distal) of a single major coronary artery through the native coronary circulation are reported with one code.
- PCI performed during the same session in additional recognized branches of the target vessel should be reported using the applicable add-on code (such as 92921).
- If a single lesion extends from one target vessel (major coronary artery, coronary artery bypass graft, or coronary artery branch) into another target vessel, but be revascularized with a single intervention bridging the two vessels, this PCI should be reported with a single code despite treating more than one vessel.

Code 92928 is reported for transcatheter stenting of a single coronary vessel. This code is only reported once per vessel even when multiple stents are placed. Code 92929 is an add-on code that can be used for stenting of additional vessels.

Example:

Physician performs balloon angioplasty (PTCA) with insertion of drug-eluting stent in the right coronary artery. The correct code would be 92928–RC.

Drug-eluting stents coated with medication are used to prevent build-up of new tissue that would reclog the artery.

Web Resources

MedlinePlus is a government website, sponsored by the U.S. National Library of Medicine, that contains a variety of tutorials and videos that can help coders understand surgical terms and techniques. For example, the following screenshot in figure 9.5 displays a link to a video explaining the surgical procedure Percutaneous Transluminal Coronary Angioplasty (PTCA). Note the website's breadcrumb trail to the resource page: Home > Videos & Tools > Health Videos. On the Videos & Tools page, you will also see a link to Surgery Videos.

Figure 9.5. MedlinePlus screenshot

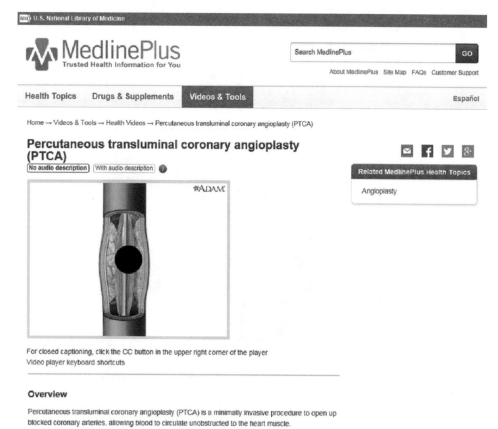

Source: U.S. National Library of Medicine. "Percutaneous transluminal coronary angioplasty (PTCA)." Digital Image. MedlinePlus. June, 2012. Accessed October, 2017. https://medlineplus.gov/ency /anatomyvideos/000096.htm.

Thrombectomy

Code 92973 should be reported when a percutaneous transluminal coronary thrombectomy (for example, with AngioJet catheter) is performed in conjunction with stenting or angioplasty. Code 92973 is considered an add-on code. Figure 9.6 illustrates an AngioJet procedure.

Brachytherapy

Code 92974 should be reported for a transcatheter placement of a radiation delivery device for intravascular brachytherapy. This procedure is used to

Figure 9.6. AngioJet

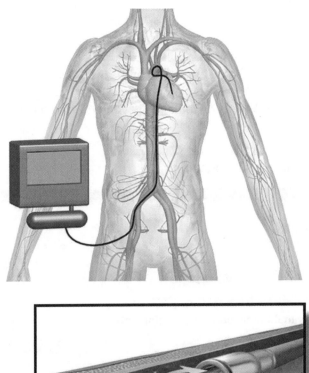

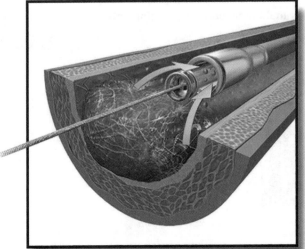

Source: Blaus, Bruce. "AngioJet." Digital Image. Wikimedia Commons. February, 2014. Accessed September, 2018. https://commons.wikimedia.org/wiki/File:Blausen_0024_Angiojet.png.

prevent repeat stenosing of the cardiac arteries. Code 92974 is an add-on code and does not include the radiation oncology service for brachytherapy.

Cardiography

The next two series of codes involve diagnostic cardiography (93000–93278), which includes electrocardiograms (EKGs) and stress tests, and echocardiography (93303–93352), which includes echocardiograms (ultrasounds of the heart).

Cardiovascular Monitoring Services: Implantable, Insertable, and Wearable Cardiac Device Evaluations

The coding selection in this section identifies cardiovascular services using both in-person and remote technology to assess device therapy and cardiovascular physiologic data. The Notes section preceding code 93264 is extensive and provides definitions and instructions for use of the implantable, insertable, and wearable code device evaluations codes. In addition to the specific description of the device and frequency of reporting, the codes can be differentiated by "in-person" and "remote."

Cardiac Catheterization

Cardiac catheterization (93451–93461) is a diagnostic procedure that can identify diseases in the coronary arteries (see figure 9.7). For a routine cardiac catheterization, only one code is required because the combination code includes associated procedures such as placement, intraprocedural injections for coronary angiography, and imaging (supervision and interpretation). According to the CPT definition, a cardiac catheterization includes the following procedures and services:

- Introduction, positioning, and repositioning of catheter(s)
- Recording of intracardiac and/or intravascular pressure
- Final evaluation and report of procedure

> If the operative report described a left heart catheterization (figure 9.7), the CPT code assignment would be 93452.

Figure 9.7.   Cardiac catheterization

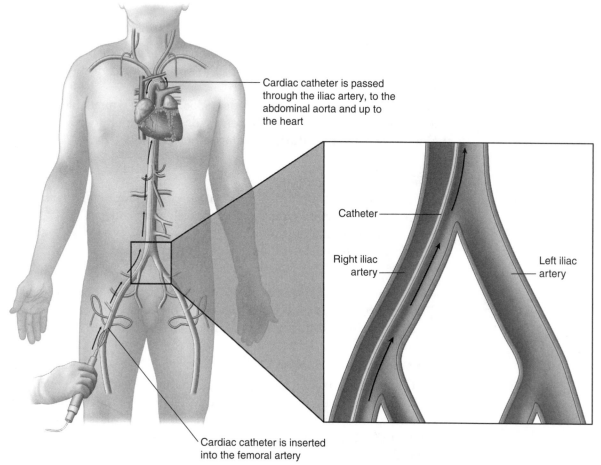

Cardiac catheter is passed through the iliac artery, to the abdominal aorta and up to the heart

Catheter

Right iliac artery

Left iliac artery

Cardiac catheter is inserted into the femoral artery

Source: ©AHIMA

The following cardiac catheterization procedures are the most common procedures:

- *Right-heart catheterization (93451):* The thin hollow tube (catheter) is inserted through a vein, typically in the neck or groin. With radiological guidance, the physician threads the catheter along the vein, through the heart and into the blood vessels going to the lungs. During the procedure, the physician can check blood pressure in the chambers of the heart. In addition, the oxygen levels of the blood can be measured.

- *Left-heart catheterization (93452):* The catheter is introduced into the artery in the groin and threaded into the heart's left ventricle. The physician can test the strength of the heart muscles, check blood pressure inside the heart, and examine the valves.

- *Combined right and left (93453):* This single code describes a procedure that is both a right-heart catheterization and a retrograde left-heart catheterization.

Example:

Physician performs percutaneous left and right cardiac catheterization with injection for left ventriculography. From the Medicine section, the facility would assign the following codes:

93453   Left and right heart catheterization (injection procedure bundled with code)

Note that there are other codes for unusual techniques, including direct ventricular puncture and puncture of the septum between the left and right atrium.

A family of injection procedure codes (93563–93568) is available for reporting "other" types of injections for right ventricular, right atrial, aortic, or pulmonary angiography performed during cardiac catheterization.

Example:

Physician performs a left cardiac catheterization with supravalvular ascending aortography. The facility would report the following codes:

93452   Left heart catheterization
93567   Supravalvular ascending aortography

The *CPT Professional Edition* provides an extensive reference table for linking cardiac catheterization procedures with add-on procedure codes such as the injection procedure (93567) referenced in the above example.

Swan-Ganz Catheterization

Swan-Ganz catheterization is the passing of a thin tube (catheter) into the right side of the heart. The procedure is done to see blood movement through the heart and to monitor the heart's function. Code 93503 is assigned to report placement of a Swan-Ganz catheter for monitoring purposes. This procedure is typically performed on patients who are critically ill or undergoing major surgery.

Infusion during Cardiac Catheterization Procedure

Physicians often infuse medications such as nitroglycerine during cardiac catheterization procedures. The January 1998 issue of *CPT Assistant* states that infusion of medications should be considered an intrinsic part of the catheterization procedure.

Intracardiac Electrophysiological Procedures and Studies

Electrophysiological testing is performed on patients with cardiac arrhythmias that result in palpitations, near syncope, or syncope with cardiac arrest. Intracardiac electrophysiological procedures, which may be diagnostic or therapeutic, are reported with codes from the range 93600 through 93662. The services described in codes 93600 through 93652 include the insertion and repositioning of catheters.

Codes 93600 through 93612 include diagnostic electrophysiological procedures that provide only recording and pacing from a single site. Codes 93619 through 93622 describe a comprehensive electrophysiological evaluation that may be reported when recording and pacing are performed from multiple sites.

Exercise 9.5 Cardiovascular Services

Answers to odd-numbered questions can be found in appendix C of this book. The answers to even-numbered questions are located in the instructor materials and are available to approved instructors.

Assign the appropriate CPT code(s) for each of the following procedures/services.

1. Patient with ventricular arrhythmia undergoes a microvolt T-wave alternans test

   _____

2. For twenty days, the physician monitors the patient's pulmonary artery pressure sensor, with weekly downloads of recording, interpretation, and report/trend analysis.

   _____

3. Coronary thrombolysis by IV infusion

   _____

4. Cardiac stress test via treadmill performed under physician supervision with interpretation and report

   _____

5. PTCA with atherectomy of left circumflex (assign HCPCS modifier)

   _____

(Continued on next page)

Exercise 9.5   (Continued)

6. PTCA of left anterior descending artery with placement of two drug-eluting stent (assign HCPCS modifier)

_____

7. A routine electrocardiogram (12 leads) was performed including interpretation and report

_____

8. Left-heart catheterization with intraprocedural injection for left ventriculography

_____

Pulmonary Services

Pulmonologists and hospitals use codes from the pulmonary subsection for pulmonary testing. When E/M services are provided separately, a code from the E/M section also should be assigned. Codes 94010 through 94799 include the performance of laboratory procedures and the interpretation of the test results.

Exercise 9.6   Pulmonary Services

Answers to odd-numbered questions can be found in appendix C of this book. The answers to even-numbered questions are located in the instructor materials and are available to approved instructors.

Assign the appropriate CPT codes for the following procedures/services.

1. Continuous positive airway pressure ventilation (CPAP) (initiation and management)

_____

2. Spirometry for bronchodilator response evaluation

_____

3. Hypoxia response curve

_____

Allergy and Clinical Immunology

The allergy and clinical immunology subsection includes the categories of allergy testing and allergen immunotherapy. The codes for allergy sensitivity tests include the performance and evaluation of selective skin and mucus tests in association with the patient's history and physical examination.

Immunotherapy (desensitization, hyposensitization) involves the parenteral administration of allergenic extracts as antigens at periodic intervals, usually on a higher dosage than a maintenance dosage. The CPT code book provides more complete definitions.

Codes from the E/M services section should be used to report visits with the patient involving the use of mechanical and electronic devices such as air conditioners, air filters, and humidifiers; climatotherapy; and physical, occupational, and recreational therapy.

Allergy testing (95004–95071) is further divided by type of test: percutaneous, intracutaneous, patch or application, and so on. For most of the codes in this series, the number of tests performed should be reported on the CMS-1500 form under item 24G.

Example:

Ten percutaneous tests with allergenic extracts were performed. The following should be reported: 95004 with 10 (to identify the number of tests) in item 24G of the CMS-1500 form or in the units field (FL 46) on the CMS-1450 form.

Allergen immunotherapy (95115–95199), more commonly referred to as allergy shots, includes the professional services related to the immunotherapy. A separate office visit code(s) should not be reported unless some other identifiable service was provided during the visit.

Exercise 9.7   Allergy and Clinical Immunology

Answers to odd-numbered questions can be found in appendix C of this book. The answers to even-numbered questions are located in the instructor materials and are available to approved instructors.

Assign the appropriate CPT code(s) for each of the following procedures/services.

1. Scratch test performed to determine allergy to bees, wasps, and yellowjackets

_____

2. Allergy shot for grass pollen (includes extract)

_____

Neurology and Neuromuscular Procedures

Consulting neurologists and hospitals generally use the range of codes in the subsections classifying neurology and neuromuscular procedures and central nervous system tests to report such procedures, assessments, and tests. Sleep testing, nerve conduction studies, and developmental testing are classified to this area of the medicine section of the CPT code book.

Adaptive Behavior Services

This new section in CPT 2019 identifies assessment and treatment for deficient adaptive behavior, maladaptive behaviors or other impaired functioning. This specialty section codes are time-based and code branching based on whether the service was provided by a physician (or other qualified health care professional) or technician.

Central Nervous System Assessments/Tests

This section of the code book has been significantly revised for 2019. The central nervous system assessments include those related to memory, language, and problem-solving ability. Due to the complexity of coding this section, CPT has provided a table for decision-making. The table categorizes three major areas of testing: Assessment of Aphasia and Cognitive Performance Testing, Development/Behavioral Screening and Testing, and Psychological/ Neuropsychological Testing. As with most specialty areas, coding professionals would need to enlist physicians or technicians to help design a strategy for coding these services.

Health and Behavior Assessment and Intervention

The focus of health and behavior assessments and interventions (beginning with code 96150) is not on mental health, but on the biopsychosocial factors affecting physical health problems and treatments (that is, patients with chronic illnesses). The codes can be reported by clinical social workers, advanced practice nurses, psychologists, and other healthcare professionals who have training in health and behavior assessment and intervention procedures. Physicians performing these services are directed to report E/M or preventive medicine codes.

Hydration, Therapeutic, Prophylactic, Diagnostic Injections and Infusions, and Chemotherapy and Other Highly Complex Drug or Highly Complex Biologic Agent Administration

It is important for coding professionals to carefully read the detailed guidelines preceding each of the coding subsections or subcategories. For example, the Notes section preceding the Injection/Infusion codes differentiates between reporting requirements for *physicians or other qualified healthcare professional* and *facilities*. CPT provides the following guidance for reporting these codes:

For physicians: The initial code that best describes the key or primary reason for the encounter should always be reported, irrespective of the order in which the infusions or injections occur.

For facility reporting: Instructions include the following hierarchy:

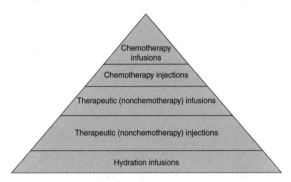

The hierarchy is used to determine the *initial* service for facilities. If there is only one service, the decision-making is simple, such as with the example below:

Facility Example:

Patient seen in the Emergency Department for severe dehydration. An IV infusion of fluids is ordered for hydration. The infusion was concluded in two hours. The following codes would be reported:
96360   IV infusion, hydration; initial, 31 minutes to 1 hour
96361   each additional hour

If multiple injections/infusions are given, then the hierarchy above is applied for coding. The bottom of the pyramid is hydration infusions and the top are chemotherapy infusions. If the patient receives hydration along with chemotherapy infusion, the initial service code for chemotherapy is assigned first, followed by an additional code for hydration.

Hierarchy Example:

Patient receives chemotherapy 1 hour infusion in the hospital. To prevent nausea and vomiting the patient receives an injection of Phenergan, 40 mg IV push. Applying the hierarchy, chemotherapy infusion is at the top and would determine the initial service. Phenergan is a therapeutic (nonchemotherapy) injection and would be assigned an add-on code.
Initial service based on hierarchy ---- 96413 Chemotherapy infusion (up to 1 hour)
IV push Phenergan ---- 96375 (additional sequential IV push of new substance/drug
(in addition, HCPCS National code J2550 would be assigned to represent the drug Phenergan)

Note that the following services are included if performed to facilitate the infusion or injection:

- Use of local anesthesia
- IV start
- Access to indwelling IV, subcutaneous catheter or port
- Flush at conclusion of infusion
- Standard tubing, syringes, and supplies

If it is elected during the patient encounter to administer multiple infusions, injections, or combinations, only one "initial" service code should be reported, unless medical protocol requires that two separate IV sites be used. This section of coding is complex and requires close examination of payers' guidelines. For Medicare guidelines, coders are encouraged to review Chapter 4, section 230.2 of the *Medicare Claims Processing Manual*, located on the CMS website.

Hydration

Two codes are provided for hydration IV infusion: code 96360 for the initial (31 minutes to 1 hour) infusion and 96361 for each additional hour. Hydration codes are to be submitted when reporting hydration IV infusion that consists of a prepackaged fluid and/or electrolyte solutions (for example, normal saline, D5-1/2 normal saline+30mEq KC1/L) but are not to be used to report infusion of drugs or other substances.

Example:

Patient with severe gastroenteritis is seen in the emergency department. Physician orders IV infusion for hydration (total of 1 hour, 45 minutes). Code assignment would be:

  96360   Intravenous infusion, hydration; initial, 31 minutes to 1 hour
+96361   each additional hour

CPT Notes guide the coding professional to report 96361 for hydration if provided as a secondary or subsequent service after a different initial service (96360, 96365, 96374, 96409, 96413) is administered through the same IV access.

Therapeutic, Prophylactic, and Diagnostic Injections and Infusions (Excluding Chemotherapy and Other Highly Complex Drug or Highly Complex Biologic Agent Administration)

CPT codes from this section (beginning with 96365) are used to describe administration of substances and/or drugs. The fluid used to administer the drug(s) is incidental hydration and is not reported with a separate CPT code.

The codes are differentiated according to the route of administration, such as IV, and the injection status (initial, sequential, concurrent).

The specific substance injected must be reported with another code. For Medicare cases, a Level II *Healthcare Common Procedure Coding System* (HCPCS) code (J series) is reported with the identification of the specific substance or drug; for non-Medicare cases, code 99070 may be reported (HCPCS Level II codes [J codes] are discussed in chapter 10 of this book). This series of codes is not to be used for allergy injections or immunizations; specific CPT codes are available for these services.

The payment policies of individual payers (including Medicare) differ and should be reviewed carefully to ensure appropriate payment.

Use the *CPT QuickRef app* or *CPT Assistant* to review the article "Infusion Reporting," published in the December 2011 issue of *CPT Assistant.*

Example:

Patient with a wound infection undergoes a one-hour infusion of Vancomycin HCl 1000 mg. The correct code assignment would be:

>   96365   Intravenous infusion, for therapy, prophylaxis, or diagnosis (specify drug); initial, up to 1 hour
>
> J3370 × 2   Vancomycin 500 mg

Chemotherapy and Other Highly Complex Drug or Highly Complex Biologic Agent Administration

The administration of chemotherapy is reported with codes beginning with 96401. The codes further identify the mode of administration: subcutaneous or intramuscular, intralesional, intravenous, or intra-arterial. The codes describing intravenous and intra-arterial administration are further subdivided to identify the technique—infusion or push—and length of time. Codes beginning with 96440 describe the administration of chemotherapy to specific body sites: pleural or peritoneal cavity, or central nervous system. Codes 96521 and 96522 describe the maintenance and refilling of portable or implantable pumps or reservoirs.

Although preparation of the chemotherapy agent is included in the administration, provision of the chemotherapy drug is not. For Medicare claims, a code from the J series of the Level II HCPCS should be reported to identify the specific drug administered. Codes describing the placement of pumps, catheters, or reservoirs can be found in the surgery section of the CPT code book.

Example:

Patient with lung cancer is seen in the hospital outpatient department for chemotherapy treatment. The patient receives Cisplatin 50 mg IV for one hour. The following should be reported:

96413   Chemotherapy administration, infusion, first hour

J9060   Cisplatin, per 10 mg (bill would reflect 5 units because 50 mg was administered)

When additional services are provided on the same day as the chemotherapy and are independent of the chemotherapy, the physician may bill the additional services separately (for example, an E/M office visit).

Exercise 9.8   Injections and Infusions

Answers to odd-numbered questions can be found in appendix C of this book. The answers to even-numbered questions are located in the instructor materials and are available to approved instructors.

Assign the appropriate CPT code(s) for each of the following procedures/ services. Do not assign HCPCS Level II codes for this exercise.

   1. Intramuscular vitamin B_{12} injection

(Continued on next page)

Exercise 9.8   (Continued)

2. IV infusion of Cisplatin (chemotherapy) administered for two hours

_____

3. IV infusion hydration for one hour

_____

4. Patient seen in outpatient department for antibiotic intravenous piggyback (IVPB) infusion for a severe infection, given at one-hour intervals at 9:00 a.m., 3:00 p.m., and 10:00 p.m. on the same day.

_____

5. Intra-arterial chemotherapy administration, IV push

_____

6. Patient receives 40 minutes of hydration prior to a 1-hour chemotherapy infusion.

_____

Special Dermatological Procedures

Services such as actinotherapy and photochemotherapy are found in the special dermatological procedures subsection of CPT. Generally, these codes are used by consulting dermatologists.

Physical Medicine and Rehabilitation

The number of physical medicine and rehabilitation services available to patients continues to expand as new modalities and therapeutic procedures are developed. The CPT codes for these services (97161–97799) are used by the physiatrists and physical therapists who provide physical therapy services to patients recovering from injuries, strokes, and other debilitating conditions. Test and measurement codes can be reported to document the use of prosthetic devices and physical performance testing apparatus. No special coding guidelines apply to this section. Physiatrists use the E/M section for professional service billing.

Active Wound Care Management

In the Integumentary System, wound debridement codes were identified with codes beginning with 11042. There is an important note under code 11012 that states:

> (For debridement of skin Iie, epidermis and/or dermis only] see 97597, 97598)

This note helps to distinguish between the use of debridement codes in Integumentary and those in the Medicine chapter. According to CPT coding

Use the *CPT QuickRef* app or *CPT Assistant* to review guidelines and examples for coding debridement found in the March 2012 and May 2011 issues of *CPT Assistant*.

guidelines, the wound care management codes should *not* be reported in addition to the debridement codes (11042–11047) included in the integumentary system subsection of the Surgery section.

The wound care management codes can be described as either selective or nonselective. Codes 97597 and 97598 are assigned for the selective technique, which includes the use of scalpels, scissors, and forceps to cut and remove the necrotic tissue. Other selective debridement includes the use of high-pressure water jets, enzyme applications, and autolysis. Code 97602 is assigned for nonselective techniques, which include the gradual removal of loosely adherent areas of necrotic tissue achieved by irrigating the wound and hydrotherapy.

Codes 97605-97607 are used to report negative pressure wound therapy, which is often described as a vacuum-assisted closure. This system encourages wound closure by applying localized negative pressure to the surface and margins of the wound. Negative pressure therapy is applied to a special dressing positioned in the wound cavity or over a flap or graft. The pressure-distributing wound dressing helps drain fluids from the wound.

Exercise 9.9   Physical Medicine and Rehabilitation

Answers to odd-numbered questions can be found in appendix C of this book. The answers to even-numbered questions are located in the instructor materials and are available to approved instructors.

Assign the appropriate CPT code(s) for each of the following procedures or services.

1. TENS unit applied by therapist for patient with low back pain, 30 minutes visit

   _____

2. Thirty minutes of water aerobic exercises with therapist for treatment of arthritis

   _____

3. The therapist provides wet-to-moist dressings to promote healing of a necrotic wound of the leg

   _____

4. Physician orders a re-evaluation of a knee injury following a course of athletic training. The 20-minute evaluation included an assessment of the patient's current functional status and a revised plan of care.

   _____

5. The epidermis and dermis wound surface of the arm (approximately 5 sq cm) was debrided with Versajet.

   _____

6. The wound surface, down to the muscle of the arm (approximately 5 sq cm) was debrided with Versajet

   _____

Manipulative Treatment

Osteopathic physicians and chiropractic physicians as well as other physicians trained in manipulation techniques use the codes found in the osteopathic manipulative treatment and chiropractic manipulative treatment subsections. E/M service codes are to be reported separately only when the services are significant and separate from the manipulative treatments. In these cases, modifier 25, Significant, Separately Identifiable Evaluation and Management Service by the Same Physician on the Same Day of the Procedure or Other Service, may be appended to the E/M code to communicate the circumstances on a claim form.

Non-Face-to-Face Nonphysician Services

There are two subcategories for assessment and management of patient services via the telephone or with internet communication. The selection of codes 98966–98969 is designated for use by qualified healthcare professionals (physicians are to use codes 99441–99444 from the E/M section). Guidelines are summarized below:

- Initiated by established patient (or guardian)
- If the telephone call ends with the decision to see the patient within 24 hours (or next available urgent appointment), then the code is not reported
- If call refers to a service performed within previous seven days or within the postoperative period, then the telephone services are considered part of the previous service or procedure; therefore *not* reported

The above guidelines also pertain to the internet services. The online communication must be maintained in permanent storage, either electronically or in hard copy.

Special Services, Procedures, and Reports

The special services and reports subsection (99000–99091) of the CPT Medicine section describes certain procedures and services or reports that the physician may add to other basic services. Codes 99050 through 99060 describe special services provided to a patient beyond the basic service, such as those requested between 10 p.m. and 8 a.m. (code 99052). Because a third-party payer may or may not reimburse these services, a review of each payer's policies might be informative. However, coded information is also used in many activities unrelated to reimbursement, and so assigning the codes for nonreimbursable services may be desirable from a data management perspective.

CPT code 99070 may be reported when the physician submits claims for supplies and other materials to an insurance plan that does not recognize Level II HCPCS codes. For Medicare claims, coding professionals should remember that, in most cases, a more specific code describing a particular supply may exist in Level II of HCPCS, and routine supplies associated with professional services are not reimbursed separately.

Qualifying Circumstances for Anesthesia

Four CPT codes (99100–99140) may be used to report qualifying circumstances or additional information on patients undergoing anesthesia who show greater risk of complications. For example, codes describing patients of extreme age (elderly or newborn), with total body hypothermia or controlled hypotension, or with possible emergency conditions, may need to be reported in addition to the code describing the anesthesia service.

Moderate (Conscious) Sedation

These codes (99151–99157) are available to report moderate (conscious) sedation, a technique used during a number of endoscopic and other procedures. CPT provides criteria for use of these codes that include Preservice, Intraservice, and Postservice Work. The codes can be differentiated by the age of the patient, time and whether or not the physician is also performing the diagnostic/therapeutic procedure or not.

Other Services and Procedures

The Medicine section of CPT also provides codes for several miscellaneous procedures that are performed by physicians but do not fit into the other sections of CPT. One example is hyperbaric oxygen therapy supervision. Another is the administration of ipecac and observation of the patient until the stomach is emptied of poison. Such codes are located in the other services and procedures subsection.

Home Health Procedures and Services

Codes from the section on home health procedures and services (99500–99600) are used by nonphysician healthcare professionals who provide medical services in the homes of patients. Physicians use codes from the E/M section for coding the home health services they provide. Healthcare professionals who are authorized to use E/M home visit codes (99341–99350) may report codes from the range 99500 through 99512 with the E/M code when a patient's condition requires significant evaluation and management services beyond the home health service or procedure. In such cases, modifier 25 may be appended to the E/M code.

Home Infusion Procedures/Services

Codes from the home infusion procedures section (99601 and 99602) include a code for home visits by nonphysician healthcare professionals and a code for all the necessary solutions, equipment, and supplies required to deliver a therapeutic service in one visit. Drugs are excluded from this code and should be reported separately.

Medication Therapy Management Services

CPT codes 99605–99607 are codes to report for face-to-face medication therapy management services (MTMS) by a pharmacist. The code selection is based on new versus established patient and time. Guidelines specify that MTMS documentation include the following:

- Review of pertinent patient history, medication profile
- Recommendations for improving health outcomes
- Treatment compliance

Chapter 9 Review

Answers to odd-numbered questions can be found in appendix C of this book. The answers to even-numbered questions are located in the instructor materials and are available to approved instructors.

Assign the appropriate code(s) from the CPT Medicine section as well as modifiers, when appropriate, for each of the following non-Medicare cases. **Do not assign HCPCS National codes.**

1. Patient (42 years old) diagnosed with ESRD requires home dialysis for the month of April.

   _____

2. A 30-year-old male is given a subcutaneous injection of live varicella virus vaccine by the nurse practitioner.

   _____

3. The surgeon performs percutaneous transcatheter closure of a mitral valve (paravalvular) leak, initial

   _____

4. MDI (metered dose inhaler) treatment for patient with asthma

   _____

5. Bundle of His electrography recording performed to evaluate patient with syncope

   _____

6. Physician treats plaque psoriasis of arms and legs with use of laser (250 sq cm)

   _____

7. Nurse makes a home visit for newborn care and assessment

   _____

8. IV chemotherapy infusion lasting two hours

   _____

9. Percutaneous transluminal coronary atherectomy with balloon angioplasty of left posterior descending and left obtuse marginal arteries

   _____

10. Speech audiometry with threshold and recognition, both ears

    _____

11. Percutaneous thrombectomy of right coronary artery and angioplasty with placement of drug-eluting stent, left circumflex (apply HCPCS anatomic modifiers)

_____

12. Pharmacist spends 30 minutes providing medication therapy management services to an established patient.

_____

13. EMG of three extremities and related paraspinal areas

_____

14. Leg prosthetic training for 30 minutes by a physical therapist

_____

15. In addition to E/M services, a physician provided a medical service on July 4 to fulfill a patient's request for the service.

_____

16. Due to an allergic reaction, patient receives 1-hour hydration along with IV push of Benadryl.

_____

17. Osteopathic manipulation; head, cervical, thoracic, and lumbar spine

_____

18. Complete duplex scan of the lower extremity arteries, bilateral

_____

19. Esophageal acid reflex test

_____

20. Individual patient interactive psychotherapy for 37 minutes provided in the outpatient setting

_____

21. Sleep study including EKG, recordings of breathing, and O_2 saturation, performed by a technician

_____

22. Photodynamic therapy session using a Photofrin® (drug) and external light to destroy esophageal premalignant lesion.

_____

Anesthesia

10

Learning Objectives

- Apply qualifying-circumstances and physical-status codes to anesthesiology services.
- Differentiate between the types of anesthesia.

- Identify the two common methods for reimbursement of anesthesiology services.
- Given an operative statement, successfully assign a CPT code.

Current Procedural Terminology (CPT) codes in this section can be reported under the condition that the procedures/services were performed by, or under the responsible supervision of, a physician or a certified registered nurse anesthetist (CRNA). Coding professionals should keep in mind that they are selecting an anesthesia code based on the surgical procedure performed. The anesthesia section of the CPT code book includes codes that describe general and regional anesthesia services, and supplementation of local anesthesia or other supportive services. These services should be reported by the physician who provides or supervises the anesthesia. The anesthesia services (00100–01999) in this section include:

- Usual preoperative and postoperative visits
- Anesthesia provided during the procedure
- Administration of fluids and/or blood
- Usual monitoring services, such as EKG, temperature, blood pressure, oximetry, capnography, and mass spectrometry (unusual monitoring, such as intra-arterial, central venous, or Swan-Ganz, is not included and should be reported separately)

The codes in the Anesthesia section are arranged first by body site and then by specific surgical procedure performed (except for Radiological Procedures and

Other Procedures at the end of the chapter). They may be found in the alphabetic index of the CPT code book by referencing the main entries of Anesthesia or Analgesia.

For anesthesia services, it is important to review third-party payer rules and regulations before submitting CPT codes.

Types of Anesthesia

There are several methods of administering anesthesia.

* *Local anesthesia:* This method involves an injection of a numbing agent directly into the area of the body, which will block pain in minor procedures.
* *Regional anesthesia:* This method involves an injection, but the anesthetic is applied to a larger area of body surface. For example, a peripheral nerve block injected near a specific nerve will block the sensation for a group of nerves supplied by the injected nerve. This type of technique is often used for procedures on hands, feet, arms, and legs. Another example of a regional anesthesia is an epidural or spinal block.
* *General anesthesia:* This method requires that the anesthetic be administered intravenously or by inhalation. The patient is unconscious during the surgery.

CPT Format

The anesthesia section is primarily organized by anatomic site (with a few exceptions). Closer examination of the code descriptions will reveal that several procedures may be assigned to one anesthesia code. For example:

00770	Anesthesia for all procedures on major abdominal blood vessels

Note the following format for anesthesia codes:

Anatomic site →

Knee and Popliteal Area
01380 Anesthesia for all closed procedures on knee joint
01382 Anesthesia for diagnostic arthroscopic procedures of knee joint

Coding Procedure

Using the surgical procedure, diagnostic arthroscopy of the knee, apply the following procedure for correct coding assignment.

In the alphabetic index of CPT, locate the main term **Anesthesia**.
Refer to the subterm **Arthroscopic Procedures** and scan for **Knee**.
Note the code selection of 01382, 01400.
Refer to both codes and you will determine that the best CPT code is 01382.

To illustrate another method of locating the correct code, locate the main term **Anesthesia** and refer to subterm **Knee**. There is a large range of codes to reference and the coding process will take significantly longer but the correct code is among this range.

Conscious Sedation

Conscious sedation produces a level of consciousness that retains the patient's ability to independently and continuously maintain an airway and respond appropriately to physical stimulation or verbal command. CPT codes 99151–99153 are used to report moderate conscious sedation provided by a physician (or other qualified healthcare professional) who is also performing the procedure. Additional code selections are available for a physician (or other than the healthcare professional) performing the diagnostic or therapeutic service that the conscious sedation supports (99155–99157).

Time Reporting

Time may be reported for reimbursement of services, if preferred by the local carrier. Counting anesthesia time should begin with preparation of the patient by the anesthesiologist for induction of anesthesia (usually in the operating room) and end when the anesthesiologist no longer is in attendance.

Anesthesia Modifiers

When reporting anesthesia services, a physical status modifier code should be used to distinguish between various levels of complexity of the anesthesia service provided. The anesthesiologist usually provides physical status modifiers on the anesthesia record. The ranking of patient physical status by the American Society of Anesthesiologists (ASA) is consistent with the following modifiers:

P1   A normal, healthy patient
P2   A patient with mild systemic disease
P3   A patient with severe systemic disease
P4   A patient with severe systemic disease that is a constant threat to life
P5   A moribund patient who is not expected to survive without the operation
P6   A declared brain-dead patient whose organs are being removed for donor purposes

Under certain circumstances, other modifiers may be assigned. The following modifiers are commonly used with codes from the anesthesia section.

22   **Increased Procedural Services**: Modifier 22 may be reported to identify that the service provided was greater than that usually required for a particular service. Supportive documentation may need to be submitted to the third-party payer to justify use of modifier 22.

23   **Unusual Anesthesia**: Modifier 23 may be reported when anesthesia is administered for a procedure that usually requires local anesthesia or none at all. This modifier would be reported along with the appropriate code describing the anesthesia service.

51 Multiple Procedures: Modifier 51 may be reported to identify that multiple anesthesia services were provided on the same day or during the same operative episode. The first procedure listed should identify the major or most resource-intensive service provided. Subsequent or secondary services should be appended with modifier 51.

53 Discontinued Procedure: Modifier 53 is appropriate for circumstances when the physician or other qualified healthcare professional elects to terminate or discontinue a procedure, usually because of risk to the patient's well-being. However, this modifier is not meant to report the elective cancellation of a procedure before the patient's surgical preparation or induction of anesthesia. Also, the appropriate ICD-9-CM code should be assigned to identify the reason for the procedure's termination or discontinuation.

59 Distinct Procedural Service: Modifier 59 may be used to identify that a procedure/service was distinct or independent from other services provided on the same day.

Modifier 47, Anesthesia by Surgeon, is never used as a modifier for the anesthesia procedures in the CPT code book (00100–01999).

HCPCS Level II Modifiers

The following National Code modifiers are applicable to anesthesia services:

AA   Anesthesia services performed personally by anesthesiologist

AD   Medical supervision by a physician: more than four concurrent anesthesia procedures

G8   Monitored anesthesia care (MAC) for deep complex, complicated or markedly invasive surgical procedures

G9   Monitored anesthesia care for a patient who has a history of a severe cardiopulmonary condition

GC   This service has been performed in part by a resident under the direction of a teaching physician

GF   Nonphysician (e.g., nurse practitioner, certified registered nurse anesthetist, certified registered nurse, physician assistant) services in a critical access hospital

QK   Medical direction of two, three, or four concurrent anesthesia procedures involving qualified individuals

QS   Monitored anesthesia care service

QX   CRNA service; with medical direction by a physician

QY   Medical direction of one certified registered nurse anesthetist (CRNA) by an anesthesiologist

QZ   CRNA service; without medical direction by a physician

The assignment of modifier QK indicates that the anesthesiologist provided medical direction to at least two, but not more than four, certified nurse anesthetists.

Qualifying Circumstances

When anesthesia services are provided under difficult circumstances because of the patient's condition, operative conditions, or unusual risk factors, an additional code may be reported along with the code describing the basic anesthesia service. Codes 99100 through 99140 can never be reported alone. Located in the medicine section of the CPT code book, these codes (99100–99140) are described as follows:

- 99100 Anesthesia for patient of extreme age, under 1 year and over 70 years
- 99116 Anesthesia complicated by utilization of total body hypothermia
- 99135 Anesthesia complicated by utilization of controlled hypotension
- 99140 Anesthesia complicated by emergency conditions

When code 99140 is reported, a separate report must be submitted describing the type of emergency. According to the CPT code book, an emergency exists when delay in treatment of the patient would significantly increase the threat to life or body part.

Application of Anesthesia Codes in the Hospital Setting

Because the anesthesia codes were developed to represent the professional services provided by anesthesiologists, the anesthesia codes cannot be reported by hospitals unless the hospitals perform billing services for the anesthesiologists.

Chapter 10 Review

Answers to odd-numbered questions can be found in appendix C of this book. The answers to even-numbered questions are located in the instructor materials and are available to approved instructors.

Assign the appropriate codes and physical status modifiers to describe the anesthesia services for the following Medicare claims. The anesthesia codes should be assigned from the Anesthesia section.

1. Anesthesia services for radical mastectomy with internal mammary node dissection; patient has diabetes mellitus well controlled with American Dietetic Association (ADA) diet

   _____

2. Anesthesia services for cervical cerclage; patient is 25 years old and in good health

   _____

(Continued on next page)

Chapter 10 Review   (Continued)

3. Anesthesia services for CABG surgery of five vessels with pump oxygenator; patient has severe coronary artery disease as well as hypertensive end-stage renal disease requiring hemodialysis

   _____

4. Anesthesia services for open repair for malunion fracture of humerus; patient is 85 years old but healthy

   _____

5. Anesthesia services for transurethral resection of prostate, 54-year-old patient is otherwise healthy

   _____

6. Anesthesia services for partial nephrectomy in a patient with renal cell carcinoma; 45-year-old patient also has mild coronary artery disease and hypertension treated with medication

   _____

7. Anesthesia services for heart transplant secondary to congenital heart defect; patient is 3 weeks old and requires a transplant to survive

   _____

8. Anesthesia services for blepharoplasty; patient is in good health

   _____

9. Anesthesia services for carotid thromboendarterectomy with patch graft for severe carotid artery stenosis; patient is 89 years old and has had recurrent carotid artery stenosis; patient also has a pacemaker for control of atrial fibrillation

   _____

10. Anesthesia services for left lobectomy due to lung carcinoma; patient also has severe chronic obstructive pulmonary disease and emphysema treated with bronchodilators

    _____

11. Anesthesia services for ERCP

    _____

12. Anesthesia services radical orchiectomy, inguinal approach

    _____

HCPCS Level II

Learning Objectives

- Identify the structure of HCPCS Level II codes.
- Describe the use of HCPCS Level II modifiers.
- Successfully apply general guidelines for HCPCS Level II coding assignment.
- Given a procedural statement, assign the correct CPT codes and/or HCPCS code.
- Validate coding assignments.

Developed by the Centers for Medicare and Medicaid Services (CMS), Level II *Healthcare Common Procedure Coding System* (HCPCS) also is referred to as the National Codes. The National Codes were designed to report physician and nonphysician services such as drugs, chiropractic services, dental procedures, durable medical equipment, and other selected procedures. These National Codes are updated periodically, published annually, and can be found on the CMS website (figure 11.1).

Use of Codes by Payer

Although the National Codes were developed for Medicare, they also are used by commercial payers. Coding professionals should note that some Medicare carriers mandate the use of Level II codes rather than specific *Current Procedural Terminology* (CPT) codes. HCPCS Level II code G0268 (Removal of impacted cerumen, one or both ears) should be reported for the earwax removal procedure performed by a physician on the same date of service as audiologic function testing. CPT code 69209 is used to report removal of impacted cerumen using irrigation/lavage, unilateral. Bulletins from Medicare carriers announce such mandates. Some Medicaid programs and private insurance carriers also may accept or mandate the use of National Codes. It is important to note that the existence of an HCPCS Level II code doesn't necessarily indicate that it will be reimbursed. For example, code A4267 is an HCPCS Level II code for male condoms and this is not payable by Medicare. Most coding professionals use software to help determine what is a covered procedure or equipment.

The American Hospital Association (AHA) and the Centers for Medicare and Medicaid Services (CMS) have joined together in establishing the AHA

Figure 11.1. CMS website links to HCPCS files

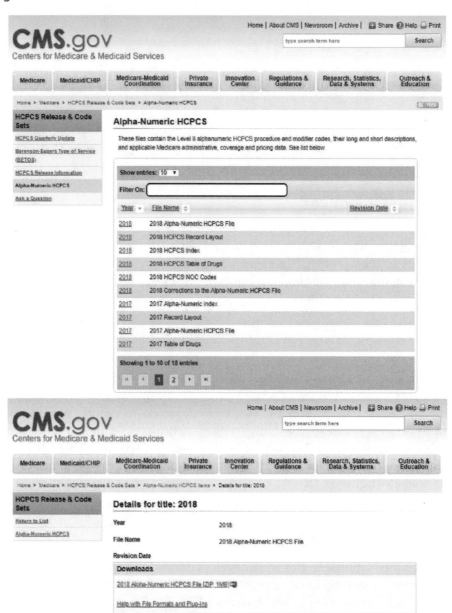

Source: CMS.gov. "Alpha-Numeric HCPCS." Digital Image. Centers for Medicare and Medicaid Services. Accessed October, 2018. https://www.cms.gov/Medicare/Coding/HCPCSReleaseCodeSets/Alpha-Numeric-HCPCS.html.

clearinghouse to handle coding questions on established HCPCS usage. The American Health Information Management Association (AHIMA) also provides input through the Editorial Advisory Board. In addition to publishing a *Coding Clinic* for ICD-10-CM, AHA also publishes a *Coding Clinic* specifically for HCPCS.

The HCPCS Level II codes included in this publication are current as of October 1, 2018.

The Coding Process

The first step for finding HCPCS codes begins with the Alphabetic Index. For example, if a patient was provided with a compression burn garment (custom fabricated glove to wrist), the range of HCPCS codes to verify can be found in the Alphabetic Index as displayed below:

Composite dressing, A6200–A6205
Compressed gas system, E0424–E0480
Compression bandage, A4460
→Compression burn garment, A6501–A6512
Compression stockings, A6530–A6549

CMS Numeric File

From the Alphabetic Index, code descriptions for A6501–A6512 would be reviewed in the CMS numeric file in order to select the appropriate code of A6504 (Compression burn garment, glove to wrist, custom fabricated) as noted below:

A6501, Compression burn garment, bodysuit (head to foot), custom fabricated
A6502, Compression burn garment, chin strap, custom fabricated
A6503, Compression burn garment, facial hood, custom fabricated
→A6504, Compression burn garment, glove to wrist, custom fabricated
A6505, Compression burn garment, glove to elbow, custom fabricated
A6506, Compression burn garment, glove to axilla, custom fabricated
A6507, Compression burn garment, foot to knee length, custom fabricated
A6508, Compression burn garment, foot to thigh length, custom fabricated
A6509, Compression burn garment, upper trunk to waist including arm openings (vest), custom fabricated
A6510, Compression burn garment, trunk, including arms down to leg openings (leotard), custom fabricated
A6511, Compression burn garment, lower trunk including leg openings (panty), custom fabricated
A6512, Compression burn garment, not otherwise classified

CMS Alphabetic Index File

Earlier, we displayed drug code J2360 Injection, orphenadrine, citrate, up to 60 mg. In order to locate this code, the HCPCS Table of Drugs would be referenced as noted below:

Ormazine, see Chlorpromazine HCl

→ Orphenadrine citrate up to 60 mg IV, IM J2360

Orphenate, see Orphenadrine citrate

Orthovisc OTH J7324

Or-Tyl, see Dicyclomine

Oxacillin sodium up to 250 mg IM, IV J2700

Oxaliplatin 0.5 mg IV J9263

Oxymorphone HCl up to 1 mg IV, SC, IM J2410

Oxytetracycline HCl up to 50 mg IM J2460

Oxytocin up to 10 units IV, IM J2590

Ozurdex, see Dexamethasone, intravitreal implant

Along with the drug name, the table provides dosage and routes of administration. For orphenadrine citrate, the dosage is listed up to 60 mg and routes of administration include IV (intravenous) and IM (intramuscular). The following abbreviations are used to designate the route of administration:

IA   Intra-arterial
IT   Intrathecal
IV   Intravenous
IM   Intramuscular
SC   Subcutaneous
INH   Inhalant solution
VAR   Various routes
ORAL   Oral
OTH   Other routes

Reporting HCPCS Codes

Typically, HCPCS codes for hospitals are maintained in an electronic charge-master file that automatically assigns the majority of HCPCS codes. In the physician office setting, coding professionals take on a more active role in assigning HCPCS codes. The offices report the HCPCS codes in the same field (24D) as CPT codes on the CMS-1500 claim form as indicated in the excerpt below:

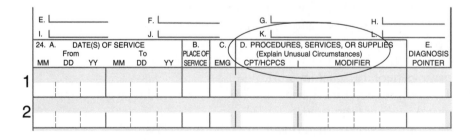

Exercise 11.1 Auditing HCPCS Level II Codes

Answers to odd-numbered questions can be found in appendix C of this book. The answers to even-numbered questions are located in the instructor materials and are available to approved instructors.

Using HCPCS Level II code book or Excel file of HCPCS codes (downloaded from CMS website), validate the HCPCS code with the documentation of a supply or service. Determine if the HCPCS code is correct or not. If there is an error, assign the correct code.

1. The patient was provided with a table heat lamp that included the bulb.

24. A. DATE(S) OF SERVICE From MM DD YY To MM DD YY	B. PLACE OF SERVICE	C. EMG	D. PROCEDURES, SERVICES, OR SUPPLIES (Explain Unusual Circumstances) CPT/HCPCS | MODIFIER	E. DIAGNOSIS POINTER
1			E0205	

2. The patient was provided with nasogastric tubing with stylet.

24. A. DATE(S) OF SERVICE From MM DD YY To MM DD YY	B. PLACE OF SERVICE	C. EMG	D. PROCEDURES, SERVICES, OR SUPPLIES (Explain Unusual Circumstances) CPT/HCPCS | MODIFIER	E. DIAGNOSIS POINTER
1			B4082	

3. The patient received an implantable single chamber non-rate responsive pacemaker.

24. A. DATE(S) OF SERVICE From MM DD YY To MM DD YY	B. PLACE OF SERVICE	C. EMG	D. PROCEDURES, SERVICES, OR SUPPLIES (Explain Unusual Circumstances) CPT/HCPCS | MODIFIER	E. DIAGNOSIS POINTER
1			C2620	

4. The patient received an IM injection of 75 mg of Hydrocortisone succinate sodium.

24. A. DATE(S) OF SERVICE From MM DD YY To MM DD YY	B. PLACE OF SERVICE	C. EMG	D. PROCEDURES, SERVICES, OR SUPPLIES (Explain Unusual Circumstances) CPT/HCPCS | MODIFIER	E. DIAGNOSIS POINTER
1			J1720	

5. The patient was provided full-length bed side rails.

24. A. DATE(S) OF SERVICE From MM DD YY To MM DD YY	B. PLACE OF SERVICE	C. EMG	D. PROCEDURES, SERVICES, OR SUPPLIES (Explain Unusual Circumstances) CPT/HCPCS | MODIFIER	E. DIAGNOSIS POINTER
1			E0305	

Exercise 11.2 HCPCS Level II Codes

Answers to odd-numbered questions can be found in appendix C of this book. The answers to even-numbered questions are located in the instructor materials and are available to approved instructors.

Using the HCPCS Level II code book or Excel file of HCPCS codes (downloaded from CMS website), assign HCPCS Level II codes for the following. If using the Excel file, click "Edit" and use the "Find" function to locate the correct codes.

1. Battery, heavy duty, replacement for patient-owned ventilator

_____

2. Healthcare professional conducts a (non-medical) family planning session

_____

3. Screening cervical PAP smear, (3 smears) interpreted by the physician

_____

4. Capecitabine, oral 500 mg

_____

5. Speech screening

_____

6. Mastectomy bra, bilateral with integrated breast prosthesis form

_____

7. A 200-mg injection of mesna

_____

8. Synthetic sheepskin pad

_____

9. Cervical collar, molded to patient model

_____

10. Congo red blood chemistry/toxicology test

_____

HCPCS Level II Modifiers

The modifiers used in HCPCS Level II were developed to serve the same purpose that modifiers serve in the CPT code book. The assignment of a modifier may indicate that a service or procedure was modified in some way, but with no change to its basic definition. HCPCS modifiers can be used to indicate the following types of information:

- The service was supervised by an anesthesiologist.
- The service was performed by a healthcare professional other than a physician, such as a clinical psychologist, a nurse practitioner, or a physician assistant.
- The service was provided as part of a specific government program.
- The service was provided to a specific site of the body.
- Equipment was purchased or rented.
- Single or multiple patients were seen during nursing home visits.

In the coding of Medicare claims, HCPCS Level II modifiers may be used with the National Codes or with CPT Category I codes.

The HCPCS modifiers consist of one or two characters and are appended to the appropriate HCPCS Level II or CPT Category I codes. The following are examples of HCPCS Level II modifiers (a complete list of modifiers can be located on the CMS website):

A1	Dressing for one wound
AA	Anesthesia services personally furnished by the anesthesiologist
AH	Clinical psychologist
AJ	Clinical social worker
AM	Physician, team member service
AS	Physician assistant, nurse practitioner, or clinical nurse specialist services for assistant at surgery
BO	Orally administered nutrition, not by feeding tube
GA	Waiver of liability statement issued as required by payer policy, individual case
JC	Skin substitute used as a graft
RR	Rental

Example:

A patient is recovering at home after having surgery for a hip fracture. The durable medical equipment (DME) provider rents the patient a rigid adjustable-height walker for 30 days. The DME provider would report the following HCPCS Level II code and modifier:

E0130-RR   (The HCPCS Level II modifier RR is for rental.)

Chapter 11 Review

Answers to odd-numbered questions can be found in appendix C of this book. The answers to even-numbered questions are located in the instructor materials and are available to approved instructors.

Use the HCPCS Level II code book to answer the following questions.

1. What is the code for an air pressure mattress?

   _____

2. What Level II code would indicate that the patient received a below-the-knee surgical stocking?

   _____

3. If a patient was given a vitamin B_{12} injection (1000 mcg) in the office, what HCPCS code would be assigned for the actual substance?

   _____

4. What code would be assigned to identify a bedside drainage bag provided to a patient?

   _____

5. If a patient was given an IM injection of 30 mg of hydrocortisone sodium phosphate, what HCPCS code would be assigned for this drug?

   _____

Assign HCPCS Level I (CPT) code(s) and HCPCS Level II code(s) to the following procedures.

6. Patient was treated for a sprained ankle; strapping was applied, and the patient was given crutches (a pair of adjustable, underarm wood crutches with pads, tips, and handgrips).

   CPT code for procedure: _____

   HCPCS code for crutches: _____

7. The physician inserted a temporary indwelling Foley catheter.

   CPT code for procedure: _____

   HCPCS code for catheter supply (bladder irrigation tubing):

   _____

8. Surgeon performed a robot-assisted thoracoscopic insertion of epicardial electrode lead.

   CPT code for procedure: _____

   HCPCS code for robotic surgical system: _____

In addition to HCPCS Level I (CPT) codes, assign HCPCS Level II modifiers for the following procedures, if applicable.

Chapter 11 Review   (Continued)

9. Patient is seen in the emergency department for a wood splinter embedded in the left upper eyelid. The ED physician removes the splinter.

_____

10. Avulsion of nail bed of left great toe and left second toe

_____

11. Release of trigger finger, right ring finger

_____

CPT and Reimbursement

12

Learning Objectives

- Describe the function of Medicare Code Editor (MCE).
- List the three elements used to calculate physician payment.
- Using the Physician Fee Schedule Look-Up Tool, retrieve reimbursement information.
- Given a coding scenario, audit the coding that was performed and calculate reimbursement.

CPT was developed as a communication tool between providers and payers. Although it is used for a variety of data purposes, it is the key to reimbursement for outpatient services. Reimbursement methodologies may change from payer to payer, but reporting a CPT code based on knowledge of the nomenclature is vital for appropriate reimbursement. However, another aspect of reimbursement is dependent on payer's policies and procedures, contracts negotiated with individual payers and in some cases, quality metrics.

The purpose of this chapter is to determine the impact of coding decisions on reimbursement.

Coding Meets Reimbursement

It is not uncommon to hear the phrase that correct coding equals appropriate reimbursement. Unfortunately, it is not that easy. The healthcare reimbursement system is complicated and varies by the type of service and payer. As an illustration, Medicare's homepage offers links to the many payment system. Figure 12.1 provides a screenshot of just a few.

Each of the hyperlinks from this Medicare-Fee-for-Service Payment list provides payment rates and downloadable documents for a better understanding of the individual payment systems. In addition, the individual hyperlink pages offer another layer of links for reference material to coding. For example, the Related Links under Hospital Outpatient PPS has another link to HCPCS Coding Questions (figure 12.2). From this page, under Related Links, note the first link in figure 12.2 for Outpatient Code Editor (OCE).

Figure 12.1. Snapshot of Medicare payment systems

Medicare Fee-for-Service Payment

Fee Schedules - General Information

Prospective Payment Systems - General Information

Accountable Care Organizations (ACO)

Acute Inpatient PPS

Ambulance Fee Schedule

Ambulatory Surgical Center (ASC) Payment

Clinical Laboratory Fee Schedule

DMEPOS Competitive Bidding

Durable Medical Equipment, Prosthetics/Orthotics, and Supplies Fee Schedule

ESRD PPS

Federally Qualified Health Center PPS

Home Health PPS

Hospice

Hospital-Acquired Conditions (Present on Admission Indicator)

Hospital Outpatient PPS

Source: CMS.gov. "Medicare." Digital Image. Centers for Medicare and Medicaid Services. Accessed November, 2017. https://www.cms.gov/Medicare/Medicare.html.

Figure 12.2. Related links

Related Links

Outpatient Code Editor (OCE)

Advisory Panel on Hospital Outpatient Payment

Consolidated Billing

HCPCS Coding Questions

PC Pricer

Hospital Center

CMS-1442-N (Published April 20, 2012)

Source: CMS.gov. "Hospital Outpatient PPS." Digital Image. Centers for Medicare and Medicaid Services. November 2017. Accessed November, 2017. https://www.cms.gov/Medicare/Medicare-Fee-for-Service-Payment/HospitalOutpatientPPS/index.html.

Medicare Outpatient Code Editor

CMS carefully evaluates the procedural and diagnostic data submitted with ambulatory claims. The agency requires Medicare Administrative Contractors (MACs) (organizations that process Medicare claims under contracts with the CMS) to use a tool known as the Medicare Outpatient Code Editor (OCE) (also referred to as the Integrated Outpatient Code Editor). The goal is to weed out incomplete or incorrect outpatient facility claims.

The OCE performs four basic functions:

- Editing data on the claim for accuracy
- Specifying the action the MAC should take when specific edits occur
- Assigning ambulatory payment classifications (APCs) to the claim for each service covered under the Outpatient Prospective Payment System (OPPS)
- Assigning an ambulatory surgical center (ASC) payment group for services on claims from certain non-OPPS hospitals.

Routine edits for age and sex inconsistencies are performed on all claim forms. All claims (facility and professional) are subject to National Correct Coding Initiative (NCCI) edits. The NCCI edits identify combinations of procedures that are unacceptable combinations. The goal is to control improper coding leading to inappropriate payment. When an edit occurs, the MAC may take one of six different actions:

- *Claim rejection:* When a claim is rejected, the provider may correct and resubmit the claim, but it cannot appeal the MAC's decision.
- *Claim denial:* The provider cannot resubmit the claim, but it may appeal the MAC's decision.
- *Claim returned to provider (RTP):* The provider may correct and resubmit the claim.
- *Claim suspension:* Payment is delayed for MAC determination; the MAC may need additional information before it can make a decision.
- *Line item rejection:* The claim is paid, but one of the line items is rejected; the provider may correct and resubmit the claim, but the MAC's decision cannot be appealed.
- *Line item denial:* The claim is paid, but some line items are denied; the provider cannot resubmit the claim, but the MAC's decision can be appealed.

Reimbursement and record processing efficiency are seriously compromised when incomplete or error-ridden claims are returned to the provider for correction and resubmission. Most insurance carriers accept only "clean claims," that is, claims that have passed OCE scrutiny.

Medicare Claims Manual and Coding

CMS also publishes a Medicare Claims Processing Manual dedicated primarily to billing but in some cases, coding guidance is provided.

Remember that the NCCI Policy Manual for Medicare Services provides a significant amount of guidance for correct coding in Chapter 1. Search the CMS website for the manual.

One of the many chapters, in the Medicare Claims Processing Manual, addresses physician services. Chapter 12 (Physicians/Nonphysician Practitioners) provides some CPT coding guidance related to billing practices. For example, section 30.2.A relates to cystourethroscopy with ureteral catheterization (code 52005):

Code 52005 has a zero in the bilateral field (payment adjustment for bilateral procedure does not apply) because the basic procedure is an examination of the bladder and urethra (cystourethroscopy), which are not paired organs. The work RVUs assigned take into account that it may be necessary to examine and catheterize one or both ureters. No additional payment is made when the procedure is billed with bilateral modifier -50. Neither is any additional payment made when both ureters are examined and code 52005 is billed with multiple surgery modifier -51. It is inappropriate to bill code 52005 twice, once by itself and once with modifier -51, when both ureters are examined.

Editing software will help navigate payer rules. In addition to standard Medicare/Medicaid edits, software packages have the ability to customize editing to take in consideration commercial payer requirements. Because of the complexity of healthcare billing, it is not unusual for billing companies and large facilities to purchase "scrubbing" software in attempt to produce a clean claim.

Reimbursement for Hospital Outpatient Services to Medicare Patients: An Overview

As mentioned previously, the Medicare-Fee-for-Service Payment links from the CMS website provide files to focus on each payment method. Hospital Outpatient Prospective Payment System (OPPS) files outline payment groups that include CPT and HCPCS codes. Hospital services are divided into ambulatory payment classification (APC) groups. The groups have similar clinical characteristics and similar costs. Each APC may include multiple CPT and HCPCS codes but they are clinically similar and require comparable resources. Packaging is an important feature in the OPPS. For example, services for routine supplies, anesthesia, operating room time, some imaging and diagnostic studies are packaged into the payment and not paid separately. Payment rates are updated annually and published on the CMS website.

Reimbursement for Physician Services to Medicare Patients: An Overview

Payment for physicians is based on a formula that includes work, practice expense, and malpractice expense. The formula also includes a geographic and conversion factor. This system is called resource-based relative value scale (RBRVS). The relative value unit is based on CPT codes and are updated and published yearly. The standard relative units per procedure include the following elements:

- *Physician work:* Technical skill, physical and mental effort; level of risk; and related stress
- *Practice expense:* The cost of supplies and equipment, wages for employees, and other overhead expenses, such as rent and utilities (there are currently values for facility and nonfacility physician practice expenses in the RBRVS system; services rendered at a facility have a lower RVU associated with them than nonfacility or office-based services)
- *Malpractice expense:* The average cost of malpractice insurance

Physician Fee Schedule Look-Up Tool

The CMS website offers an online software program called the Physician Fee Schedule Look-Up to identify pricing information for carriers by a HCPCS code. For this illustration, HCPCS code 19000 (drainage of breast lesion) revealed the following: (as shown in table 12.1).

Table 12.1.   HCPCS code 19000 (National Carrier)

MAC	Non-Facility Price	Facility Price
0000000	$115.20	$45.36

In this illustration, the file differentiates between a non-facility price and a facility price. A non-facility price represents the physician's costs related to providing the service in the physician's office, patient home, or other non-facility setting. Expenses may include staff, supplies, equipment, and such. Therefore, if the physician drained the breast lesion in his office, the non-facility price ($115.20) would be applicable. Facility pricing represents the provider's cost of providing the service in the facility setting (such as a hospital ambulatory care center). If the surgeon drained the breast lesion in the local hospital, the reimbursement would be significantly lower.

For the following exercise, access the Physician Fee Schedule Look-Up Tool and default to the criteria settings as seen in the screen snapshot in figure 12.3. For the purposes of this exercise, a National Payment Amount is used.

Figure 12.3. Physician Fee Schedule Look-Up Tool

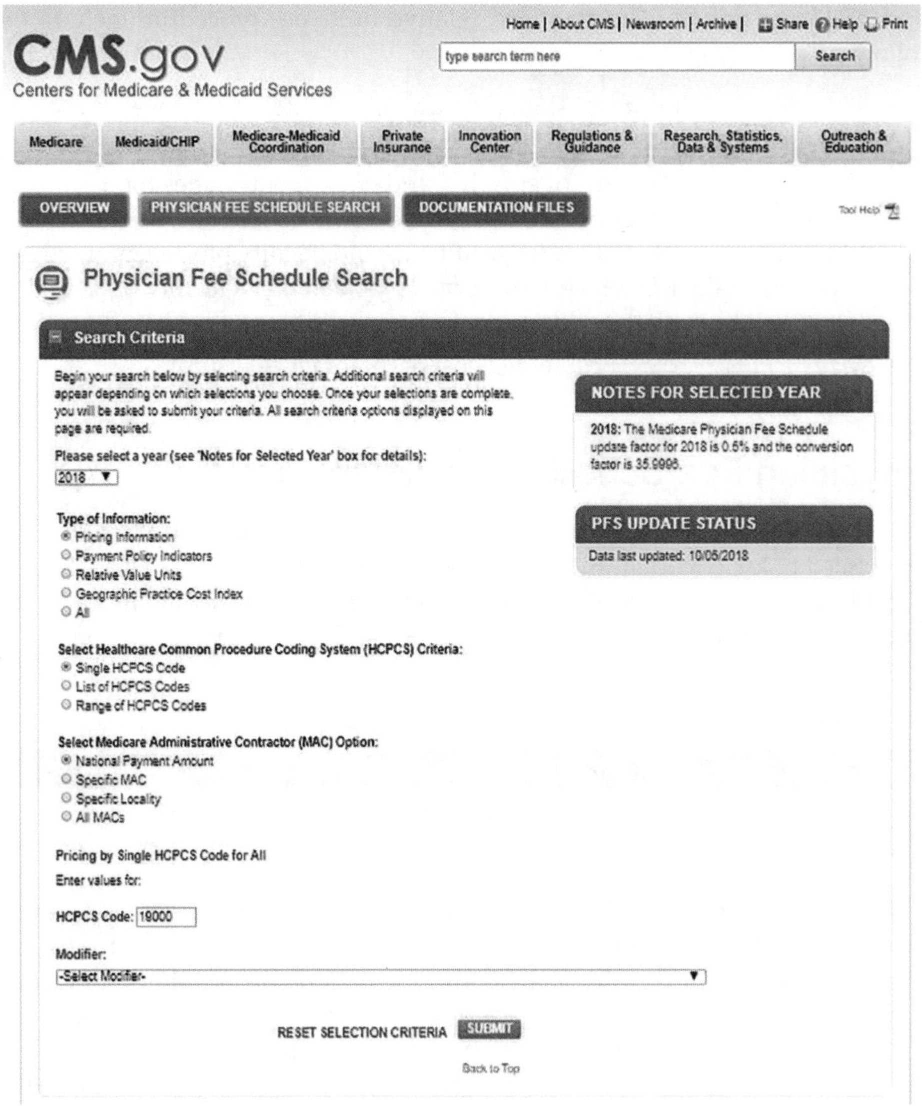

Source: CMS.gov. "Physician Fee Schedule Search." Digital Image. Centers for Medicare and Medicaid Services. October 2017. Accessed October, 2018. https://www.cms.gov/apps/physician-fee-schedule/search/search-criteria.aspx.

Chapter 12 CPT and Reimbursement Exercise: Cost of Errors

Answers to odd-numbered questions can be found in appendix C of this book. The answers to even-numbered questions are located in the instructor materials and are available approved instructors. The answer key amounts are correct as of November 2018.

Review the following scenarios and the codes suggested for reporting the services on the CMS-1500 billing form. For those codes that are incorrect, identify the correct CPT code. The ICD-10-CM codes are provided for reference only.

Payment component: For each exercise, use the Physician Fee Look-Up Tool, document the price for the code listed on the billing form and then document the price based on the code you selected. Note whether the exercise specifies Non-Facility Price or Facility Price.

1. At a local hospital, the gynecologist performed a total abdominal hysterectomy with bilateral salpingo-oophorectomy (uterus 260 gr). The pathological diagnosis was submucous leiomyoma of the uterus.

   Facility Price for 58262

   Your CPT Coding Assignment:

   Facility Price for your CPT Code:

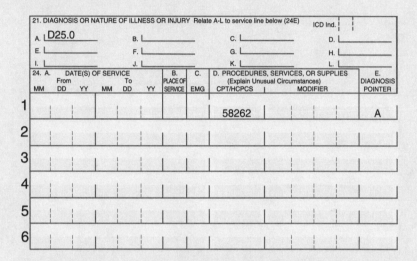

2. At the hospital's ambulatory surgery center, the patient underwent a diagnostic colonoscopy to determine the reason for abnormal bowel movements. Using a snare, the physician removed a benign polyp of the cecum.

   Facility Price for 45388

   Your CPT Coding Assignment:

   Facility Price for your CPT Code:

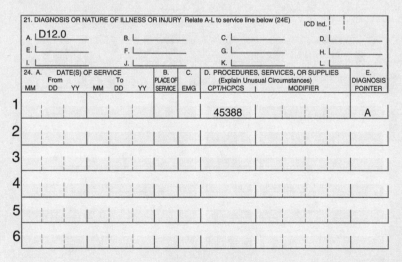

(Continued on next page)

Chapter 12 CPT and Reimbursement Exercise: Cost of Errors   (Continued)

3. At the hospital's outpatient surgery center, the patient was seen for removal of 2.0-cm basal cell carcinoma of the left arm. The surgeon excised the lesion with 0.5-cm margins around the diameter of the skin tumor.

<u>Facility</u> Price for 11403

Your CPT Coding Assignment:

Facility Price for your CPT Code:

21. DIAGNOSIS OR NATURE OF ILLNESS OR INJURY Relate A-L to service line below (24E)			ICD Ind.	
A. C44.619	B.	C.	D.	
E.	F.	G.	H.	
I.	J.	K.	L.	

24. A. DATE(S) OF SERVICE From To MM DD YY MM DD YY	B. PLACE OF SERVICE	C. EMG	D. PROCEDURES, SERVICES, OR SUPPLIES CPT/HCPCS MODIFIER	E. DIAGNOSIS POINTER
1			11403	A
2				
3				
4				
5				
6				

4. A 35-year-old male is seen at the hospital outpatient center for a recurrent left inguinal hernia. The surgeon performs a laparoscopic herniorrhaphy.

<u>Facility</u> Price for 49505:

Your CPT Coding Assignment:

Facility Price for your CPT Code:

21. DIAGNOSIS OR NATURE OF ILLNESS OR INJURY Relate A-L to service line below (24E)			ICD Ind.	
A. K40.91	B.	C.	D.	
E.	F.	G.	H.	
I.	J.	K.	L.	

24. A. DATE(S) OF SERVICE From To MM DD YY MM DD YY	B. PLACE OF SERVICE	C. EMG	D. PROCEDURES, SERVICES, OR SUPPLIES CPT/HCPCS MODIFIER	E. DIAGNOSIS POINTER
1			49505 LT	A
2				
3				
4				
5				
6				

5. The patient was seen in the emergency department for facial lacerations. The on-call plastic surgeon performed simple repairs on a 3.0-cm laceration on the forehead, a 2.8-cm laceration of the left upper eyelid, and a 1.0-cm laceration of the right upper eyelid.

<u>Facility</u> Price for 12053

Your CPT Coding Assignment:

Facility Price for your CPT Code:

21. DIAGNOSIS OR NATURE OF ILLNESS OR INJURY Relate A-L to service line below (24E)			ICD Ind.	
A. S01.81XA	B. S01.112A	C. S01.111A	D.	
E.	F.	G.	H.	
I.	J.	K.	L.	

24. A. DATE(S) OF SERVICE From To		B. PLACE OF SERVICE	C. EMG	D. PROCEDURES, SERVICES, OR SUPPLIES (Explain Unusual Circumstances) CPT/HCPCS | MODIFIER	E. DIAGNOSIS POINTER
MM DD YY MM DD YY					
1				12053	A, B, C
2					
3					
4					
5					
6					

6. At the hospital, the patient presents with a right breast mass. Under ultrasound guidance, a localization wire was inserted and a percutaneous breast biopsy was performed.

21. DIAGNOSIS OR NATURE OF ILLNESS OR INJURY Relate A-L to service line below (24E)			ICD Ind.	
A. N63	B.	C.	D.	
E.	F.	G.	H.	
I.	J.	K.	L.	

24. A. DATE(S) OF SERVICE From To		B. PLACE OF SERVICE	C. EMG	D. PROCEDURES, SERVICES, OR SUPPLIES (Explain Unusual Circumstances) CPT/HCPCS | MODIFIER	E. DIAGNOSIS POINTER
MM DD YY MM DD YY					
1				19085 RT	A
2					
3					
4					
5					
6					

(Continued on next page)

Chapter 12 CPT and Reimbursement Exercise: Cost of Errors (Continued)

7. At the hospital, the surgeon removed a 2.0-cm fibroma from the intramuscular area of the left foot.

<u>Facility</u> Price for 11402

Your CPT Coding Assignment:

Facility Price for your CPT Code:

21. DIAGNOSIS OR NATURE OF ILLNESS OR INJURY Relate A-L to service line below (24E)			ICD Ind.	
A. D21.22	B.	C.	D.	
E.	F.	G.	H.	
I.	J.	K.	L.	

24. A. DATE(S) OF SERVICE From MM DD YY To MM DD YY	B. PLACE OF SERVICE	C. EMG	D. PROCEDURES, SERVICES, OR SUPPLIES (Explain Unusual Circumstances) CPT/HCPCS	MODIFIER	E. DIAGNOSIS POINTER
1			11402		A
2					
3					
4					
5					
6					

8. At the hospital, a patient is seen for a displaced distal left fibular fracture. The surgeon performed an open reduction with internal fixation.

<u>Facility</u> Price for 27784:

Your CPT Coding Assignment:

Facility Price for your CPT Code:

21. DIAGNOSIS OR NATURE OF ILLNESS OR INJURY Relate A-L to service line below (24E)			ICD Ind.	
A. S82.832A	B.	C.	D.	
E.	F.	G.	H.	
I.	J.	K.	L.	

24. A. DATE(S) OF SERVICE From MM DD YY To MM DD YY	B. PLACE OF SERVICE	C. EMG	D. PROCEDURES, SERVICES, OR SUPPLIES (Explain Unusual Circumstances) CPT/HCPCS	MODIFIER	E. DIAGNOSIS POINTER
1			27784	RT	A
2					
3					
4					
5					
6					

9. At the hospital, the surgeon performed a cystourethroscopy for insertion of a urethral stent for stricture.

<u>Facility</u> Price for 52332

Your CPT Coding Assignment:

Facility Price for your CPT Code:

21. DIAGNOSIS OR NATURE OF ILLNESS OR INJURY Relate A-L to service line below (24E)			ICD Ind.	
A. N35.9	B.	C.	D.	
E.	F.	G.	H.	
I.	J.	K.	L.	

24. A. DATE(S) OF SERVICE From MM DD YY To MM DD YY	B. PLACE OF SERVICE	C. EMG	D. PROCEDURES, SERVICES, OR SUPPLIES (Explain Unusual Circumstances) CPT/HCPCS | MODIFIER	E. DIAGNOSIS POINTER
1			52232	A
2				
3				
4				
5				
6				

10. At the hospital, A pregnant patient in her second trimester has polyhydramnios; therefore, the physician performs amniocentesis.

<u>Facility</u> Price for 59000

Your CPT Coding Assignment:

Facility Price for your CPT Code:

21. DIAGNOSIS OR NATURE OF ILLNESS OR INJURY Relate A-L to service line below (24E)			ICD Ind.	
A. O40.2XX0	B.	C.	D.	
E.	F.	G.	H.	
I.	J.	K.	L.	

24. A. DATE(S) OF SERVICE From MM DD YY To MM DD YY	B. PLACE OF SERVICE	C. EMG	D. PROCEDURES, SERVICES, OR SUPPLIES (Explain Unusual Circumstances) CPT/HCPCS | MODIFIER	E. DIAGNOSIS POINTER
1			59000	A
2				
3				
4				
5				
6				

Computer-Assisted Coding

13

Learning Objectives

- Define *computer-assisted coding*.
- Identify coding skills for using CAC technology.

- Given a simulated CAC exercise, successfully review documentation and determine the correct CPT coding assignment.

Computer-assisted coding (CAC) is a general phrase associated with technology that provides coding options based on software that scans health record documentation and applies logic rules to produce a suggested code(s). Depending on the software features, a highlighted phrase in the operative report generates suggested codes, such as the example in figure 13.1. It is up to the coding professional to verify the suggested code and agree or disagree to the code assignment. If the code is correct, a simple click of the mouse will add the code to the potential coding profile for billing submission. Similar to spell check functionality, the coder will have the option to click "ignore" or "change." CAC provides a link between documentation and a suggested code. For example, if the operative note states that a repair of incomplete circumcision was performed, the computer software compares this phrase to stored CPT phrases and descriptions and assigns CPT code 54163. If the coding professional reads the operative report and determines that it was the correct code, then it saves the time of searching for the code.

Search the internet for video demonstrations of software tools.

Role of Coding Professionals in CAC

The impact of software programs will continue to have a significant impact on the coding profession. The CAC is a tool and coding professionals will take on the role of auditor and the ultimate decision about code assignment is still made by the coder. Coders will spend much less time on assigning highly repetitive codes (such as those for chest x-rays) and will concentrate on validation of the coding assignment. If the repetitive (rote) coding diminishes, coders will have more time to focus on the difficult surgical procedures.

Figure 13.1. Simulation of computer-assisted coding screen

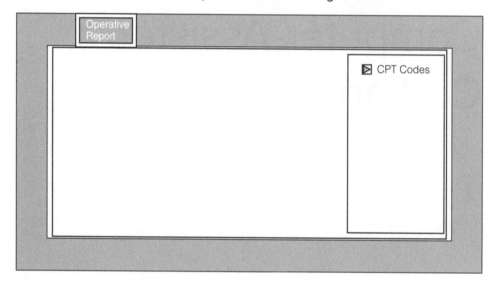

Preparing for the Future

Just as word processing did not require individuals to relearn how to spell or create sentences, CAC does not require coding professionals to relearn how to code. Rather it allows coders to apply their analytical coding knowledge. Validation of the CPT coding assignment in CAC will require integration of the following knowledge and skills:

- Knowledge of clinical foundations related to anatomy and physiology
- Knowledge of how surgical procedures are performed
- Translating physician documentation into CPT terminology
- Knowledge of CPT structure
- Application of coding guidance (Notes, *CPT Assistant*)
- Skill in working with the technology

In summary, coding professionals must make a commitment to lifelong learning. Integrating new and prior skills builds a coding professional's confidence in an ever-changing healthcare landscape.

The following exercise allows you to integrate your CPT coding skills and practice working in a simulated CAC environment.

Chapter 13 CAC Simulation for CPT Coding Exercise

Answers to odd-numbered questions can be found in appendix C of this book. The answers to even-numbered questions are located in the instructor materials and are available to approved instructors.

Read the following operative report excerpts and compare the documentation to the suggested CPT codes on the right-hand side of the screen. Circle the code(s) that you agree should flow to the coding summary. Write any codes you wish to add to the case in the same area. Do not assign modifiers for this exercise.

Case 1

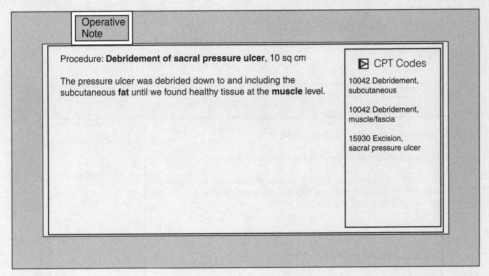

Operative Note

Procedure: **Debridement of sacral pressure ulcer**, 10 sq cm

The pressure ulcer was debrided down to and including the subcutaneous **fat** until we found healthy tissue at the **muscle** level.

▷ CPT Codes

10042 Debridement, subcutaneous

10042 Debridement, muscle/fascia

15930 Excision, sacral pressure ulcer

Case 2

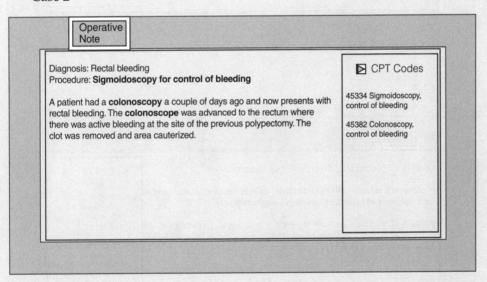

Operative Note

Diagnosis: Rectal bleeding
Procedure: **Sigmoidoscopy for control of bleeding**

A patient had a **colonoscopy** a couple of days ago and now presents with rectal bleeding. The **colonoscope** was advanced to the rectum where there was active bleeding at the site of the previous polypectomy. The clot was removed and area cauterized.

▷ CPT Codes

45334 Sigmoidoscopy, control of bleeding

45382 Colonoscopy, control of bleeding

Case 3

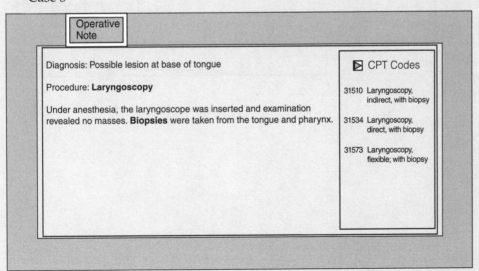

Operative Note

Diagnosis: Possible lesion at base of tongue

Procedure: **Laryngoscopy**

Under anesthesia, the laryngoscope was inserted and examination revealed no masses. **Biopsies** were taken from the tongue and pharynx.

▷ CPT Codes

31510 Laryngoscopy, indirect, with biopsy

31534 Laryngoscopy, direct, with biopsy

31573 Laryngoscopy, flexible; with biopsy

(Continued on next page)

Chapter 13 CAC Simulation for CPT Coding Exercise (Continued)

Case 4

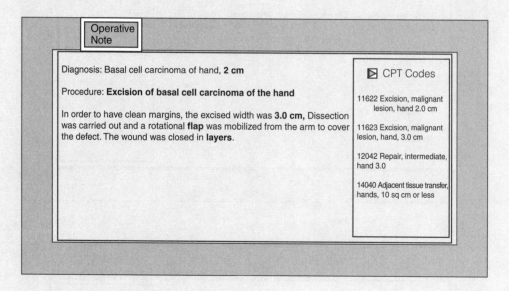

Operative Note

Diagnosis: Basal cell carcinoma of hand, **2 cm**

Procedure: **Excision of basal cell carcinoma of the hand**

In order to have clean margins, the excised width was **3.0 cm,** Dissection was carried out and a rotational **flap** was mobilized from the arm to cover the defect. The wound was closed in **layers**.

▷ CPT Codes

11622 Excision, malignant lesion, hand 2.0 cm

11623 Excision, malignant lesion, hand, 3.0 cm

12042 Repair, intermediate, hand 3.0

14040 Adjacent tissue transfer, hands, 10 sq cm or less

Case 5

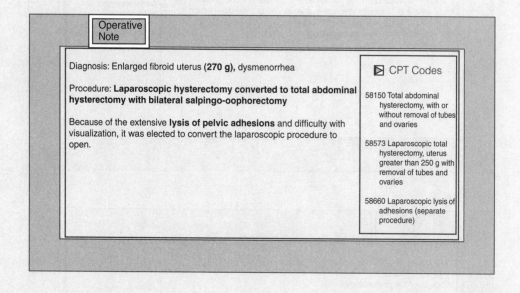

Operative Note

Diagnosis: Enlarged fibroid uterus **(270 g),** dysmenorrhea

Procedure: **Laparoscopic hysterectomy converted to total abdominal hysterectomy with bilateral salpingo-oophorectomy**

Because of the extensive **lysis of pelvic adhesions** and difficulty with visualization, it was elected to convert the laparoscopic procedure to open.

▷ CPT Codes

58150 Total abdominal hysterectomy, with or without removal of tubes and ovaries

58573 Laparoscopic total hysterectomy, uterus greater than 250 g with removal of tubes and ovaries

58660 Laparoscopic lysis of adhesions (separate procedure)

Case 6

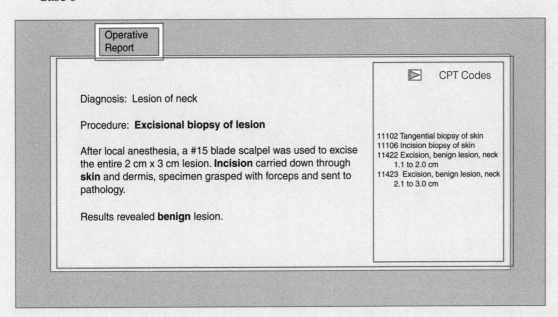

Operative Report

Diagnosis: Lesion of neck

Procedure: **Excisional biopsy of lesion**

After local anesthesia, a #15 blade scalpel was used to excise the entire 2 cm x 3 cm lesion. **Incision** carried down through **skin** and dermis, specimen grasped with forceps and sent to pathology.

Results revealed **benign** lesion.

CPT Codes

11102 Tangential biopsy of skin
11106 Incision biopsy of skin
11422 Excision, benign lesion, neck
        1.1 to 2.0 cm
11423 Excision, benign lesion, neck
        2.1 to 3.0 cm

References and Bibliography

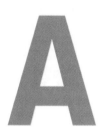

American Academy of Family Physicians. http://www.aafp.org.

American Hospital Association. *AHA Coding Clinic for HCPCS*. Chicago: AHA.

American Medical Association. 2019. *Current Procedural Terminology 2019*. Chicago: AMA. http://www.ama-assn.org.

American Medical Association. 1989–2018. *CPT Assistant*. Chicago: AMA.

American Medical Association. 2018. http://www.ama-assn.org.

Centers for Disease Control and Prevention. http://www.cdc.gov.

Centers for Medicare & Medicaid Services. http://www.cms.gov.

Contributing Authors. 1990–2018. Coding Notes and Clinical Notes. *Journal of AHIMA*. Chicago: AHIMA.

National Uniform Billing Committee. http://www.nubc.org.

Smith, G.I. and J. Bronnert. July 2010. Transitioning to CAC: The Skills and Tools Required to Work with Computer-assisted Coding. *Journal of AHIMA* 81(7): 60–61.

Society of Cardiovascular and Interventional Radiology, et al. 2009. *Interventional Radiology Coding User's Guide*, 5th ed. Fairfax, VA: Society of Cardiovascular and Interventional Radiology, American College of Radiology, Radiology Business Management Association, American Health Radiology Administrators.

U.S. Preventive Services Task Force. http://www.uspreventiveservicestaskforce.org.

Additional Practice Exercises

B

Assign the appropriate CPT code(s) for each of the cases. Assign only anatomic modifiers (such as LT, RT, E1) and modifier 59 if appropriate. Do not append modifier 51. If you wish to practice assigning codes by body system, the following reference will help.

Practice Exercises Indexed by Surgical Section

Integumentary System
Case #1   Excisional Biopsy
Case #2   Shaving of Lesion
Case #5   Excisional Biopsy
Case #7   Excision Lesion of Nose
Case #12   Excision of Cyst
Case #17   BKA Amputation
Case #25   Repair of Laceration
Case #27   Excision of Lipoma
Case #33   Breast Mass
Case #34   Debridement
Case #43   Excision of Cyst
Case #50   Laceration of Leg
Case #54   Excision of Carcinoma
Case #64   Repair of Multiple
            Lacerations
Case #68   Mastectomy
Case #74   Breast Augmentation
Case #76   Excision Cyst

Musculoskeletal System
Case #4   Reduction of Shoulder
            Dislocation
Case #20   Excision of Lipoma

Case #22   Mumford Procedure
Case #26   Arthroscopic Meniscectomy
Case #44   Injury to Toes
Case #45   Lipoma of Shoulder
Case #47   Fracture of Metacarpals
Case #60   Stab Wound
Case #62   Release of Trigger Finger
Case #70   Zygomatic Fracture

Respiratory System
Case #13   Laryngoscopy
Case #41   VATS
Case #55   Laryngoscopy with Vocal
            Cord Lesion
Case #61   Bronchoscopy
Case #71   Microlaryngoscopy

Cardiovascular System
Case #15   Carotid
            Thromboendarterectomy
Case #18   Creation of AV Fistula
Case #31   Placement of Catheter
Case #48   Pacemaker
Case #52   Thrombectomy
Case #73   Thrombectomy

Hemic and Lymphatic Systems
Case #38   Excision of Lymph Nodes

Digestive System
Case #3   Endoscopy
Case #5   Cholecystectomy
Case #11   Parotidectomy
Case #14   PEG Tube Placement
Case #19   Colonoscopy
Case #23   Endoscopy
Case #24   EGD with biopsy
Case #30   Sigmoidoscopy
Case #32   Repair of Hernia
Case #42   Tonsillectomy
Case #46   Colonoscopy
Case #53   Endoscopy with Dilatation
Case #56   Colonoscopy with Polyp

Urinary System
Case #51   Cystoscopy and Fulguration
Case #59   Cystoscopy with Dilation
Case #69   ESWL
Case #75   Removal of Ureteral Stent

Male/Female Genital System
Case #8   Tubal Ligation
Case #9   Transurethral Resection of Prostate
Case #16   Cerclage Placement
Case #28   Biopsy of Prostate
Case #36   Keratosis of Penis Procedure
Case #39   Dilation and Curettage
Case #63   D&C with Hysteroscopy
Case #65   Colposcopy
Case #67   Hysterectomy

Maternity Care and Delivery
Case #66   Amniocentesis

Endocrine System
Case #29   Thyroidectomy

Nervous System
Case #6   Nerve Stimulator
Case #35   Carpal Tunnel Release
Case #37   Epidural Block
Case #57   Nerve Block
Case #58   Steroid Injection

Eye and Ocular Adnexa
Case #21   Ptosis of Eyelid
Case #40   Foreign Body in Eye
Case #49   Nasolacrimal Duct Procedures
Case #72   Excision of Chalazion

Surgical Case #1

Physician Office Surgical Note

Diagnosis: Actinic keratosis, 1.0 cm of the chest

Procedure: Excisional biopsy of actinic keratosis of chest

Chest was prepped and with the use of #15 blade scalpel, the skin lesion was shaved it its entirety. Closed in one-layer technique.

Code(s): _____

Surgical Case #2

Physician Office Surgical Note: Dermatology

Diagnosis: Raised lesion of the chin, suspicious in nature.

Patient complains that the lesion on his chin gets nicked every time he shaves and wishes to have it removed. He explained that it occasionally bleeds and has been changing in shape lately. The raised, irregular 9 mm shiny dark red lesion is suspicious for basal cell carcinoma. The decision was to perform a biopsy to determine further treatment.

After local anesthesia was administered, the top of the lesion was shaved for pathological analysis. The specimen was sent to pathology for evaluation. Patient will return to discuss the results and further treatment.

Code(s): _____

Surgical Case #3

Operative Report

Procedure:	Esophagogastroduodenoscopy
Instrument Used:	Olympus GIF-100
Premedication:	The patient was premedicated with a total of Fentanyl, 50 mcg, and Versed, 4 mg, intravenously.
Indications:	The patient has presented with recurrent dysphagia. She has a history of a Schatzki's ring, which has been dilated in the past.
Procedure:	The endoscope was inserted from the mouth into the esophagus without difficulty. The esophageal mucosa was normal. A reformed Schatzki's ring was located at the Z line, which was at approximately 29 cm. The endoscope could be inserted through this area with no resistance. The ring was located above a 3-cm hiatal hernia. The stomach, duodenal bulb, and descending duodenum were all normal. After the endoscope was withdrawn, a #60 French Maloney dilator was passed with very mild resistance. The patient tolerated the procedure well, and there were no immediate complications.
Impression:	1. A reformed Schatzki's ring, which was dilated
	2. A 3-cm hiatal hernia

Code(s): _____

Surgical Case #4

Emergency Department Record

Chief Complaint:	Right shoulder dislocation
History of Present Illness:	The patient is a 53-year-old man who has dislocated his right shoulder three previous episodes. Today, he was kayaking and dislocated his shoulder while paddling.
Past Medical History:	Previous right shoulder dislocation
Medications:	Vitamins
Allergies:	Sulfa
Physical Examination:	Alert male in no acute distress
Right Upper Extremity:	He has obvious deformity with loss of the right shoulder prominence with a palpable anterior dislocation of the humeral head. He has good distal pulses with the remainder of his arm being nontender.
Emergency Department Course:	X-ray of his right shoulder shows an anterior dislocation.
Procedure:	Reduction of the shoulder dislocation. The patient was placed on a monitor with continuous pulse oximetry. He was given Demerol and Phenergan IV for pain control. In-line traction and reduction was accomplished after three attempts. Reduction films showed good position of the shoulder. He had good distal neurovascular status after reduction. He tolerated the procedure well.
Diagnosis:	Anterior dislocation, right shoulder
Disposition and Plan:	Sling and swathe for two to three days. Vicodin #30. Follow up with Dr. Smith in one to two days or call for an orthopedic referral. The patient states he has been avoiding any potential surgery at this point and would prefer to avoid it. I explained to him that he should follow up with Dr. Smith or an orthopedist. He should not use the shoulder in the next several days until reevaluation.

Code(s): _____

Surgical Case #5

Operative Report

Preoperative Diagnosis: Cholecystitis with cholelithiasis

Postoperative Diagnosis: Cholecystitis with cholelithiasis

Procedure Performed: Laparoscopic cholecystectomy with operative cholangiogram

Anesthesia: General

Bleeding: None

Complications: None

Description of Procedure: The patient was brought to the OR, placed in the supine position, and given general anesthesia. The skin over the abdomen was prepped with DuraPrep and draped in the sterile fashion. A 1-cm incision was made above the umbilicus, and the Veress needle was introduced into the abdominal cavity obtaining pneumoperitoneum. A 10-mm trocar was inserted and a laparoscope introduced. The patient had significant cholecystitis. Direct exploration of the abdomen was normal. Other trocars were inserted into the subcostal space under direct vision. Lysis of adhesions was performed. Exposure to the gallbladder bed was obtained, and the cystic artery and the cystic duct were isolated. The common duct was of normal size. The cystic duct was ligated distally and proximally and was opened. We inserted the biliary catheter and obtained a cholangiogram that showed a normal biliary tree. The catheter was removed and the cystic duct double ligated with hemoclips and divided. The gallbladder was removed through the upper trocar and dissected with electrocautery. The area was irrigated with saline solution. The trocars were removed under vision and pneumoperitoneum decompressed. The skin was closed with subcuticular #4-0 Vicryl, and a sterile dressing was applied. The patient tolerated the procedure well.

Code(s): _____

Surgical Case #6

Operative Report

Preoperative Diagnosis: Neurogenic bladder with an implanted sacral nerve stimulator

Postoperative Diagnosis: Neurogenic bladder with an implanted sacral nerve stimulator

Procedure Performed: Removal of InterStim sacral nerve stimulator

Indications for Procedure: This patient is a 96-year-old female with a history of neurogenic bladder with recurrent urinary tract infections due to poor emptying. She is here for removal of her sacral nerve stimulator, which had subsequently quit working. After all the risks, benefits, and expected outcomes were explained, she agreed to proceed.

Details of Procedure: The patient was brought to the operative suite, given a light intravenous anesthetic, and laid in the prone position. The area overlying the InterStim neurostimulator was infiltrated using 1% lidocaine mixed with 0.35% Marcaine. Once this was done, an incision was made over this and dissection was carried down to the InterStim neurostimulator. The device was removed from its pouch. The leads, which were tunneled down to the S3 foramina, were identified and with careful manipulation we were able to remove in their entirety. Once this was done, hemostasis was obtained. The wound was copiously irrigated using antibiotic solution. The 3-0 Vicryl pop-offs were used to close the subcutaneous tissue, 4-0 Monocryl was used to close the skin. Benzoin, Steri-Strips, and Tegaderm were applied. She tolerated the procedure well and was taken to the recovery room in stable condition.

Code(s): _____

Surgical Case #7

Operative Report

Preoperative Diagnosis: Subepidermal nodular 1.0-cm lesion of the left side of the nose

Operation: Excision, lesion of nose

Procedure: Under local anesthesia, we excised the 1.0-cm lesion with 0.5 cm margins on all sides of the defect. The lesion was excised in fragments and submitted to pathology along with an ellipse of skin margins. Bleeding was controlled with electrocautery, and the wound was closed with four vertical mattress sutures of 5-0 nylon. Polysporin and dressing were applied.

Pathological Diagnosis: Well-organized basal cell carcinoma with no significant increase in activity or dysplasia of the cells

Code(s): _____

Surgical Case #8

Operative Report

Procedure: Laparoscopic tubal ligation with application of Falope rings; dilatation and curettage (D&C) and removal of intrauterine device

Diagnosis: Multiparity, voluntary sterilization; removal of retained intrauterine device

Anesthesia: General

Technique: Placed in the supine lithotomy position, the patient was prepped and draped in the usual manner for a laparoscopic and D&C procedure. A D&C was performed to gain access to a deeply embedded IUD. This was curetted up and eventually removed with some difficulty. Both the IUD and the curetted endometrial tissue were submitted to pathology.

A two-puncture laparoscopy was performed in the usual manner of insufflation through a Veress needle inserted infraumbilically. Through a first puncture, a trocar insertion infraumbilically was followed by the laparoscope and a second trocar insertion suprapubically in the midline was followed by, first, a probe and, then, a Falope ring applicator. Both tubes were ligated in their midsegment. On the right side, two rings were applied because of the round position of the Falope ring director. The left tube was ligated singly. The procedure was performed with no complications. After the operation, the trocar sites were closed with subcuticular sutures of 2-0 Vicryl, and the patient was transferred to the recovery room in satisfactory condition.

Code(s): _____

Surgical Case #9

Operative Report

Procedure: Transurethral resection of the prostate

Diagnosis: Bladder outlet obstruction; benign prostatic hypertrophy

Anesthesia: General

Technique: The patient was placed under general anesthesia and in the dorsolithotomy position. Two grams of Claforan parenterally were used. The Iglesias resectoscope was introduced through the obturator, and this was followed by the working element connected to the Olympus video camera. The obstructive prostatic tissue was appreciated mainly anteriorly and to the left lateral lobe. Resection was started at the bladder neck down to the level of the verumontanum and toward the capsule, as necessary, in all directions. Bleeders were fulgurated, with satisfactory patency with coagulation having been secured. Dissected tissues were removed using the Ellik evacuator. A size 24 three-way Foley catheter was retained with a 30-cc balloon inflation. Minimal blood loss was appreciated. The patient tolerated the procedure well and was transferred to the recovery room in stable condition.

Code(s): _____

Surgical Case #10

Operative Report

Preoperative Diagnosis: Critical vascular ischemia, right lower extremity

Postoperative Diagnosis: Critical vascular ischemia, right lower extremity

Procedure: Femoral-popliteal bypass using stripped saphenous vein

Details: The patient was taken to the OR. General anesthesia was administered and antibiotics were given. An incision was made in the skin of the right leg overlying the greater saphenous vein. The greater saphenous vein was isolated from adjacent critical structures from the upper thigh to the level of the knee. Vessel clamps were affixed above and below the site of the anastomosis to the femoral and popliteal arteries. All side branches of the saphenous vein were tied off. All valves within the vessel were destroyed. The upper end of the saphenous vein was divided and sutured into the femoral artery end-to-side. The lower end was divided and sutured into the popliteal artery end-to-side. The clamps were removed, and blood flowed backward toward the foot, perfusing well. When the procedure was complete, the skin incision was repaired with a layered closure.

Code(s): _____

Surgical Case #11

Operative Report

Procedure: Lateral lobe parotidectomy with facial nerve preservation

Diagnosis: Warthin's tumor of the parotid gland

Anesthesia: General

Findings: The patient has a long history of a right parotid mass that apparently has grown and fluctuated in size. An office examination revealed the nose, nasopharynx, larynx, and neck to be normal. She is status post thyroidectomy with a well-healed thyroidectomy incision. The parotid mass is overlying the mandible approximately 2 × 3 cm in diameter, and there is a possibility of another mass or lymphadenopathy in the lower aspect of the parotid gland. Facial nerve functions are normal.

Technique: Placed in the supine position, the patient was given general endotracheal anesthesia. Her neck was positioned, and the whole right side of her face and neck was prepped and draped in the usual manner.

The modified Blair type of incision was made in the preauricular area vertically and then curved behind and below the earlobe and extended as a curved submandibular incision. The bleeders were electrocoagulated and the dissection deepened in the lower part to the platysma. The dissection and front of the tragus were done by both sharp and blunt dissection until the external ear canal cartilage was identified and palpated. The dissection was pushed through this and inferiorly, identifying the anterior border of the sternocleidomastoid muscle, mastoid process, and, subsequently, the main trunk of the facial nerve, which was preserved from trauma. The major lower and inferior subdivisions were followed, identifying the cervical, mandibular, and buccal branches, as well as the upper division.

The cystic mass was bluish in color. The lateral lobe of the parotid gland was removed and given for frozen section, and this was reported as a benign cystic mass. No lobe was encountered with suspicion of malignancy, and no other masses were in the deep lobe. Hemostasis was obtained by electrocautery on the superficial oozing points and ligature of the small vessels. The wound was washed, and afterward the main trunk and subdivisions of the facial nerve again were identified and verified to be intact.

The lower Hemovac drain was placed. The wound was closed with 3-0 chromic catgut, interrupted, involving both the subcutaneous tissue and the platysma muscle with continuous and interrupted mattress sutures using 5-0 silk. The wound was cleaned, Bacitracin ointment was applied, and a dry sterile occlusive dressing was placed over it. After the procedure was terminated, the patient was extubated and brought to the recovery room in good condition.

Code(s): _____

Surgical Case #12

Operative Report

Preoperative Diagnosis: Dermal cyst of right breast

Postoperative Diagnosis: Dermal cyst of right breast

Procedure Performed: Excision of dermal cyst of right breast

Description of Procedure: Erythematous dermal cystic area of the right breast was marked out with an elliptical incision, anesthetized with local anesthesia, and prepped and draped sterilely.

Incision was made elliptically, including the whole cyst down through the fatty tissue. On palpation afterward, no abnormalities were noted. Then the area had hemostasis obtained with electrocautery. The incision was closed with interrupted 3-0 Vicryl sutures.

The skin was closed with interrupted 5-0 nylon sutures. Steri-Strips and a sterile dressing were applied over it. The patient tolerated the procedure well and was sent to the recovery room with instructions to be discharged home with follow-up appointment given.

Code(s): _____

Surgical Case #13

Operative Report

Preoperative Diagnosis:	Bilateral vocal cord neoplasm
Postoperative Diagnosis:	The same, with right postprocedural pharyngeal bleed
Procedures:	1. Laryngoscopy with bilateral vocal cord stripping with use of operating microscope
	2. Control of oral pharyngeal hemorrhage, less than 20 cc
Indications for Surgery:	This 65-year-old woman presented to the ENT service with a two-year history of hoarseness. Upon evaluation, she was noted to have bilateral vocal cord neoplasms. The patient also has a history of smoking. A decision for the above-stated procedures was made for definitive diagnosis.
Procedure:	The patient was brought to the operating suite, given a general anesthetic, and properly prepared and draped. It was noted that her teeth were not in good repair, and that the lateral incisor was already loose on the right side. However, teeth guards were put into place. The Jako laryngoscope was carefully introduced into the oral cavity with attention not to injure the lips, gums, or teeth. The base of the tongue, vallecula, epiglottis, paraform sinuses, and false and true vocal cords all were visualized. The laryngoscope was fixed into place with microsuspension. The vocal cords were well visualized. There were polypoid-type neoplasms bilaterally. These were grasped anteriorly, stripped to the posterior bilaterally, and sent to pathology. Hemostasis was obtained with an adrenaline cotton ball and silver nitrate. After good hemostasis was obtained, the scope was removed. However, upon removal, she was noted to have a pooling of blood in the posterior pharynx and that the blood was coming from the right tonsillar fossa. Apparently, this had been abraded with the laryngoscope upon insertion. Therefore, a self-retaining mouth gag was carefully introduced into the oral cavity. The patient did not have good extension of the mandible, but after this was visualized, the right pharyngeal wall was noted to have oozing and some irritation. This was controlled with the help of silver nitrate and suction cautery. After good hemostasis was obtained, the oral cavity was irrigated with a saline solution. When the patient exhibited good hemostasis, she was taken out of anesthetic and transferred to the recovery room in stable condition.

Code(s): _____

Surgical Case #14

Operative Report

Procedure: Percutaneous endoscopic gastrostomy (PEG) tube placement

Diagnosis: Old cerebrovascular accident with inanition and need for supplemental nutritional support with no contraindication to enteral access

Technique: After anesthetization of the gag reflex, the gastroscope was introduced. There was no abnormality of the esophagus, stomach, pylorus, or duodenum. The abdomen had been prepped and draped as a sterile field. The light was found to transilluminate in the left upper quadrant. The skin was anesthetized with 1% Xylocaine. A blunt needle was used to access the stomach percutaneously and a guide wire inserted. The guide wire was grasped with a snare and brought through the mouth, along with the gastroscope. The feeding tube was threaded over the guide wire and brought through the abdominal wall with a small stab incision made along the guide wire. The gastroscope was reinserted and the PEG tube photo-documented. There was no evidence of bleeding or undue tension as a result of tube placement. Air was suctioned from the stomach, and the gastroscope was removed with no other findings. The Silastic fastener was placed on the PEG tube near the skin entrance. The PEG tube then was connected to dependent drainage. The patient tolerated the procedure well and was taken to the recovery area with stable vital signs.

Code(s): _____

Surgical Case #15

Operative Report

Procedure: Right carotid thromboendarterectomy and vein patch angioplasty

Diagnosis: Right carotid artery stenosis with hemorrhagic plaque

Anesthesia: General

Technique: Under general anesthesia, the right side of the patient's neck was prepared and draped in a sterile fashion. An incision was made along the sternocleidomastoid muscle, and a sharp dissection was carried down to expose the common internal and external carotid arteries. Care was taken to avoid injury to the hypoglossal, vagus, and ansa cervicalis nerves. The vessels were inserted with elastic tapes. The patient was heparinized, and an arteriotomy was made. A very high-grade stenosis estimated at 1.5-mm opening was present at the origin of the internal carotid artery, and there was evidence of significant hemorrhage and degeneration in the plaque. A shunt was placed for cerebral perfusion, and then the endarterectomy was done in the usual fashion. The vessel was picked free of any debris or other plaque and then closed with a patch angioplasty using saphenous vein from the left groin. This was sutured in place with 6-0 Prolene. Flow was first directed into the external carotid to allow any possible air or debris to escape and then restored to the internal carotid. The wound was packed open until the end of the procedure and after the heparin was reversed. Then the wound was closed with 3-0 Vicryl in the subcutaneous and platysma muscle and 4-0 Vicryl for a subcuticular skin closure. The patient left the operating room in satisfactory condition.

Code(s): _____

Surgical Case #16

Operative Report

Procedure: McDonald's cerclage placement

Diagnosis: Intrauterine pregnancy at 12 weeks, history of cervical incompetence

Anesthesia: Epidural

History: The patient is a 36-year-old gravida 3 para 2 with a last menstrual period (LMP) on January 28. Positive HCG was noted on March 1. Intrauterine pregnancy was determined to be at 12 weeks by time of LMP and at first trimester by ultrasound. She has a history of cervical incompetence in a previous pregnancy that was brought to term with a cerclage. She also has a history of diethylstilbestrol exposure and of cerclage placement times 2, D&C times 2, and umbilical herniorrhaphy.

Findings and Technique: Preoperatively, her internal os was approximately 1 cm dilated. The posterior cervix was approximately 2 cm long, and the interior cervix was approximately 1 cm long. At the end of the procedure, the knot could be felt at the 12 o'clock position and the internal os was closed to digital examination.

The patient was in the dorsal lithotomy position. She had internal and external perineal preps and was draped for the procedure. A Mersilene band on two needles was used with one needle placed in at the 6 o'clock position and brought out at 3 o'clock, and replaced at the same position and brought out at 12 o'clock. The other needle was taken in at 3 o'clock and brought out at 9 o'clock, and then replaced and brought out at 12 o'clock. The Mersilene band then was tied at the 12 o'clock position until the internal os was closed. It was palpable at the end of the procedure, and the two ends were cut long. The patient received perioperative antibiotics, and her heart tones were Dopplerable before the procedure. The procedure was without complications, and the patient was taken to the recovery room in stable condition.

Code(s): _____

Surgical Case #17

Operative Report

Preoperative Diagnosis: Gangrene of the distal foot. Osteomyelitis of the left foot.

Postoperative Diagnosis: Gangrene of the distal foot. Osteomyelitis of the left foot.

Procedure: BKA Amputation

Procedure: Under satisfactory spinal anesthesia, the left lower member was prepped and draped in the usual manner. A fish mouth incision was made at the junction of the distal third, and proximal and middle third of the leg. A posterior flap was made along with a proximal flap and the muscles and soft tissue were divided sharply. The tibia was amputated with the power saw, doubled anteriorly and rasped. The fibula was amputated about an inch shorter than the tibia. The tibial and perineal nerves were amputated sharply proximal to the soft tissue incision. Hemostasis was achieved with knives and 3-0 Vicryl and running 0-Vicryl. Skin was closed with staples. Skin was tissue thin and tore very easily making the closure difficult. A sterile dressing was applied and injected with antibiotic. The patient tolerated the procedure well and was transferred to the Recovery Room in satisfactory condition.

Code(s): _____

Surgical Case #18

Operative Report

Preoperative Diagnosis: Chronic renal failure with limited vascular access

Postoperative Diagnosis: Chronic renal failure with limited vascular access

Procedure: Right upper arm arteriovenous graft

Operation: The patient was taken to the operating room, positioned, prepped, and draped appropriately. Local anesthesia was given to the antecubital site and the axillary site. Incision was made and the fascia was divided. Axillobrachial vein was identified, dissected, and controlled. Incision was made in the antecubital site, through the subcutaneous tissue and brought down to the fascia. This was divided. The brachial artery was identified and dissected and controlled. The 6-mm Gore-Tex graft was anastomosed to the vein end-to-side. Then the graft was tunneled subcutaneously and brought to the antecubital site and anastomosis with brachial artery was performed with #5-0 Prolene. Hemostasis was achieved and closure was done in layers.

Code(s): _____

Surgical Case #19

Operative Report

Procedure: Colonoscopy

History and Indications: The patient is a 30-year-old woman who has had complaints of abdominal pain, altered bowel habits, and a 2- to 3-g documented decline in her hemoglobin level. Her stools have been heme negative, but there is significant suspicion that she may have pathology in the colon.

Technique: The patient was sedated with 1.5 mg Versed and received antibiotics prior to the procedure per the recommendations of the cardiology service. She is status post heart transplant with significant cardiac complications.

In the endoscopy suite with appropriate monitoring of pulse, oxygenation, temperature, blood pressure, and other vital signs, a digital rectal examination was performed. Following the examination, the Pentax video colonoscope was inserted through the anus and advanced to the cecum. There was no evidence of malignancy. The scope was withdrawn.

Code(s): _____

Surgical Case #20

Operative Report

Preoperative Diagnosis: Sebaceous cyst, right posterior neck

Postoperative Diagnosis: Lipomatous lesion, approximately 1.5 cm, right posterior neck, intramuscular

Procedure: Excision of lipoma, right posterior neck

Technique: The patient was brought to the operating suite and was placed in the prone position on the operating table. The patient's right neck was then prepped and draped in a sterile fashion. At this point, we suspected the patient to have a cyst. We subsequently decided to do a circumferential incision around what was thought to be the puncta. The incision was marked, and the area was prepped and draped with a local anesthetic. A skin incision was made. The incision was carried down to the subcutaneous tissue. At this point, we realized that it was not a cyst but, rather, a lipoma, which was actually deep into the muscle area. We excised the skin, dissected down through the capsule of the lipoma, and then were able to harvest this from its capsule within the muscle fibers. This was done with sharp dissection. Bleeding was controlled with cautery. The wound was closed with 3-0 Vicryl subcutaneous sutures, and a 4-0 Vicryl subcuticular stitch was placed. The wound edges were painted with Benzoin and Steri-Strips applied. The patient tolerated the procedure well and was taken to the recovery area in stable condition.

Code(s): _____

Surgical Case #21

Operative Report

Preoperative Diagnosis:	Ptosis, left upper eyelid
Postoperative Diagnosis:	Same
Procedure:	Frontalis ptosis, left upper eyelid
Anesthesia:	Local

Description of Procedure: Topical Tetracaine was applied to both eyes. The left upper lid and brow were infiltrated with Xylocaine with epinephrine and Marcaine with Wydase. The patient was prepared and draped in the usual fashion for oculoplastic surgery. Incisions were made in the medial and lateral thirds of the lid, 3 mm above the lash line. Stat incisions were made at the medial and lateral thirds of the brow, approximately 5 mm above the brow and a single incision was made in the middle of the brow, approximately 1 cm higher than the previous two incisions. A 3-0 Prolene suture was passed from the lateral lid incision to the medial lid incision beneath the orbicularis, just above the tarsus. Suture was then passed beneath the brow and frontalis to emerge from the medial and lateral brow incisions respectively. Each end of the suture was then passed beneath the frontalis to emerge through the central brow incision. The suture was tied and tension was adjusted so that the lid level was just above the papillary border. The brow incisions were closed with interrupted sutures of 6-0 Prolene, the eye was dressed with Ocumycin ointment. The patient tolerated the procedure well and left the OR in good condition.

Code(s): _____

Surgical Case #22

Operative Report

Preoperative Diagnosis: Arthritis of right acromioclavicular joint

Postoperative Diagnosis: Same

Operation: Mumford procedure, right shoulder

Procedure: The patient was brought to the operating room after general anesthesia. The patient was placed in the lounge chair position, the right shoulder was sterilely scrubbed and draped in the usual manner. Routine incision was taken down to the distal clavicle. The distal clavicle was identified subperiosteally. Retractors were put in place. At this time the clavicle was osteotomized using a saw, and the distal end of the clavicle was removed. The wound was then irrigated. Marcaine with epinephrine was injected. The periosteum was closed with 0 Vicryl, subcutaneous, with 2-0 Vicryl, and the skin with staples. Dry sterile dressings were applied, and the patient was sent to the recovery room in good condition.

Code(s): _____

Surgical Case #23

Operative Report

Procedure: Endoscopy

Preoperative Diagnosis: Abdominal pain, possible peptic ulcer disease

Patient has upper abdominal pain, unresponsive to H2 blockers.

Postoperative Diagnosis:
1. Hiatal hernia
2. Moderate reflux esophagitis
3. Healing prepyloric gastric ulcer
4. Normal sigmoidoscopy

Findings: Endoscopy was performed with the Olympus video panendo-scope, which was easily introduced into the esophagus. This was normal to the proximal midportion of the esophagus, but at the GE junction, there was evidence of a moderate degree of reflux esophagitis with several small superficial erosions at the location and also isolated erosions several centimeters above. The endoscope was advanced into the stomach and turned in a retrograde direction. The cardiac and fundic areas were examined and found to be otherwise normal. The antrum showed normal peristalsis and mucosa. In the immediate prepyloric area, a small defect was thought to represent scarring from a previous ulcer, which was still healing. Biopsies were obtained. The duodenum, including the second portion, was normal. Subsequently, the endoscope was withdrawn, and the patient turned onto his left side. Flexible sigmoidoscopy then was carried out to the lower descending colon. A biopsy of the sigmoid was obtained. Patient tolerated the procedure well.

Code(s): _____

Surgical Case #24

Operative Report

Procedure: Esophagogastroduodenoscopy with biopsy

Diagnosis: Gastritis and duodenitis

Technique: The patient was premedicated and brought to the endoscopy suite where his throat was anesthetized with Cetacaine spray. He then was placed in the left lateral position and given 2 mg Versed, IV.

An Olympus gastroscope was advanced from the mouth into the esophagus, which was well visualized with no significant segmental spasms. Subsequently, the scope was advanced into the distal esophagus, which was essentially normal. Then the scope was advanced into the stomach, which showed evidence of erythema and gastritis. The pylorus was intubated and the duodenal bulb visualized. The duodenal bulb showed severe erythema, suggestive of duodenitis. Multiple biopsies were taken. The scope was withdrawn, and the patient tolerated the procedure well.

Code(s): _____

Surgical Case #25

Emergency Department Report

Chief Complaint:
Lacerations, left face

History of Present Illness:
Patient is a 26-year-old man who was driving a car with the window down when another car moving in the opposite direction hit his mirror. Glass from the broken mirror flew into his face, and he sustained two small lacerations. There were no other injuries.

Past Medical History:
Unremarkable

Medications:
None

Allergies:
None

Physical Examination:

General:
Alert male in no acute distress

HEENT:
Pupils are equal and reactive to light. Extraocular muscles intact. Nose is clear. Oropharynx negative. Two lacerations are on left cheek region. The uppermost laceration is below the eye laterally and is about 2.25 cm in length. Full-skin thickness. The second laceration is 1.25 cm in length directly below the upper laceration. Full-skin thickness. No palpable foreign bodies.

Procedure:
Local injection with a total of 3 cc 1% lidocaine with epinephrine. Prepped and routine exploration performed. The upper laceration is only about 5 mm deep. No foreign bodies noted. No neurovascular injuries. It was closed with three 6-0 nylon sutures. The lower laceration was approximately 12 to 15 mm deep. I could not palpate any foreign bodies. There are no obvious neurovascular injuries. Closed in single layer with five 6-0 nylon sutures. Polysporin ointment was applied.

Laboratory Data:
X-ray to rule out foreign body negative

Diagnosis:
1. Simple facial laceration, 2.25 cm
2. Simple facial laceration, 1.25 cm

Disposition and Plan:
Wound care instructions given; sutures out in five to seven days

Code(s): _____

Surgical Case #26

Operative Report

Procedure: Arthroscopic partial medial meniscectomy

Diagnosis: Torn left medial meniscus

Anesthesia: General

Technique: After induction with general anesthesia, a standard three-portal approach of the knee was evaluated. Mild synovitic changes were noted in the suprapatellar pouch. No chondromalacia changes were noted in all three compartments. The anterior cruciate ligament was intact, as was the lateral meniscus; and there were only slight synovitic changes in the anterior compartment. The anterior portion of the medial meniscus had a flap tear, which was debrided with an aggressive resector.

After all instruments were withdrawn, 4-0 nylon horizontal mattress stitches were used to close the wound, and pressure dressings were applied. The patient was awakened and removed to the recovery room in good condition.

Code(s): _____

Surgical Case #27

Operative Report

Preoperative Diagnosis: Right arm lipoma

Postoperative Diagnosis: Same

Procedure Performed: Excision of right arm lipoma

Anesthesia: Local

Indications for Procedure: The patient is a 48-year-old woman who presents with a 4.0-cm mass on her right arm. She has had the mass for several months, and it is getting larger. She now presents for an excisional biopsy.

Description of Procedure: The patient was brought to the OR and placed on the operating table in the supine position. Her right arm was prepared and draped in the usual sterile fashion, and anesthetized with 1% lidocaine with bicarbonate. A longitudinal incision was made measuring 3 cm and carried down through the skin and subcutaneous tissues, and the underlying lipoma was dissected away from the surrounding tissues and removed. Parts of the lipoma were intermingled with surrounding tissues, requiring these areas to be pulled out. Hemostasis then was ensured and the wound closed with layered Vicryl, followed by Benzoin, Steri-Strips, and a Tegaderm dressing. The patient tolerated the procedure well and was taken to the recovery room in stable condition.

Pathological Diagnosis: Forearm, right: lipoma

Gross: The specimen consists of nine pieces of soft, predominantly fatty yellow tissue ranging from 0.9 cm to 3 cm in greatest diameter; representative sections were submitted in one cassette.

Code(s): _____

Surgical Case #28

Operative Report

Preoperative Diagnosis: Elevated PSA of 16.6 and bladder outlet obstruction

Postoperative Diagnosis: Same

Procedure: Cystoscopy and transrectal needle biopsy of the prostate

Anesthesia: General

Procedure: This man was taken to the operative suite, placed in the dorsolithotomy position after being administered anesthesia, and sterilely prepped and draped in the normal fashion. A needle was used to take multiple transrectal biopsies of his prostate under ultrasound guidance. After this, a cystoscopy was performed and bladder outlet obstruction and BPH were noted. The urethra was normal, and the bladder was moderately trabeculated. There was no evidence of neoplasm, infection, or calculus; and the ureters were normal in position, effluxing clear urine. The bladder was emptied, and the patient was sent to the recovery room in satisfactory condition.

Code(s): _____

Surgical Case #29

Operative Report

Preoperative Diagnosis: Right thyroid mass

Postoperative Diagnosis: Right thyroid mass

Procedure Performed: Excision of thyroid mass

The patient has a family history of thyroid cancer.

Procedure in Detail: The patient was taken to the operating room and general endotracheal anesthesia with orotracheal intubation was performed. The neck was prepped and draped in the usual fashion and locally injected with 4 cc of 0.5% lidocaine, plus 1:200,000 of epinephrine. Incision was made and superior and inferior subplatysmal flaps were elevated and the strap muscles were divided in the midline, and dissection was carried down to the thyroid isthmus. The mass on the right was identified and capsular dissection around the mass was performed using the harmonic scalpel in regions near the nerve. The superior vessels were isolated and ligated with 2-0 silk and the inferior vessels were ligated in a similar fashion. The recurrent laryngeal nerve was identified and followed superiorly up to its insertion, and the ligament was taken down with the nerve under direct visualization.

The mass was submitted for frozen section. Doctor called back stating grossly the nodule was not suspicious for papillary cancer. He felt frozen section would likely be of low yield so the specimen was submitted for permanent pathology.

A medium Blake was placed. The platysma, strap muscles, and skin were closed with Caprosyn suture. The patient was awakened, extubated, and transported to the recovery room in good condition.

Code(s): _____

Surgical Case #30

Operative Report

Procedure: Sigmoidoscopy

Indications for Procedure: The patient is 75 years old. She has had an alteration in her bowel pattern and is being evaluated with a sigmoidoscopy.

Description of Procedure: She was given Fleet's enema preparation. She required no sedation. The CF100L video colonoscope was inserted and passed without difficulty to 50 cm. The mucosa were normal. No diverticulosis was observed. Some scybalous stool was present, but this was minimal. The patient tolerated the procedure well.

Code(s): _____

Surgical Case #31

Operative Report

Diagnosis: Hodgkin's disease, nonsclerosing type

Operation: Placement of right subclavian Hickman catheter

Indications: The patient is a 35-year-old woman with the diagnosis of Hodgkin's disease. Her indication for a Hickman catheter was chemotherapy infusion.

Procedure: The patient was taken to the operating room and placed in the supine position. The right chest and subclavian area, neck, and shoulder were prepped and draped in routine manner. A total of 48 cc of 1% Carbocaine without epinephrine was used for anesthesia. The subcutaneous area below the right clavicle was numbed with the lidocaine down to the periosteum. The subclavian vein was stuck with the needle. Good blood flow was returned. The guide wire was passed. At this time, a 2-cm incision was made below the clavicle at the middle aspect. The Hickman catheter was then placed over the guide wire into the superior vena cava. This was documented with fluoroscopy. A second incision was made 3 cm below the first distance of 2 cm transverse. The area between the two incisions was then tunneled with a curved six. The distal aspect of the catheter was brought out through the second inferior incision. The Teflon Hickman catheter was trimmed to the appropriate length with Teflon coating at the skin incision. The superior skin incision was closed with interrupted #3-0 nylon, as was the inferior skin incision. The patient tolerated the procedure well.

Code(s): _____

Surgical Case #32

Operative Report

Preoperative Diagnosis: Ventral hernia

Postoperative Diagnosis: Ventral hernia

Operation Performed: Laparoscopic repair of ventral hernia

Anesthesia: General

Details of Procedure: The patient was taken to the operating room, placed in the supine position. The abdomen was prepped and draped in the usual sterile fashion. A Veress needle was then inserted in the left lateral abdominal wall. The abdomen was insufflated with CO_2 gas. A 10-mm Surgiport was then placed. The laparoscopic camera was then inserted. Additional 5-mm Surgiports were placed under direct vision, one in the left lower quadrant of the abdomen, the other in the left upper quadrant of the abdomen.

The 5-mm harmonic scalpel was used along with the dissecting forceps to take down the adhesions from within and around the hernia sac. There were a number of adhesions, primarily involving the omentum. These were all removed.

Two hernia defects were noted, one just above the umbilicus, perhaps 3 to 4 cm in diameter, and another toward the upper aspect of the midline incision, that had not been previously recognized.

It was elected to place an 18 3 24-cm segment of Gore-Tex dual mesh. #1 Prolene was sewn at each of the corners of this as well as in between, at the midpoint of each of the sides. Suitable locations were chosen for tying the anchoring sutures. The patch then was rolled around a grasper and inserted into the abdominal cavity through the 10-mm port. The patch was then unrolled and the orientation placed with the smooth side down against the bowel. An endoclose device was used to grasp each of the sutures and bring out through the previously placed incisions for the anchoring sutures. The patch was anchored at each of the six locations as noted previously. Then, an auto suture Protac was placed around the periphery of the patch. Additional staples were placed within the inner aspect of the patch using an Ethicon tacking stapler. The patch was noted to be quite taut and applied closely to the abdominal wall to prevent any movement of the patch. The abdomen was then desufflated and the ports withdrawn. Each of the skin incisions was closed with 4-0 clear PDS subcuticular suture and Steri-Strips. Tegaderm dressings were then applied. The patient tolerated the procedure well with no apparent difficulty. She was then taken to the postanesthesia recovery room for further postoperative care.

Code(s): _____

Surgical Case #33

Operative Report

Preoperative Diagnosis: Left breast mammographic abnormality

Postoperative Diagnosis: Same

Procedure: Breast biopsy

Indications: This is a 53-year-old woman who presented with a nonpalpable left breast mammographic abnormality. A stereotactic biopsy was recommended. Possible perioperative risks and complications and alternatives were discussed with her prior to surgery.

Details of Procedure: After informed consent was obtained from the patient, she was taken to the OR and placed on the table in the supine position. Under stereotactic guidance, a localization needle was inserted. The breast was prepped with Betadine solution and draped sterilely. Sedation was administered by anesthesia. Local anesthesia was achieved with 1% lidocaine and 0.5% Marcaine with epinephrine. A 14-gauge core biopsy needle was used to remove the tissue. This was forwarded to the radiology department, which confirmed the presence of the previously marked mammographic abnormality within the specimen. It was then forwarded to pathology.

Wound was inspected for hemostasis, which was excellent. The deep tissues were approximated with interrupted 3-0 Vicryl, and a running 4-0 Monocryl subcuticular stitch was used to approximate the skin edges. Benzoin, Steri-Strips, and dry sterile dressing were applied. The patient was then awakened from anesthesia and returned to the recovery room in stable condition.

Code(s): _____

Surgical Case #34

Operative Report

Preoperative Diagnosis: Pressure ulcer, right hip

Postoperative Diagnosis: Same

Procedure: Debridement of ulcer

The patient was taken to the operating room and administered general anesthesia. The skin was prepped and draped in the usual sterile fashion.

An incision was made over the hip joint. The size of the debrided area was approximately 15 sq cm. The skin was sharply debrided down through and including subcutaneous tissue. The wound was inspected and hemostasis achieved. The wound was then packed with sterile Kerlix. The patient had no complications.

Code(s): _____

Surgical Case #35

Operative Report

Preoperative Diagnosis: Carpal tunnel compression, left, severe

Postoperative Diagnosis: Same

Operation: Release, left carpal tunnel

Procedure: After successful axillary block was placed, the patient's left arm was prepared and draped in the usual sterile manner. Tourniquet was inflated. A curvilinear hypothenar incision was made and the palmaris retracted radially. The carpal tunnel and the transverse carpal ligament were then opened and completely freed in the proximal directions. It was noted to be severely tight in the palm with flattening and swelling of the median nerve. The carpal tunnel was opened distally in the hand and noted to be clear, out to the transverse palmar crease. The wound was then closed with 4-0 Dexon in subcuticular tissues. Sterile bulky dressing was applied, and the patient was awakened and taken to the recovery room in satisfactory condition.

Code(s): _____

Surgical Case #36

Operative Report

Preoperative Diagnosis: Keratosis of glans penis

Postoperative Diagnosis: Same

Procedure: The penis was prepared and draped in the usual manner. Along the distal portion of the penis on the right side and adjoining the urinary meatus was a well-defined, firm area suggesting a keratosis. The entire lesion was excised and submitted for pathological examination. The pathologist confirmed the diagnosis of keratosis. The glans penis was then approximated with black silk. The patient returned to the recovery room in satisfactory condition.

Code(s): _____

Surgical Case #37

Operative Report

Preoperative Diagnosis: Herniated disc at L4-L5, L5-S1; good relief with previous two epidural blocks

Postoperative Diagnosis: Same

Operation: Therapeutic epidural block injection

Procedure: The patient is kept on the left lateral side. The back is prepared with Betadine solution, and 1% Xylocaine is infiltrated at the L5-S1 interspace. Deep infiltration is carried out with a 22-gauge needle, and a 17-gauge Touhy needle is used and an interlaminar epidural is performed. After careful aspiration, which was negative for blood as well as for cerebrospinal fluid, about 80 mg of Depo-Medrol then were injected along with 5 cc of 0.25% Marcaine and 1 cc of 50 mcg of fentanyl citrate. The injection was done in a fractionated dose in a slow fashion. The patient was examined and evaluated following the block and found to have excellent relief of pain. The patient is advised to continue physical therapy and to come back in one month for further evaluation.

Code(s): _____

Surgical Case #38

Operative Report

Procedure: Excision of left axillary lymph nodes

Indications for Procedure: This female patient had a lumpectomy for a breast lesion approximately 2.5 years ago. She presents with palpable adenopathy in the left axilla.

Description of Procedure: The patient was brought into the operating room and placed on the OR table in the supine position. The left axilla was prepared and draped in the usual sterile fashion. After an adequate level of general anesthesia had been achieved, a knife with a #10 blade was used to make a curvilinear incision in the skin overlying the adenopathy.

This incision was carried down deep through the subcutaneous tissue using a Bovie knife. Babcock forceps were used to grasp the area of tissue surrounding the lymph node, which was carefully dissected from the surrounding tissues using a Bovie knife and scissors. All vessels encountered were either Bovied or clipped.

The wound was irrigated and carefully examined for bleeders. The subcutaneous tissue was closed using a Vicryl suture placed in interrupted fashion, and the skin was reapproximated using staples. Drainage was achieved with a Jackson-Pratt drain brought out through a separate wound. Sterile dressings were applied, and the patient was taken to the recovery room in a stable postoperative condition.

Code(s): _____

Surgical Case #39

Operative Report

Preoperative Diagnosis: Incomplete abortion

Postoperative Diagnosis: Same

Operation: Dilatation and curettage

History: This 22-year-old female, gravida IV, para II, AB I, comes in today because of abdominal pain and passing fetus on the sidewalk just outside the hospital. Apparently, her last menstrual period was two months ago. She had been doing well, and this problem just started today.

Procedure: The patient was placed on the operating table in the lithotomy position, and prepped and draped in the usual manner. Under satisfactory intravenous sedation, the cervix was visualized by means of a weighted speculum and grasped in the anterior lip with a sponge forceps. Cord was prolapsed through the cervix and vagina, and a considerable amount of placental tissue was in the vagina and cervix. This was removed. A sharp curet was used to explore the endometrial cavity, and a minimal amount of curettings was obtained. The patient tolerated the procedure well.

Code(s): _____

Surgical Case #40

Emergency Department Physician Report

Chief Complaint:	Left eye, foreign body x two days
History of Present Illness:	The patient is a 29-year-old man who presents to the emergency room after having a piece of metal fly into his left eye yesterday. Since that time, he still continues to have the metal present. He denies any major disturbance in vision, although he states that his vision is slightly more blurry and irritated. He does complain of some pain.
Past Medical History:	Hypertension
Allergies:	None
Immunizations:	Unknown for tetanus
Social and Family History:	Noncontributory
Physical Examination of Eyes:	Reveals the left eye to have some periorbital erythema, but minimal swelling of the lids. PERRLA: No papilledema. EOMs intact. Vision intact. Inspection of the left eye shows a foreign body that resembles a piece of metal at the 6 o'clock position. At this time, Tetracaine was applied. The foreign body was successfully removed with the bevel of a 22-gauge needle. Two more drops of Tetracaine were applied, followed by Homatropine and Polysporin ophthalmic ointment.
Assessment:	Foreign body of left eye, removed. The patient understood all instructions and agreed with the plan, at which time he was discharged.

Code(s): _____

Surgical Case #41

Operative Report

Preprocedure Diagnosis:	Left lower lobe lung nodule
Postprocedure Diagnosis:	Left lower lobe lung nodule
Operations Performed:	1. Left video-assisted thoracoscopy
	2. Wedge resection biopsy, left lower lobe times two
	3. Bronchoscopy with the right upper lobe, transbronchial biopsy times two

Indications for Procedure: The patient, who has been followed by both the pulmonary services as well as seen in the thoracic surgery clinic, had had a long history of smoking. His chest CT had a nodule in the left lower lobe as well as an area in the right upper lobe that was consistent with some consolidation that had not increased in size. It was decided to perform a wedge biopsy of the left lower lobe lung nodule since this is a discrete mass, and bronchoscopy for the right upper lobe. Patient understood the previously mentioned procedures and approach. Informed consent was obtained.

Procedure: Patient was brought into the operating room, placed on the operating table in the supine position. After smooth induction of general anesthesia and endotracheal intubation, a Foley catheter was placed. The double-lumen endotracheal tube was placed. Patient was then turned to the left lateral decubitus position with the left side up and right side down. We prepared and draped with Hibiclens, alcohol, and Loban. We then made a small incision in the posterior space with a scalpel, dissected down, bluntly entered into the chest cavity, and placed a 5-mm port.

We then placed an additional port and moved the camera to the anterior inferior portion and placed another 5-mm trocar posterior inferior. We then used gross inspection of the chest. There were no adhesions and no pleural fluid to sweep out. No gross masses. Using a blunt grasper, we were able to palpate the left lower lobe posteriorly and feel the mass. We then used graspers retracted to the lung specimen up, used the EndoGIA staplers to perform wedge biopsies or initial wedge biopsy. We did not have the specimen. In this second wedge biopsy, we were able to get around from the green staple load and perform the biopsy and wedge out the mass lesion. This was then placed in a EndoCatch bag and removed. We were then able to palpate the mass, but the scalpel we opened had an appearance of an infectious etiology. Gram staining was sent and then it was sent for further dissection.

We then placed a #9 French pneumocatheter anteriorly under direct vision. There was no bleeding to speak of. We removed

(Continued on next page)

Surgical Case #41 (Continued)

our trocars under direct vision. Lung was allowed to reinflate. Chest tube was placed to suction 10 cm to close the 10 3 12 site with 2-0 Vicryl and 4-0 Vicryl followed by Dermabond. Other trocar sites were closed with 4-0 Monocryl and Dermabond. Once this was completed, the patient was turned supine. We then performed a bronchoscopy. During bronchoscopy, the trachea at the right appeared normal. On the right side, the bronchus intermedius appeared normal. We were able to cannulate the right upper lobe. We were able to then use the biopsy forceps to cannulate the apical segment of the right upper lobe. We sent several specimens with biopsy forceps for cytology as well as performed a biopsy with fluoroscopic guidance times two. We then removed the biopsy forceps.

We inspected the bronchus intermedius, the right medial lobe and right lower lobe orifices appeared normal. We then removed, pulled the scope back, advanced down the left main stem bronchus. All segments and lobes appeared normal. Through the bronchoscope, this point of procedure was terminated. Patient was extubated, transferred off the operating room table, awakened stable to the SICU. Dr. Howard was present for the entire procedure. There were no complications.

Code(s): _____

Emergency Department Case #42

Operative Report

Procedure: Tonsillectomy

Diagnosis: Recurrent tonsillitis

Indications: This 10-year-old patient was found to have recurrent tonsillitis, and a tonsillectomy was planned.

Technique: The patient was placed in the supine position, and general endotracheal anesthesia was begun. The nasopharynx was inspected, revealing only a very small amount of adenoid, which was not removed. The tonsils were noted to be very large and obstructive, and were removed by dissection and snare technique. The bleeders were electrocoagulated. The inferior cuff was suture ligated with 2-0 plain catgut. The patient tolerated the procedure well and was brought to the recovery room in satisfactory condition.

Code(s): _____

Surgical Case #43

Operative Report

Preoperative Diagnosis: Epidermal cyst

Postoperative Diagnosis: Awaiting permanent section by pathology

Operation: Excision of the area

Procedure: This 91-year-old woman who resides in the Sunnybrook Nursing Home presented with a 0.75 cm enlarging tender granulomatous type lesion over the dorsum of the MCP joint of the left ring finger. Because of the patient's arthritis, she was left in the wheelchair while the procedure was done. The left hand was scrubbed for 10 minutes with sterile soap solution with Betadine, prepared with Betadine. The patient was draped with sterile towels and drapes exposing the area and then the area about the lesion was blocked with 1% lidocaine without epinephrine. Then an ellipse was outlined with long axis vertical, and the lesion was excised and submitted to pathology. The total excised lesion including margins was 1.0 cm. It was closed with five sutures of 5-0 Prolene and dressed with Polysporin and a Band-Aid. The family was instructed that the Band-Aid could be changed, and she was discharged to the home where I will follow her and remove the sutures in one to two weeks.

Pathological Diagnosis: Skin lesion, left ring finger: epidermal cyst, excised and actinic keratosis with extensive atypical basosquamous cell hyperplasia

Code(s): _____

Surgical Case #44

Emergency Department Record

Chief Complaint:	Injury to right fourth and fifth toes
History of Present Illness:	Patient states that he was running for the phone when he stubbed his toes on a piece of furniture. Did this yesterday and has marked ecchymosis noted in the fourth and fifth toes of the right foot, slight swelling also. He states he has been able to ambulate and that his foot does not hurt, except for when he walks. Denies any numbness, tingling, or loss of sensation. He does also have an abrasion noted to the distal aspect of the fourth toe. He denies any further injury.
Past Medical History:	Noncontributory
Allergies:	Patient has no known medication allergies
Current Medications:	None
Review of Systems:	Negative

Physical Examination

Vital Signs:	Blood pressure is 145/89. Temperature is 97.7° F, pulse of 76, respirations 16.
General:	Patient is alert, oriented, in no acute distress.
Extremities:	Shows marked ecchymosis noted in the fourth and fifth toes and in the dorsal aspect of the foot adjacent to the fourth and fifth toes on the right foot. The patient is tender to palpation over the fourth and fifth digits proximal. Right foot is neurovascularly intact. Sensation is intact. Patient has an abrasion noted to the distal aspect of the right fourth digit. Range of motion is intact. Patient is able to ambulate with a slight limp due to pain. Remainder of physical examination is normal.
Emergency Department Course:	An x-ray was taken of the patient's right foot with attention to the fourth and fifth toes. X-ray showed a fracture of the fourth and fifth proximal phalanx. X-ray was also reviewed by Dr. Smith, who agreed with this assessment. The patient's right fourth and fifth toes were digitally blocked with 2.5 cc of 2% lidocaine each. Abrasion on the fourth digit was prepared per protocol. Fractures were reduced in the fourth and fifth digits and buddy taped. Patient's right foot was again x-rayed. His postreduction film showed that the fractures were in better alignment. X-rays were also reviewed by Dr. Blevins, who agreed with this assessment. Patient was fitted for a postoperative shoe.
Impressions/Diagnosis:	Patient has fractured right fourth and fifth toes.

Plan:
1. Rest, ice, compress, and elevate the right foot.
2. Buddy tape 3 two weeks.
3. Follow-up with family medical doctor as needed.
4. Return if condition worsens. Patient refused any pain medication.

Disposition:
Home

Code(s): _____

Surgical Case #45

Operative Report

Preoperative Diagnosis: Lipoma of the right shoulder

Postoperative Diagnosis: Same

Procedure: Removal of lipoma

Description of Procedure: The patient was taken to the operating room and prepared and draped in the usual manner. A longitudinal incision was made centered over the palpable and visible mass, carried down through the skin. The subcutaneous layer was noted to be large lobulations, and dissection was begun around the obvious palpable 3.0 cm mass. This was dissected free and carried down through the deltoid muscle down to the level of the subscapularis tendon of the shoulder joint. Did not seem to have any major neurovascular attachments otherwise. Mass was dissected free through the muscle-slitting incision. The cephalic vein was retracted laterally.

Bleeding was controlled with hemostats and Bovie cautery. Estimated blood loss: 30 cc. The wound was then copiously irrigated after total removal was verified, and the fascia was closed with 2-0 chromic catgut, subcutaneous layer with 2-0 plain catgut and skin with 2-0 Dermalon. The patient tolerated the procedure well and left the OR in good condition after dressing was applied.

Code(s): _____

Surgical Case #46

Operative Report

Procedure: Colonoscopy

Indications for Procedure: This is a 65-year-old woman with a family history of colonic malignancy who is being evaluated for altered bowel function. When evaluated in my office prior to the procedure, her vital signs, cardiac status, pulmonary status, and mental status were stable and adequate for conscious sedation.

Description of Procedure: The patient was given Demerol 50 mg IV and Versed 3 mg IV, and the CF1OOI video colonoscope was inserted and passed without difficulty to the cecum. Its position was confirmed by the ileocecal valve. Diverticulosis was observed in the left colon. A 5- to 7-mm circular, semipedunculated polyp was observed in the cecal area. It was secured with the snare and recovered. The patient tolerated the procedure well.

Impression: She has a small cecal polyp, which has been removed. She has diverticulosis and will need reevaluation in three years.

Clinical Diagnosis: Polyp, cecum

Pathological Diagnosis: Polyp, cecum: Villotubular adenoma

Code(s): _____

Surgical Case #47

Operative Report

Preoperative Diagnosis: Displaced, rotated fractures of left index and long metacarpal shafts

Postoperative Diagnosis: Same

Procedure: Closed reduction and percutaneous pin fixation of displaced fractures of the left index and long metacarpal shafts

Description of Procedure: The patient is a 22-year-old, right-hand-dominant man who sustained left index and long metacarpal shaft fractures while playing soccer. He was referred to my office and was found to have internal rotation and shortening deformities through the index and long metacarpal shaft fractures and subsequently is scheduled for closed, possibly open, reduction and percutaneous pin fixation or possible internal fixation of the previously-mentioned fractures. The patient was placed in the supine position on the OR table and general anesthesia was administered. Left proximal arm tourniquet was placed, and the left upper extremity was prepared and draped in the usual sterile fashion. The arm was exsanguinated with an Esmarch bandage and the tourniquet inflated to 250 mm Hg. Sterile finger traps and ropes were then applied to the left index and long fingers, and 10 lb of weight were then applied over the end of the hand table. The fractures were then gently manipulated and multiple fluoroscopic views were obtained, which revealed satisfactory alignment. Attention was then turned to the index metacarpal shaft fracture, which was percutaneously pinned from its radial to ulnar aspect with excellent purchase being obtained on both sides. X-rays were then taken and revealed anatomic alignment. Attention was then turned to the long metacarpal shaft fracture, which was still slightly distracted and displaced. Additional manipulation was performed. A pin was initially inserted from radial to ulnar, which resulted in further distraction of the fracture. The pin was removed, and another pin was inserted from ulnar to radial. This appeared to close the fracture gap and held the fracture in better alignment. A second pin was then placed just proximal and parallel to the original pin with resultant satisfactory alignment. There was still some slight gapping at the fracture site, but the rotation and angulation were corrected. The finger traps were removed, and the fingers were flexed to the same degree. All fingertips appeared to point to the distal pole of the scaphoid without any evidence of angulation or rotation malalignment. The pins were trimmed and bent over at 90-degree angles. The pin sites were irrigated, and Xeroform dressings were applied. Sterile gauze, lightly compressive hand dressing was then applied, reinforced with plaster splint with the hand placed in the intrinsic plus position and the PIP joint left free. The patient tolerated the procedure well and was sent to recovery in satisfactory condition.

Code(s): _____

Surgical Case #48

Operative Report

Preoperative Diagnosis: Symptomatic third-degree heart block

Postoperative Diagnosis: Same

Operation: Placement of permanent pacemaker with transvenous electrode

Anesthesia: Local infiltration of lidocaine 1%, total volume 13 cc

Complications: None

Indications: This 74-year-old man was admitted with a diagnosis of third-degree heart block complicated by congestive cardiac failure. Patient is scheduled for placement of a permanent pacemaker today.

Procedure: With the patient supine on the operating table with a shoulder roll placed beneath the thoracic spine, the chest was prepared and draped in a sterile fashion. In the right infraclavicular region, a subcutaneous pocket was created for containing the pulse generator. Using an introducer guide wire, a sheath technique bipolar-targeted lead was introduced into the right subclavian vein. Under fluoroscopy control, this was directed into the right ventricle. Two initial locations were not satisfactory for pacing parameters. Finally, the pacemaker was positioned in satisfactory position with the following parameters: at the threshold 0.4 volts, current 1.5 milliamps, and R wave 15. The pacing system analyzer was then turned to 10 volts output and the diaphragm observed for pulsations, which were not proven. The lead was then secured under the clavicle with a single suture of 2-0 Ethibond. It was then attached to a 5794 Medtronic low-profile VVI pacemaker programmed at 70 beats per minute. The pulse generator was then anchored in the subcutaneous pocket with a single O PDS suture. The subcutaneous tissue was then approximated with 2-0 PDS and the skin approximated with 4-0 Maxon. Sterile dressing was applied. A chest x-ray was obtained, which showed no pneumothorax and satisfactory position of the lead. The patient was then returned to the coronary care unit in good condition.

Code(s): _____

Surgical Case #49

Operative Report

Preoperative Diagnosis: Nasolacrimal duct obstruction, right eye

Postoperative Diagnosis: Same

Operation:
1. Probing right nasolacrimal duct
2. Balloon dilation, right nasolacrimal duct

Procedure: The patient was taken to the operating room and given general anesthesia by mask. The right upper punctum was then dilated and a #0 Bowman probe passed from the upper punctum into the lacrimal sac and down through the nasolacrimal duct with a small amount of resistance. A second probe was then passed under the right inferior turbinate and definite metal-on-metal contact established. The original probe was then withdrawn, and a #2 Lacricath was inserted from the upper punctum into the lacrimal sac and down through the nasolacrimal duct. Its position was confirmed in the nose. The balloon was inflated eight atmospheres for 90 seconds. It was then withdrawn 5 mm and again inflated eight atmospheres for 60 seconds. At this point, the Lacricath was withdrawn. A lacrimal cannula attached to a syringe containing normal saline dyed with fluorescein was then inserted from the upper punctum into the lacrimal sac and fluid freely irrigated into the nose and recovered with a suction catheter. A drop of a steroid antibiotic combination was then applied to the right eye, and the patient awakened and returned to the recovery room in good condition.

Code(s): _____

Emergency Department Case #50

Emergency Department Record

Chief Complaint:	A laceration to the left lower leg
History of Present Illness:	The patient is a 33-year-old man who presents to the ER today with a chief complaint of a laceration to his left lower leg. The patient states that he came to Cincinnati for a mountain bike competition, which he was in today. The patient stated that he was practicing before the competition when he accidentally cut the posterior aspect of his left leg on the pedal of his bike. The patient stated that the pedal was clean and that he had this accident on the pavement. There was no grass or dirt around at that time. The patient currently complains of pain to the area of the laceration. He is ambulatory with a limp. The patient stated that the accident happened approximately one hour prior to arrival at the emergency room. The patient denies any left calf pain. Denies any left knee pain. The patient did not have any head injury or any loss of consciousness. The patient's tetanus is up to date. The patient also denies any neck or back injury. The patient has no other complaints.
Review of Systems:	See HPI; otherwise negative
Past Medical History:	Unremarkable
Medications:	None
Allergies:	No known drug allergies

Physical Examination:

Vital Signs:	Blood pressure is 128/68; temperature is 97.8° F; pulse 77; respirations 18
General:	The patient is a 33-year-old man who is in no acute distress. The patient is alert and oriented.
Skin:	Pink, warm. Patient currently has a 5-cm gaping laceration to the posterior aspect of his left leg that is just inferior and medial to the left knee.
HEENT:	Within normal limits
Neck:	Supple, no cervical tenderness; no cervical adenopathy
Musculoskeletal:	The patient has full active range of motion of his left knee at this time. There is no edema, ecchymosis, or erythema noted to the left knee. However, the patient's posterior aspect of his left knee is indurated somewhat. The patient is nontender with palpation over the left gastrocnemius muscle. The patient's dorsalis pedis and posterior tibialis pulses are present and strong. Doppler was then used to pick up the patient's left popliteal pulse. This was present and strong, and when

(Continued on next page)

Emergency Department Case #50 (Continued)

compared to the popliteal pulse of the right leg, it was the same strength. The patient is nontender with palpation of the left quadriceps as well as over the left hamstring muscles.

ED Course:
The patient was discussed with Dr. Smith. Dr. Smith also examined the patient. X-rays were then obtained of the patient's left tib/fib as well as the patient's left knee. X-rays were reviewed by both myself and Dr. Smith and were unremarkable. The patient was then given Keflex 1 g p.o. The patient was then given Lortab 5 mg p.o.

ED Procedure:
The patient's laceration was anesthetized using 15 cc of 1% lidocaine plain. The area was then cleansed using Betadine and normal saline solution. The wound was then explored for any evidence of foreign bodies. No foreign bodies were noted. Wound edges were then well approximated and brought together using three deep-layered sutures of 4-0 Vicryl and seven mattress sutures of 4-0 nylon as well as one simple suture of 4-0 nylon. The area was then cleansed again using normal saline. Xeroform was applied as well as a Keflex wrap and Ace wrap. The patient was informed to remove the Ace wrap prior to sleeping in the evening. The patient was also given a Lortab starter pack and informed to fill his antibiotic prescription. Patient was also informed to watch for any pain to his left calf. The patient understood this and stated that he would return if any pain occurred.

Impression/Diagnosis:
1. A 5-cm laceration, left posterior leg, which was repaired

Plan:
1. Keep area clean and dry

2. Suture removal 10 to 12 days by primary care physician

3. Wound care instructions: Watch for infection

4. Keflex 500 mg #20 no refills

5. Lortab 5 mg #10 no refills

6. Return with any worsening symptoms

Code(s): _____

Surgical Case #51

Operative Report

Preoperative Diagnosis: Rule out bladder tumor

Postoperative Diagnosis: Same

Procedures: Cystoscopy, biopsy, and fulguration of bladder

Anesthesia: Spinal

Indications: This is a 68-year-old white woman with a history of grade II superficial transitional cell carcinoma of the bladder. Cystoscopy showed a suspicious erythematous area on the right trigone. She presented today for cystoscopy, biopsy, and fulguration.

Findings: The urethra was normal, the bladder was 1+ trabeculated, the mid and right trigone area were slightly erythematous and hypervascular, no papillary tumors were noted, no mucosal abnormalities were noted.

Description of Procedure: The patient was placed on the table in supine position, satisfactory spinal anesthesia was obtained. She was placed in the dorsolithotomy position and prepared and draped in the usual manner. A #22 French cystoscopy sheath was passed per urethra in atraumatic fashion. Cup biopsy forceps were placed and three biopsies were taken of the suspicious areas of the trigone. For hemostasis, these areas were fulgurated with the Bugby electrode. There was no active bleeding seen. The scope was removed, and the patient was returned to recovery in satisfactory condition.

Pathology Report:

Bladder biopsy: chronic cystitis (cystica) with squamous metaplasia

Code(s): _____

Surgical Case #52

Operative Report

Preoperative Diagnosis: Thrombosis, right forearm, Gore-Tex graft

Postoperative Diagnosis: Same

Operation: Thrombectomy

Indications: This 73-year-old woman has a right forearm graft used for dialysis that has developed an arterial occlusion.

Procedure: The patient was placed in the supine position and prepared and draped in the normal fashion. A transverse incision was made at the outflow tract of the vein and the Gore-Tex graft anastomosis. A complete thrombectomy was performed. The area was fully irrigated with saline and heparin lock. There was satisfactory pulse through the graft, and the incisions were closed with 3-0 Dexon and running 4-0 Prolene. The patient tolerated the procedure well.

Code(s): _____

Surgical Case #53

Endoscopy Report

Procedure: Gastroenterology consultation/gastroscopy/esophageal dilatation

Indications: This is a 72-year-old woman who has had dysphagia for solids for some time. Barium swallow showed a smooth stricture at the LES. She is generally in good health otherwise except for hypertension. Because of her dysphagia, upper GI endoscopy is done today.

She was premedicated with Versed. Conscious sedation was monitored in the usual fashion. The Olympus video endoscope was introduced from the mouth into the esophagus. The distal esophagus has a tight stricture at the LES. The stomach, pyloric channel, duodenal bulb, and second part of the duodenum were normal. The scope was withdrawn, and she was serially dilated using Maloney dilators.

Code(s): _____

Surgical Case #54

Operative Report

Preoperative Diagnosis: Squamous cell carcinoma of the left forearm, 8 mm

Postoperative Diagnosis: Same

Procedure: Excision of the same with layered primary closure

Anesthetic: Local

Brief Clinical History: The patient had a biopsy-proven squamous cell carcinoma of the left forearm. After explanation of the risks, benefits, and alternatives, she agreed to re-excision and closure. She understood that there would be a scar as a result.

Details of Procedure: The patient was taken to the outpatient operating area. An ellipse was taken around the primary lesion with 5-mm margins for excision around the lesion. The area was infiltrated with 0.5% Xylocaine with 1:200,000 epinephrine and approximately 5 cc was used. The area was prepared with Betadine paint and draped in a sterile manner. The lesion was elliptically excised and closed in layers with 4-0PDS. The deep subcutaneous layer was closed separately and then a running subcuticular layer was performed. She tolerated the procedure well. She was given instructions for local care and will return in nine days for a checkup and suture removal.

Code(s): _____

Surgical Case #55

Operative Report

Preoperative Diagnosis:

Right true vocal cord lesion

Postoperative Diagnosis:

Same

Operative Procedure:

Direct laryngoscopy with excision of right true vocal cord lesion

Findings:

Firm right true vocal cord lesion and some scarring on the right true vocal cord, otherwise normal laryngoscopy

Indication for the Procedure:

This is a 51-year-old man who had a history of anterior commissure nodule that was biopsied in 2001 and came back as benign. He was lost to follow-up, but returned with increasing hoarseness and was found on flexible laryngoscopy to have a mid-right-sided true vocal cord lesion. He was brought to the operating room today for laryngoscopy and removal of this lesion.

Details of the Procedure:

He was placed in the supine position on the operating room table and mask anesthesia was induced. Once deeper anesthesia had been achieved, the table was turned toward the laryngoscopy instrumentation. A Dedo laryngoscope was placed carefully into the mouth after the upper gums were protected using wet gauze. The lingual surface of the epiglottis appeared normal as did the vallecula. The laryngeal surface of the epiglottis also appeared completely normal as did the arytenoids and false vocal cords bilaterally. The true vocal cords were bilaterally mobile. They were slightly edematous and there was an approximately 1.5 cm whitish nodule on the right vocal cord in the middle third of the cord. There was a small area of heaped mucosa near the anterior commissure that was slightly hard, but deemed normal and another one at the vocal process that again had normal mucosa, but was slightly firm as if some scarring was present. Again, the left true vocal cord was completely normal except for slight edema. The posterior commissure area appeared normal. Again, the arytenoids were visualized and were thought to be completely normal. At this point, an LTA was sprayed and the patient was intubated. Completion of the direct laryngoscopy revealed a normal piriform sinus on the left normal postcricoid area and a normal right piriform sinus. At this point, the laryngoscope was replaced such that the right vocal cord was easily visualized and palpated. It was suspended at this time. Next, the operating microscope was brought into place, through the #400 lens, and the vocal cord was easily inspected and palpated. A right biting forceps was used to retract the mid third of the right vocal cord and a leftward scissors was used to dissect the area where this lesion was noted on the vocal cord. This did include the medial aspect of the true cord on that side. Once this was excised in toto, it was sent off for permanent pathology. There was minimal bleeding at the site. The microscope and Dedo laryngoscope were taken out of the field, and the patient was returned to the anesthesia department for reawakening, extubation, and transported to the postanesthesia care unit in a stable condition. Dr. Fowler was present for this entire case.

Pathology Report

Specimen:	Right true vocal cord lesion
Gross description:	One specimen is received in formalin labeled with demographics and "right true vocal cord." It consists of a 0.2 3 0.1 3 0.1 cm white tissue fragment. The specimen is stained with eosin and entirely submitted in one cassette.
Microscopic Examination/Diagnosis:	Squamous mucosa with focal moderate dysplasia

Code(s): _____

Surgical Case #56

Operative Report

Preoperative Diagnosis: Previous history of polyps

Postoperative Diagnosis: Descending colon polyp

Operation: Colonoscopy total and polypectomy of descending colon polyp

Procedure: Patient was placed in the left lateral position. After adequate sedation the 168-cm videoscope was passed through the rectum, through the sigmoid colon, through the descending colon, through the transverse colon to the right colon. The position of the cecum was confirmed. The cecum and the right colon were found to be normal. The transverse colon was found to be normal. In the descending colon there was a small 3-mm polyp. This was removed with use of cold knife forceps. The polyp was then given out for histopathology. The base of the polyp was electrocoagulated. The remainder of the colon was found to be normal except for diverticulosis involving sigmoid colon. The rectum was found to be normal except for hypertrophied anal polyp. The scope was removed. The patient tolerated the procedure well and was transferred to the recovery room in fair condition.

Code(s): _____

Emergency Department Record Case #57

Operative Report (Emergency Room)

Diagnosis: Post Herpetic Neuralgia

Procedure: Nerve Block

Procedure: After the consent was obtained, the patient was placed in the right lateral position. A pillow was placed under her trunk on the right side. It was then cleansed with Betadine solution. Intercostal blocks were performed at the T8, T9, and T10 level using Marcaine 0.5% with Epinephrine 1:200,000. A 5 cc solution was injected at each site after careful aspiration. The needle was a 23 gauge 1.5 inch needle.

She tolerated the procedure very well. There was no suggestion of pneumothorax or lung puncture during the procedure. A chest x-ray was obtained; after which it confirmed that there was no pneumothorax. She has been given an instruction sheet and will be discharged home in stable condition. I will schedule an appointment for her to return in two to three days to assess her response and either repeat the intercostal block or perform an epidural block, depending upon her response.

Code(s): _____

Surgical Case #58

Operative Report

PreProcedure:	1. Backache, unspecified
Diagnosis(es):	2. Related back and leg pain
Procedure(s) Performed:	Lumbar epidural steroid injection L5–S1 interspace
Indications for Procedure:	The patient is a 41-year-old man with severe work-related back and leg pain, more left than right. The patient understands the reasons for the procedure and the risk associated with it. The patient is anxious and needed IV sedation and tolerated the pain associated with injection.
Details of Procedure:	For the procedure, the patient was placed prone on the fluoroscopy table with a pillow under his abdomen. We identified the sacral hiatus. We prepared the skin with alcohol and DuraPrep and applied drapes and anesthetized the skin with xylocaine.
	Next, we used fluoroscopy to guide the 17-gauge needle into the spinal canal through the sacral hiatus. This was advanced under AP and lateral fluoroscopic guidance with loss of resistance. We verified proper depth and placement with myelography injection.
	The lumbar myelography injection was extradural in the lumbosacral area and consisted of 2 cc of Isovue 300. This showed we were in the spinal canal and highlighting the nerve roots at the lumbosacral region.
	Next, we placed the catheter to the L5-S1 interspace. Through the catheter we injected steroid solution that contained 80 mg of Depo-Medrol, 3 cc of 0.75% marcaine, and 4 cc of Omnipaque 300. This was injected under fluoroscopy, visualizing the nerve roots well throughout the lower lumbar area, more left than right. We cleared the catheter and needle of solution and removed them from the back. Permanent films were taken, and the patient was taken to the recovery room where he recovered in good condition.
Interpretation of Permanent Films:	The permanent films afterward verified the myelography and steroid solution were in the proper areas. On AP and lateral views, the solution highlighted the nerve roots at the lower lumbar area but scar tissue is preventing the spread of medication throughout the entire region. Nerve roots do highlight in the lower lumbar spine. No evidence of dural puncture.

Code(s): _____

Surgical Case #59

Operative Report

Preoperative Diagnosis: Bladder neck contracture, status post radical retropubic prostatectomy

Postoperative Diagnosis: Same

Procedure: Cystoscopy with dilation

Indications for Procedure: The patient is a 58-year-old man who underwent a radical prostatectomy in 2004. Postoperatively, he has had problems with bladder neck contractures requiring dilation. His last dilation was done in November 2004. He had been performing intermittent catheterization following this with good results of continence. Unfortunately, over the past several months, he had been unable to pass this catheter and appeared to be in urinary retention. He was scheduled for cystoscopy and dilation of bladder neck contracture accordingly. All alternative treatment options as well as risks and benefits and expected outcomes of the procedure were explained to the patient prior to the procedure and he understood these and wished to proceed.

Findings: Severe bladder neck contracture was noted. It was approximately #5 French in diameter.

Details of Procedure: After informed consent was obtained and the patient received 1 g of ampicillin and 100 mg of gentamicin IV, the patient was brought to the operating theater and placed in supine fashion. After adequate sedation, the patient was placed in the dorsal lithotomy position; his genitalia and perineum were prepared and draped in the usual sterile fashion. Using a #22.5 French sheath, a scope was inserted into the patient's urethra and subsequently into the bladder. A long filiform was passed through the bladder neck contracture. Subsequent dilation from #8 French to #20 French was carried out. After approximately #16 French, it is very difficult to pass the dilator and therefore this was determined at the #20 French dilation. Another attempt at placing the filiform or followers was discontinued at approximately #14 French because of difficulty in passing the followers.

The filiform was then removed, and under direct visualization, an Amplatz super stiff guide wire was inserted into the bladder with the aid of a Pollack catheter to the #5 French open-ended catheter. The renal Amplatz dilators were then used to dilate the bladder neck contracture to #18 French. A #18 French Councill catheter was then inserted over the guide wire into the bladder. 10 cc was inflated into the balloon and the wire was removed. Irrigation confirmed that this was in the bladder. Patient was taken to the recovery room in satisfactory condition.

Code(s): _____

Surgical Case #60

Operative Report

Preoperative Diagnosis: Stab wound, left thigh

Postoperative Diagnosis: Stab wound, left thigh with arterial bleeders secondary to branches off the deep femoral artery

Procedures Performed: Exploration of left thigh stab wound with control of bleeding and repair of rectus femoris muscle

Indications for Procedure: This 24-year-old man was stabbed in the left anteromedial thigh earlier this morning. He presented to the emergency department, and the examination revealed a 1-cm stab wound about 20 cm below the inguinal ligament in the mid-thigh anteromedial. Posterior tibial pulses were equal bilaterally. There was no swelling in his foot or calf. The wound was explored in the emergency room, and it was obvious that there was a huge cavity within the rectus femoris muscle. Nothing further was done there and he was brought to the operating room.

Details of Procedure: The patient was placed on the operating table in the supine position. General endotracheal anesthesia was induced, and endotracheal tube was used. Left leg was prepared with Betadine and then draped. Enlarged the stab wound medial and laterally in oblique fashion, carried it down to the muscle, opened up the anterior fascia of the rectus femoris, got into a large cavity within it that went down almost to the femur. At the base of this there were two small pumping vessels that were electrocoagulated, which pretty much controlled the bleeding. There were then multiple small bleeders within the muscle belly itself that we coagulated. The wound was copiously irrigated, rechecked, and little bleeders Bovied and the bleeding was controlled. We evacuated all the hematoma that was present. Cleaned it out, irrigated it again, rechecked it, and no further bleeding was noted. The anterior fascia was closed with interrupted 2-0 Vicryl, and subcutaneous tissue was irrigated and the skin closed with staples, 4 3 4 Kerlix and Ace wrap over that. The patient tolerated the procedure well. Estimated blood loss of the actual procedure was only about 50 cc. He was extubated, and taken to the recovery room in stable condition.

Code(s): _____

Surgical Case #61

Operative Report

Procedure: Fiberoptic bronchoscopy

Diagnosis: Hemoptysis with easily bruisable mucosa and bronchiectasis

Technique: The patient was brought to the endoscopy suite and placed on a stretcher. Oxygen was given via nasal cannula at 3 L/min. Local anesthetic lidocaine was given to anesthetize the upper airway. Because the nostrils had considerable blockage secondary to trauma, the oral route was used for the bronchoscopy. Following placement of a bite block and application of Cetacaine to the posterior pharynx, the fiberoptic bronchoscope was placed without difficulty into the upper airway.

The epiglottis appeared somewhat prominent, but normal. In addition, the vocal cords appeared normal. The bronchoscope was passed easily through the cords into the trachea, which also appeared normal, although somewhat easily bruisable. The carina appeared normal. The right side was entered first. The right upper lobe and its subsegments were seen very clearly, and there appeared to be bronchiectasis. The 6-mm bronchoscope would go very easily into the subsegments. No mass lesions were seen. The bronchus intermedius, right middle lobe, lower lobe, and its subsegments also were entered; and, again, bronchiectasis was noted. There appeared to be no abnormal mucosal lesions and no abnormal secretions; however, the bronchial tree was easily bruisable. The bronchoscope then was withdrawn to the carina and the left side entered.

The left main bronchus, upper lobe, lower lobe, and its subsegments were seen. There appeared to be an extrinsic compression of a subsegment of the left lower lobe; however, no mucosal lesions were seen and this area appeared pulsatile, which suggested extrinsic compression from the descending aorta. Once again, easy bruisability of the mucosa was noted. The bronchoscope was withdrawn. There were no apparent complications.

Code(s): _____

Surgical Case #62

Operative Report

Preoperative Diagnosis: Left third finger, trigger finger

Postoperative Diagnosis: Left third finger, trigger finger

Procedure Performed: Release of the left third finger, trigger finger

Indications for Procedure: Patient is an 84-year-old male who presented to our clinic with complaint of the left third finger locked up on extension. He was diagnosed with a trigger finger and was scheduled for repair.

Procedure: Patient was placed in supine position. After prep and draping, approximately 20 cc of local anesthetic consisting of 2% lidocaine, without epinephrine, was injected over the palmar aspect of the left third finger over the MCP, followed by tight wrap over the forearm and blood pressure cuff over the left forearm, then it inflated to 215 mmHg and tight wrap was then released and with the blood pressure cuff remained inflated for hemostasis. An incision was made over the palmar aspect of the left third finger at the MCP, and this incision was then carried down through the fascia to expose the tendon sheath, and the tendon sheath was then opened using sharp dissection. Hemostasis, meanwhile, obtained using electrocautery. After release was done, patient was asked to flex and extend the finger and his symptoms subsequently resolved. Compression was used for hemostasis while the tourniquet was deflated. Before closure, approximately 3 cc of Kenalog was used for steroid treatment. For closure, a #5-0 nylon was used in an interrupted fashion to approximate the skin edges in a nontension fashion. For dressing with Bacitracin was applied over the finger and the hand was wrapped and finally Ace bandage was applied. The patient tolerated the procedure well and was subsequently transferred to recovery.

Code(s): _____

Surgical Case #63

Operative Report

Preoperative Diagnosis: Menometrorrhagia and anemia

Postoperative Diagnosis: Same

Procedures: Dilatation and curettage, Hysteroscopy.

Indications for Procedure: The patient is a 53-year-old female who reports that she has had extremely heavy periods for several months. The patient had two periods lasting 10 each for the past two months.

Based on the patient's history of simple hyperplasia, anemia, and menometrorrhagia, the risks, benefits and alternatives of the D&C, hysteroscopy were thoroughly discussed with the patient who agreed to the procedure.

Description of Operation: The patient was taken to the operating room where under the effects of adequate general anesthesia, was prepped and draped in the usual sterile fashion for vaginal surgery.

A weighted speculum was placed posteriorly and the Sims anteriorly to allow visualization of the cervix. The cervix was noted to descend to the introitus. The uterus was then sounded to 10 cm. On examination under anesthesia, she had no appreciable adnexal masses. Her uterus was slightly enlarged, anteverted, mobile.

The patient's cervix was dilated to a #15 dilator. The hysteroscope was then introduced into the cervix. The endocervical canal appeared without lesions. Advancing to the uterus, there appeared to be a desynchronous endometrium with lush endometrium posteriorly and somewhat atrophic appearing anteriorly. Tissue sample were taken for pathological diagnosis.

The right tubal ostia was visualized; the left was obscured by lush endometrium. The hysteroscope was then removed.

The cervix was then dilated to #20 dilator. The sharp curet was then removed. All instruments were then removed from the patient.

All sponge, needle and instrument counts were correct at the end of the procedure.

The patient tolerated the procedure well, was taken to the postoperative recovery room in good condition.

Code(s): _____

Surgical Case #64

Operative Report

Preoperative Diagnosis: Multiple lacerations to both ears

Preoperative Diagnosis: Multiple lacerations to both ears, a laceration to the left ear and a series of four lacerations to the right ear

Anesthetic: Local anesthetic was used, 1% carbocaine plain

Indications: The patient sustained the above-named lacerations when she was involved in a hay wagon accident.

Procedure: The patient was treated in the emergency department. The right ear was treated first. The two smaller, more superficial lacerations, measuring 1.0 cm each, were closed after the wound had been infiltrated with 1% carbocaine and then cleaned copiously with Betadine, saline, and peroxide. They were closed with simple interrupted #6-0 Prolene sutures. The two other lacerations on the right ear, total of 3 cm in length, and two different lacerations were closed in the deep layer with #5-0 Vicryl suture after they had been infiltrated with 1% carbocaine, prepared and draped in the appropriate fashion using Betadine, peroxide, and saline. The superficial layers were closed with interrupted #6-0 Prolene suture. After the right ear was completed the wounds were covered with polysporin. The left ear was then treated after the 2.0-cm wound was infiltrated with 1% carbocaine. After the wound was cleaned with Betadine, saline, and peroxide, the superficial layers were closed with interrupted #6-0 Prolene suture. The wounds were then covered with polysporin.

Follow-Up: The patient was instructed to follow up and take the sutures out in six to seven days.

Code(s): _____

Surgical Case #65

....

Operative Report

Procedure: Colposcopy

Diagnosis: Class II Pap; cervicitis

History of Present Illness: The patient is a 27-year-old woman who had previously undergone a Pap smear showing class II Pap. She is admitted today for a colposcopy.

Technique: The patient was placed in the lithotomy position. Her vagina and cervix were examined and a speculum inserted; dyeing was done with acetic acid followed by gram iodine and methylene blue. Cervical biopsies were performed at indicated areas, with Monsel solution applied for cautery. There were no complications, and the patient tolerated the procedure well.

Plan: The patient is to call the office within one week for her biopsy report.

Code(s): _____

Surgical Case #66

Procedure Performed:	Amniocentesis
Reason for Procedure:	The patient is a 32-year-old white female who is gravida 5, para 1, with intrauterine pregnancy at 36-4/7 weeks gestation. She was admitted in prodromal labor. She has gestational diabetes mellitus and an ultrasound suggesting fetal weight of greater than 10 pounds. The patient has been quite uncomfortable in recent weeks and is adamant about wanting to be delivered. In view of the gestational diabetes requiring insulin I feel it important to document fetal lung maturity in a more or less elective delivery.
	I discussed amniocentesis and the risks, benefits and alternatives. After answering her questions she agreed to proceed with the procedure.
Description of the Procedure:	Under ultrasound guidance a 4 to 5 cm pocket of amniotic fluid was identified in the fundal left side. The abdomen was prepped and draped. Under ultrasound guidance a 22-gauge needle was inserted into this pocket and approximately 8 cc of fluid was obtained, which was lightly blood stained. I attempted to aspirate more using a second syringe but was unable to get further fluid so the procedure was terminated.
Assessment & Plan:	Post procedure the fetal heart tracing was obtained and fetal heartbeat was in the 150s. Biophysical profile post procedure was 10 out of 10. We will await the amniocentesis results and if the l/s (lecithin/sphingomyelin) is mature we will proceed with cesarean section.

Code(s): _____

Surgical Case #67

Operative Report

Preoperative Diagnoses:
1. Enlarged symptomatic fibroid uterus.
2. Dysmenorrhea.
3. Menorrhagia.

Postoperative Diagnosis:
1. Enlarged symptomatic fibroid uterus.
2. Dysmenorrhea.
3. Menorrhagia.

Anesthesia Type: General endotracheal tube.

Estimated Blood Loss: 300 mL.

Procedures Performed: Laparoscopic-assisted robotic hysterectomy that was converted to total abdominal hysterectomy and bilateral tube removal and lysis of adhesions.

The patient had a 12 to 14 week sized uterus with a particularly large pedunculated subserosal to intramural fibroid off the posterior aspect of the uterus. There were also significant omental adhesions. There were also adhesions of the lower uterine segment/cervix to her bladder consistent with her prior vertical C-section. She also has signs of tubal ligation noted. Both ovaries were normal. There was an ovulatory type cyst on the patient's right ovary. The appendix was not visualized. The remainder of the intra-abdominal cavity was visually normal. The uterus was also quite boggy consistent with adenomyosis.

Procedure In Detail: The patient was taken to the operating room and was placed under general anesthetic. She was prepped and draped in normal sterile fashion and beanbag gel pads for robotic surgery. A time-out was called and agreed upon by all in the room. Her uterus was examined and appeared to be larger than was suggested by ultrasound, but also seemed to be relatively fixed to the anterior wall, which would have been consistent with her prior C-sections through a vertical incision. Placement for ports was decided. The VCare apparatus of the large size was placed in the uterus and sew into the cervix and the uterus did sound to 10 cm and the device was pushed all the way to the fundus and the VCare balloon blown up.

When I was happy with placement it did seem to have adequate uterine mobility, we went from above placed our Veress needle supraumbilically in incision followed by a 10-mm disposable trocar and sheath. Intra-abdominal placement confirmed some adhesive disease in the significantly enlarged uterus but did appear to be freely mobile and no other adhesions were noted to the sides or posteriorly, so the decision to continue with robotic procedure was made. All 3 arms were used and bipolar forceps, monopolar scissors, and ProGrasp ring forceps were placed then an arm 3. The left and right fallopian tubes were cauterized to remove the ovarian ligaments and both sides were cauterized and cut. There was a significant amount of blood vessels throughout. Both cornu bled easily, but we were able to back cauterized those with the bipolar and the round ligaments were then taken down also. Both parametrial areas were opened. The right ureter was easy to be seen, however, the left one was harder to visualize, but did appear to be far down below. I then attempted to retrovert the uterus, which was quite difficult given the size of her fibroid; however, switched out my Pro-Grasper to a tenaculum in arm #3 to try and do retraction. There was significant scarring of the bladder flap, but we were able to with sharp dissection with monopolar scissors take it down to at least the level of the internal cervical os.

At this time, I tried to go back and was able to cauterize the uterine arteries on the right, however, the left is could still not be very easily skeletonized and despite manipulation with both the VCare and with the tenaculum and multiple attempts, I was having a difficult time visualizing safely the left ureter from the uterine artery pedicle. So than we anteverted the uterus, held it up again with the tenaculum to attempt to go posterior for colpotomy and despite multiple attempts, I did not feel that there was adequate enough traction between the VCare and the size of the uterus for me to safely perform a colpotomy either anterior posteriorly, so I again remanipulated the uterus and replaced the tenaculum from arm 3 to try and reevaluate the left uterine pedicle. After multiple attempts, I still did not feel that I could safely visualize the area, so in order not to compromise ureteral integrity of patient's safety, despite the fact that we were already down to the level of the external cervical os, I deemed that the safest option at this point for the patient to avoid major injury or bleeding would be to open her up.

So at this point, all of our instruments were removed from any of the uterus or anatomy. The instruments were all removed out of the robotic ports, the robotic arms were detached and the robot was undocked, all ports were removed. We repositioned the patient for abdominal hysterectomy. I did, however, prior to doing that remove the VCare and evaluate the patient on vaginal exam to see if vaginal hysterectomy would be possible, which given her uterine size and the narrow introitus did not think would be. So we made a Pfannenstiel skin incision about 2 cm above the symphysis pubis carried through the underlying fascia. The fascia was nicked in the midline and incised laterally. The rectus muscles were separated and the peritoneum was identified, elevated, and stretched open and a Balfour retractor was placed in. All the irrigant that had we placed in the patient's abdominal cavity was irrigated and suctioned out. The Balfour retractor was placed in and moist laparotomy sponges were used to hold the bowel out of away. Most of the specimen was already removed, so 2 straight clamps were placed on either side of the cornua of the cardinal ligament complex, cut and sutured.

(Continued on next page)

Surgical Case #67   (Continued)

A second grouping of straight clamps were placed down and it was noted that the patient actually at this point had a profoundly elongated cervix, almost 6 cm in and of itself. So finally were able to shell, two curved clamps were placed and we were still not able to shell out the specimen, so I did finally use a knife to tunnel out until the vaginal cuff could be opened posteriorly and the Jorgenson scissors could be placed.

At this point, the specimen was handed off the table. Allis clamps were used to hold the vaginal cuff while figure-of-eight interrupted Vicryl sutures were placed on either end and then I placed a running locked #1m Vicryl suture in the midline. The area was then copiously irrigated. The remainder of the fallopian tube segments were removed. The right and left ureter could now be directly visualized and were peristalsing and normal and then at this point to assure that there have been no bladder injury, we backfilled the bladder with almost 350 mL of methylene blue dyed sterile saline with no leakage noted into the abdomen. The bladder was unclamped. The Foley allowed to drink completely and then I cut all sutures, did one final exam to reveal no signs of bleeding noted. A piece of Interceed was placed in. All packs were removed. The Balfour was removed. The peritoneum was closed with a running 3-0 Vicryl and then the fascia was closed with two #1 Vicryl sutures starting at either end and meeting in midline. A subcuticular 0-Vicryl was used to close the skin. While I was doing this, my partner close to the other incisions with UR-6 sutures in the large ports and 4-0 Vicryl on the skin. The patient was cleansed, anesthesia was reversed, and she was taken awake and stable to the recovery room.

Code(s): _____

Surgical Case #68

Operative Report

Procedure: Modified radical mastectomy

Diagnosis: Infiltrating ductal carcinoma, left breast

Indications: The patient is a 79-year-old woman who recently noticed a left breast mass. A subsequent mammogram revealed a spiculated suspicious lesion. On examination, she had a 2.5 to 3 cm palpable mass with no obvious axillary adenopathy. After an outpatient breast biopsy performed a week ago showed the mass was positive for carcinoma, she was admitted for a mastectomy.

Technique: Under general anesthesia, the patient's left breast was prepped. A transverse elliptical incision, including the nipple, areolar complex, and the previous biopsy site were utilized. Flaps were elevated medially to the sternum, superiorly to the clavicle, laterally to the latissimus, and inferiorly to the rectus. The depressed and anteropectoral fascia were dissected from medial to lateral with cautery dissection. The axilla was entered and the axillary vein identified. The venous tributaries were clipped inferiorly and divided. The long thoracic and thoracodorsal nerves were identified and traced to their insertions; the axillary contents were swept inferiorly and laterally out with the breast specimen.

Hemostasis was obtained with a Bovie knife in addition to clips and sutures. Two Jackson Pratt drains were placed. The subcutaneous tissue was reapproximated with interrupted 3-0 Vicryl, and the skin was closed with clips. Some of the skin flaps were trimmed to make the closure more acceptable cosmetically. The patient tolerated the procedure well and was returned to the recovery area in satisfactory condition.

Code(s): _____

Surgical Case #69

Operative Report

Procedure: Extracorporeal shock wave lithotripsy of right kidney stone

Diagnosis: Right kidney stone

Anesthesia: IV sedation

Technique: Under IV sedation, the patient was placed in the supine position. The stone in the upper right kidney was positioned at F2. The extracorporeal lithotripsy was started at 19 KV, which subsequently was increased to a maximum of 26 KV at 1,600 shocks. The stone was revisualized, and repositioning was done considering the transverse colon passing right anterior to the stone. Because the stone appeared to be in the same place after the repositioning, shocks were delivered. Apparent adequate fragmentation was obtained after a total of 2,400 shocks had been administered. The patient tolerated the procedure quite well.

Code(s): _____

Surgical Case #70

Operative Report

Procedure: Open reduction of right zygomatic arch fracture

Diagnosis: Right zygomatic arch fracture

Anesthesia: General

Technique: The patient was placed on the operating table in the supine position and administered general endotracheal anesthesia. He was prepped and draped in the usual fashion. A small incision was made in the temporal scalp area and carried down through the superficial temporal fascia until the deep temporal fascia was identified. This was incised, and an elevator was passed beneath the deep fascia until it was below the zygomatic arch. The arch was reduced manually and elevated back into its anatomical position noted by palpation. The wound was irrigated and hemostasis was obtained with cautery.

The superficial temporal fascia was reapproximated using interrupted 4-0 Monocryl sutures. The skin was closed with interrupted 4-0 nylon sutures, and a sterile dressing was applied along with a metal cup to protect the zygomatic arch. The patient was extubated and transferred to the recovery room in stable condition.

Code(s): _____

Surgical Case #71

Operative Report

Procedure: Direct microlaryngoscopy under general anesthesia

Diagnosis: Dysphonia

Technique: A 40-year-old patient was taken to the OR where, under general anesthesia, the Jako laryngoscope was inserted with the operating microscope to perform a laryngoscopy. The vocal cords were found to be totally normal on both sides with no evidence of nodules or granuloma formation. The entire endolarynx was well visualized. Moreover, there was no evidence of subglottic stenosis; and as the patient was awakening, vocal cord mobility appeared to be normal. The procedure was terminated, and the patient awakened and was taken to the recovery room in good condition with stable vital signs.

Recommendation: Speech therapy

Code(s): _____

Surgical Case #72

Preoperative Diagnosis: Chalazion, left lower lid

Postoperative Diagnosis: Same

Operation: Excision of mass, left lower lid

Procedure: Under adequate topical anesthesia and block anesthesia, the eye was prepared and draped in the usual manner. Chalazion speculum was applied. The left lower lid was everted and a vertical incision made. Excision of the mass was performed using curet, and a biopsy of the capsule of this 9-mm mass was made, as requested. Patient tolerated the procedure well and left the operating room in good condition after application of Cortisporin ointment and pressure patch.

Code(s): _____

Surgical Case #73

Diagnosis: Clotted AV Graft

Procedure: Left forearm dialysis graft thrombectomy and angioplasty

Using sterile technique, ultrasound guidance, and a micropuncture set, access was obtained to the arterial side of the graft and a 7-French sheath was placed with the tip directed towards the venous anastomosis. A 7-mm balloon was then advanced across the venous anastomosis and multiple dilations were performed. The thrombus was removed from the graft using the clot buster device. Heparin was then injected into the graft.

An additional 5-French sheath was then placed in the venous side of the graft with the tip directed towards the arterial anastomosis. A 5-French Fogarty catheter was advanced across the arterial anastomosis and pulled back into the graft. The pulled thrombus was then removed.

Additional dilations were then performed in the venous side of the graft and across the venous anastomosis.

Code(s): _____

Surgical Case #74

Diagnosis: Unacceptable cosmetic appearance of the breast

Procedure Performed: Bilateral breast augmentation with silicone implants

Indications: A 42-year-old female was seen in consultation for breast augmentation and is a good candidate; therefore, she will be having the procedure.

Description of Procedure: Patient was taken to the operating room and placed in supine position where general anesthesia was established. Chest was prepped and draped via standard surgical fashion.

My attention was turned to the breasts where an inframammary fold incision was made to open pockets were then developed. Sizers in the range of 550 were placed. It was decided to move forward with 500 mL implants. The pockets were irrigated with triple antibiotic solution. 0.25% Marcaine with epinephrine was infiltrated. The permanent prostheses were placed in the inframammary folds and were secured with 2-0 PDS. The incisions were closed with 3-0 Vicryl, 4-0 Vicryl, followed by 4-0 Monocryl. The patient tolerated the procedure well.

Code(s): _____

Surgical Case #75

Operative Report

Preoperative Diagnosis: Retained right ureteral double J stent

Postoperative Diagnosis: Retained right ureteral double J stent

Procedure: Cystoscopy and removal of right double J stent

Summary: Under anesthesia, the patient's genitalia was prepped and draped in the usual manner.

A 19.5 French cystourethroscope was inserted into the bladder without difficulty. An oblique lens was used to identify the retained right ureteral double J sent. The forceps instrument was inserted through the scope to grasp the stent. It was removed without difficulty.

Surgical Case #76

Operative Report

Preoperative Diagnosis: Bilateral inclusion cysts of the cheeks

Postoperative Diagnosis: Same

Procedure: Excision of 1 cm inclusion cyst of the right cheek and 1.5 cm inclusion cyst of the left cheek.

Anesthesia: Local

Brief History: The patient had persistent recurrent cystic lesions of both cheeks and a history of previous cystic acne. After explanation of the risks, benefits, and alternatives, the patient agreed to the excision.

Details of Procedure: The patient was taken to the outpatient- operating suite. The areas of the cheek were carefully marked and infiltrated with local anesthesia and prepared with Betadine paint. The lesions were elliptically excised (excised diameters of 1 cm of the right and 1.5 cm of the left.). Both lesions required layered closure of the deeper subcutaneous and epidermis with 4-0 Vicryl and 6-0 nylon. The patient tolerated the procedure well.

Code(s): _____

Answers to Odd-Numbered Exercises

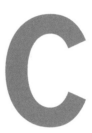

Chapter 1: Introduction to Clinical Coding

Chapter 1 Review

1. The American Medical Association (AMA) updates the CPT codes.

3. Diagnosis code set (ICD-10-CM)

5. All of the diagnoses except G83.84 Todd's paralysis would support medical necessity.

7. Procedure code 11440 is linked with diagnosis code A (D22.30). Procedure code 82951 is linked with diagnosis code B (R73.9)

   Note: Depending on the carrier, you may link more than one reference number in block 24E, whereas some payers require just one. When reporting more than one code on a CMS-1500 claim, enter the code with the highest fee in line 1 of block 24 and the remaining in descending order of charges.

Chapter 2: Application of the CPT System

Exercise 2.1 Organization of CPT

1. Anesthesia, Perineum (Category I)

3. Pathology and Laboratory, Therapeutic Drug Assay (Category I)

5. Evaluation and Management, Hospital Inpatient Services (Category I)

(Continued on next page)

Exercise 2.1 (Continued)

7. Surgery, Digestive (Category I)

9. Surgery, Maternity Care and Delivery (Category I)

11. Radiology, Nuclear Medicine (Category I)

Exercise 2.2 CPT Conventions

1. No

3. New descriptor

5. Revised descriptor

7. No

9. 40814

Exercise 2.3 Use of the Alphabetical Index

1.	23400	Green operation, *see* scapulopexy
3.	35556	Bypass graft, venous, femoral-popliteal
5.	26991	Incision and drainage, bursa, hip
7.	31526	Laryngoscopy, direct, diagnostic
9.	11055	Paring, skin lesion, benign hyperkeratotic
11.	41105	Biopsy, tongue
13.	29881	Meniscectomy, knee joint, arthroscopic
15.	65222	Removal, foreign body, cornea, with slit lamp
17.	4008F	Beta-blocker therapy, *see* Performance Measures, interventions – Performance measures, coronary artery disease, anti-hypertensive agents, Beta-Blocker therapy
19.	59001	Amniocentesis, therapeutic, amniotic fluid reduction

Exercise 2.4 CPT Coding Process

Operative Report #1

1. Colonoscopy and polypectomy

3. How was the polyp removed (hot biopsy forceps, snare, and so on)?

5. 45384

Operative Report #2

1. Excision

3. Documentation is needed to code malignant lesion, size of lesion + margins (or size of excision) (2.0 cm + 0.5 cm + 0.5 cm = 3.0 cm excision site) and site (arm).

5. 11603

Operative Report #3

1. Hernia repair

3. Age of patient; incarcerated or strangulated hernia

5. Wound closure would be an integral part of the procedure and would not be assigned a CPT code.

Exercise 2.5   *CPT Assistant* Coding Reference

1. *CPT Assistant,* January 1996, page 7, instructs the coder to assign 45380 or 45385 depending on the actual technique employed. *CPT Assistant,* January 2004, states that if a small polyp is removed via cold knife biopsy, the appropriate code is 45380. This is a good example of the need to research the most current coding advice.

Exercise 2.6   *CPT Assistant* Coding Reference

1. When a biopsy of a lesion is obtained and the remaining portion of the *same* lesion is then excised/fulgurated, only the code for the excision/fulguration should be used. When the biopsy is taken from a *different* lesion than the one excised, the biopsy code and an additional code for the removal of the separate lesion are reported. It would be appropriate to append modifier 59 to the code reported for the biopsy procedure.

Exercise 2.7   Coding References: *CPT QuickRef* App

1. Yes, the work associated with the free flap would not be reported separately.

3. Yes, code 27236 may be reported for the repair of the trochanteric fracture.

5. Unlisted code 19499 (Unlisted procedure, breast).

7. According to the guidelines and decision tree, code 45378 with modifier 53 would be reported.

9. The decision making depends on if the closure required one layer (simple) or a layered closure involving one or more deeper layers of the subcutaneous tissue and superficial (non-muscle) fascia (intermediate).

Exercise 2.8   *CPT® QuickRef App* Coding Vignettes

1. A patient who presents for removal of an atypical pigmented **nevus** on the waistline with excised diameter of 0.45 cm. Note that the waistline would be classified as trunk.

3. Patient with stenosing tenosynovitis of the right index finger treated with a steroid injection into its flexor tendon sheath.

5. A gap in the median nerve is repaired with a synthetic nerve conduit.

Chapter 2   Review

1. Bullet

3. Category III

5. 40842

7. No. The instructional note after code 43275 states to code once during the same session.

9. 43260 Diagnostic ERCP

11. 21933

13. 42320

Chapter 3:   Modifiers

Chapter 3   Review

1. 62

3. 22

5. 53

7. 19081–RT Biopsy, breast, with imaging of specimen

9. 11043–73 Debridement, muscle

11. 47562-22 Cholecystectomy, laparoscopic

13. 28485–RT Fracture, metatarsal, open treatment

15. Yes, it is appropriate

17. Modifier 59 because they describe distinct procedures.

Chapter 4:   Surgery

Exercise 4.1   Integumentary System—Debridement

1. 11042   Debridement, skin, subcutaneous tissue
3. 11011   Debridement, skin, with open fracture and/or dislocation
5. 11043   Debridement, muscle

Exercise 4.2   Integumentary System—Lesions and Skin Biopsies

1. 11421   Excision, skin, lesion, benign
   11421   Excision, skin, lesion, benign
   11402   Lesion, skin, excision, benign
3. 11642   Excision, skin, lesion, malignant; or Lesion, skin, excision, malignant
5. 11403   Lesion, skin, excision, benign
7. 11641   Lesion, skin, excision, malignant
   11640
9. 11102   Biopsy, skin lesion, tangential

Exercise 4.3   Integumentary System—Operative Reports

Operative Report #1
   11442   Excision, skin, lesion, benign; or Lesion, skin, excision, benign

Exercise 4.4   Integumentary System—Wound Repairs

1. 12032   Wound, repair, trunk, intermediate
3. 12041   Wound, repair, hands, intermediate
   12002   Wound, repair, arms and legs, simple (sum of repairs)

Exercise 4.5   Integumentary System—ED/Operative Reports

ED Report #1
   12001   Wound, repair; or Repair, wound, simple

ED Report #3
   13121   Wound, repair, scalp, complex
   13122

Exercise 4.6 Integumentary System—Skin Grafts

1. 15150 Skin Graft and Flap, tissue-cultured
3. 15200 Skin Graft and Flap, free skin graft, full thickness

Exercise 4.7 Integumentary System—Operative Reports

Operative Report #1

15120 Split Grafts

11646 Excision, skin, lesion, malignant; or Lesion, skin, excision, malignant

Exercise 4.8 Integumentary System—Operative Reports

Operative Report #1

19000–LT Breast, cyst, puncture aspiration

Operative Report #3

19120–RT Breast, excision, cyst; or Excision, breast, cyst

Note: The entire nodule was excised, not just a piece of tissue, which is implied with the term *biopsy*.

Exercise 4.9 Integumentary System Review

1. 16020 Burns, dressings
3. 12032 Wound, repair, arms, intermediate

   Note: Anatomic modifiers (LT, RT) are not appropriate for skin repair.
5. 11606 Lesion, skin, excision, malignant
7. 11750–T5 Nails, removal
9. 17272 Skin, destruction, malignant lesion

Exercise 4.10 Musculoskeletal System—Fractures

1. 25545–LT Fracture, ulna, shaft, open treatment
3. 23605–RT Fracture, humerus, closed treatment with manipulation
5. 27562–RT Dislocation, patella, closed treatment
7. 24516–RT Fracture, humerus, shaft
9. 27535-LT Fracture, tibia, open treatment

Exercise 4.11   Musculoskeletal System—ED/Operative Reports

ED Report #1

29515–RT   Splint, leg, short

Note: E/M code 99283–25 is applicable in this case.

Exercise 4.12   Musculoskeletal System—Arthroscopy

1. 29827–LT   Arthroscopy, surgical, shoulder
3. 29836–RT   Arthroscopy, surgical, elbow

Exercise 4.13   Musculoskeletal System—Operative Report

Operative Report #1

29882–RT   Arthroscopy, surgical, knee

Exercise 4.14   Musculoskeletal System Review

1. 28475–LT   Fracture, metatarsal, closed treatment
   28475–LT
3. 27769–RT   Fracture, ankle, posterior
5. 27301   Hematoma, thigh
7. 28750   Arthrodesis, metatarsophalangeal joint, great toe
9. 28108–T2   Excision, cyst, phalanges, foot
11. 22558   Spine, fusion, anterior approach
    22853   Spine Instrumentation, biomechancial device
    20937   Spine autograft, morselized

Exercise 4.15   Respiratory System—Endoscopy

1. 31255–50   Ethmoidectomy, endoscopic
3. 31233–50   Sinusoscopy, sinus, maxillary

Exercise 4.16   Respiratory System

Operative Report #1

30520	Septoplasty
31267–50	Endoscopy, nose, surgical
30140–50	Turbinate, excision

Exercise 4.17   Respiratory System—Laryngoscopy

1. 31540   Laryngoscopy, direct

3. 31541   Laryngoscopy, direct

5. 31578   Laryngoscopy, flexible, removal, lesion

Exercise 4.18   Respiratory System—Operative Report

Operative Report #1

31536   Laryngoscopy, direct

Exercise 4.19   Respiratory System—Bronchoscopy

1. 31640   Bronchoscopy, removal, tumor

3. 31625   Bronchoscopy, biopsy

31623   Bronchoscopy, brushing/protective brushing

Exercise 4.20   Respiratory System—Operative Report

Operative Report #1

31623   Bronchoscopy, brushing/protective brushing

Exercise 4.21   Respiratory System Review

1. 32663   Thoracoscopy, surgical with lobectomy

3. 30130   Excision, turbinate, inferior

5. 31257   Endoscopy, nose, surgical

7. 31576   Laryngoscopy, flexible

9. 30300   Removal, foreign body, nose

Exercise 4.22 Cardiovascular System—Operative Reports

Operative Report #1

33207 Pacemaker, heart, insertion; or Insertion, pacemaker, heart

Operative Report #3

36556 Insertion, venous access device, central

Exercise 4.23 Cardiovascular System Review

1. 33222 Pacemaker, heart, relocate, skin pocket for pacemaker
3. 33824 Ductus Arteriosus, repair
5. 36582 Venous Access Device, replacement
7. 36215 Catheterization, brachiocephalic artery
9. 33228 Pacemaker, replacement, pulse generator
11. 36569 Central Venous Catheter Placement, insertion, peripheral, without port or pump

Exercise 4.24 Digestive System—Endoscopy

1. 43202 Endoscopy, esophagus, biopsy
   43217 Endoscopy, esophagus, removal, polyp

   Note: Modifier 59 or new subset modifiers would apply.
3. 43284 Laparoscopy, esophagus, sphincter augmentation, device placement
5. 45378-53 Endoscopy, colon, exploration (the professional edition of CPT has a helpful Colonoscopy Decision Tree)
7. 45346 Sigmoidoscopy, ablation, polyp

Exercise 4.25 Digestive System—Operative Reports

Operative Report #1

43247 Endoscopy, gastrointestinal, upper, foreign body

Operative Report #3

45330 Sigmoidoscopy, exploration

Exercise 4.26   Digestive System—Hernia Repairs

1. 49500   Hernia, repair, inguinal, initial, child under 5 years
3. 49651   Laparoscopy, hernia repair, inguinal, recurrent
5. 49580   Hernia, repair, umbilicus, reducible
7. 43281   Hernia Repair, paraesophageal, hiatal, laparoscopic

Exercise 4.27   Digestive System—Operative Report

Operative Report #1

49505–LT   Hernia, repair, inguinal, child 5 years or older

Note: Mesh code is only coded with incisional and ventral hernia repairs.

Exercise 4.28   Digestive System Review

1. 46930   Hemorrhoids, destruction
3. 43245   Esophagogastroduodenoscopy, transoral, dilation of gastric/duodenal stricture
5. 45381   Colonoscopy, injection

   45385-59   Colonoscopy, removal, polyp

   (The coding for this procedure is discussed in the January 2017 (page 6) of *CPT Assistant*)
7. 42809   Removal, foreign body, pharynx
9. 46611   Anoscopy, removal, polyp

Exercise 4.29   Urinary System—Cystoscopy

1. 52332   Cystourethroscopy, insertion, indwelling ureteral stent
3. 52235   Cystourethroscopy, with fulguration, lesion
5. 52330   Cystourethroscopy, manipulation of ureteral calculus

Exercise 4.30   Urinary System—Operative Reports

Operative Report #1

52352   Cystourethroscopy, removal, calculus

52332–51–RT   Insertion, stent, ureteral

Note: Because the stent was inserted at the conclusion of the procedure, one can presume it is an indwelling ureteral stent.

Exercise 4.31 Urinary System Review

1. 51992 Sling Operation, stress incontinence
3. 52235 Cystourethroscopy, with fulguration, tumor
5. 50200 Kidney, biopsy
7. 52290 Cystourethroscopy, with ureteral meatotomy (bilateral modifier not appropriate because the code description specifies "unilateral" or "bilateral")
9. 50543 Nephrectomy, laparoscopic

Exercise 4.32 Male Genital System

1. 54057 Lesion, penis, destruction, laser surgery
3. 55845 Prostatectomy, retropubic, radical
5. 54150 Circumcision, surgical excision, neonate

Exercise 4.33 Male Genital System—Operative Reports

Operative Report #1
55875 Prostate, brachytherapy, needle insertion

Exercise 4.34 Male Genital System Review

1. 54840 Spermatocele, excision
3. 54690 Orchiectomy, laparoscopic
5. 54865 Epididymis, exploration, biopsy
7. 55700 Prostate, biopsy, needle or punch
9. 54640–50 Orchiopexy, inguinal approach

Exercise 4.35 Female Genital System

1. 58670 Laparoscopy, Ovary/Oviduct, Fulguration; Oviducts
3. 59812 Abortion, incomplete
5. 58674 Laparoscopy, uterus, ablation, fibroids
7. 58552 Hysterectomy, vaginal

Exercise 4.36   Female Genital System—Operative Reports

Operative Report #1

57461   LEEP Procedure, loop electrode conization

Exercise 4.37   Female Genital System Review

1. 57421   Colposcopy, vagina
3. 58662   Laparoscopy, destruction, lesion
5. 58674   Ablation, uterine fibroids, laparoscopic
7. 58554   Hysterectomy, vaginal
9. 58573   Hysterectomy, laparoscopic, total

Exercise 4.38   Endocrine System Review

1. 60280   Thyroglossal Duct, cyst, excision
3. 60260–50   Thyroid Gland, excision, total, removal of all thyroid tissue
5. 60300   Thyroid gland, cyst, aspiration

Exercise 4.39   Nervous System

1. 64445   Injection, nerve, anesthetic
3. 62281   Epidural, injection
5. 62164   Endoscopy, brain, excision, brain tumor
7. 63005   Laminectomy, for decompression, lumbar

Exercise 4.40   Nervous System—Operative Report

Operative Report #1

63075   Discectomy, cervical

Exercise 4.41   Nervous System Review

1. 62223   Shunt, brain, creation
3. 64782   Excision, neuroma
5. 63272   Laminectomy, for excision, intraspinal lesion, other than neoplasm
7. 63688   Neurostimulators, removal, pulse generator
9. 64408   Nerves, injection, anesthetic

Exercise 4.42   Eye and Ocular Adnexa—Operative Report

Operative Report #1

66984–LT   Phacoemulsification, removal, extracapsular cataract

Exercise 4.43   Eye and Ocular Adnexa Review

1. 65222   Removal, foreign body, cornea with slit lamp
3. 68110   Lesion, conjunctiva, excision
5. 67810–E1 Biopsy, eyelid
7. 67906–E1 Blepharoptosis, repair, superior rectus technique with fascial sling
9. 67914   Ectropion, repair, suture

Exercise 4.44   Auditory System—Operative Report

Operative Report #1

69436–50   Tympanostomy, general anesthesia (–50 for bilateral)

Exercise 4.45   Auditory System Review

1. 69910   Labyrinthectomy with mastoidectomy
3. 69642   Tympanoplasty, with mastoidectomy, with ossicular chain reconstruction
5. 69005–LT Hematoma, ear, external, incision and drainage (would expect to see documentation to explain why the procedure took an extensive amount of time)

Chapter 4   Review: Coding for Facility

1. 42305 — Incision and drainage, abscess, parotid gland
3. 57455 — Colposcopy, biopsy, cervix
5. 19342 — Prosthesis, breast insertion
7. 26750–F5 — Fracture, phalanges, distal, closed treatment,
9. 36569 — Catheterization, venous, central line *see* Central Venous Catheter Placement, Insertion, Peripheral without port or pump
11. 49507–50 — Hernia repair, inguinal, incarcerated
13. 26010–FA — Finger, abscess, incision and drainage
    26010–F1
15. 69666 — Fistula, repair, oval window ear
17. 54060 — Lesion, penis, excision
19. 59000 — Amniocentesis, diagnostic

Chapter 4   Review: Coding for Physician Services

1. 61520–62 — (physician #1)
   Cerebellopontine angle tumor, *see* brain, tumor, excision, cerebellopontine angle
   61520–62 — (physician # 2)
3. 29821–LT — Arthroscopy, surgical, shoulder
5. 43274 — Cholangiopancreatography, Endoscopic Retrograde (ERCP), with placement, stent
7. 68811–50 — Nasolacrimal duct, exploration, with anesthesia
   Note: Bilateral modifier applies because the code describes one duct.
9. 44151 — Colectomy, total, open, with ileostomy
11. 15783 — Dermabrasion
13. 21743 — Thoracoscopy, surgical, with sternum reconstruction
15. 46257 — Hemorrhoidecomy, simple, with fissurectomy
17. 62323 — Injection, steroids, spine, lumbar
19. 31571 — Laryngoscopy, flexible, injection, vocal cord

Chapter 5:   Radiology

Exercise 5.1   Diagnostic Radiology

1. 73722   MRI, *see* Magnetic resonance imaging, knee
3. 72170   X-ray, pelvis
5. 74430   Cystography, bladder
7. 74177   CT scan, with contrast, abdomen (*Note:* The note under code 74170 directs the coder to assign a code for a combined CT of abdomen and pelvis)
9. 71260   CT, with contrast, thorax

Exercise 5.2   Diagnostic Ultrasound

1. 76831   Hysterosonography, *see* Ultrasound; Sonohysterography
3. 76641–50   Ultrasound, breast
5. 76870   Ultrasound, scrotum

Chapter 5   Review

1. 73090–26   X-ray, arm, lower

   Note: Modifier 26 is reported to identify the professional component of the procedure, which includes supervising the procedure, reading and interpreting the results, and documenting the interpretation in a report.

3. 74430   Cystography, bladder

   Note: Modifier 26 was not appended to the code because the description includes supervision and interpretation.

5. 74280   Barium enema
7. 70460–TC   CT scan, with contrast, head

   Note: In this case, the radiology facility would report modifier TC to identify the technical component of the procedure, which includes performance of the actual procedure and expenses for supplies and equipment.

9. 76930   Ultrasound, guidance, amniocentesis
11. 76706   Ultrasound, aortic aneurysm screening
13. 77402   Radiation therapy, treatment delivery, single area
15. 73000   X-ray, clavicle
17. 72255   Myelography, spine, thoracic
19. 73560   X-ray, knee

(Continued on next page)

Chapter 5   Review   (Continued)

21. 76775   Ultrasound, kidney (Code 76775, limited, is for a single organ.) (see *CPT Assistant*, May 1999.)

23. 74247   X-ray, gastrointestinal

25. 70450   CT scan, without contrast, head

27. 78278   Gastrointestional Exam, nuclear medicine, blood loss study

Chapter 6:   Pathology and Laboratory Services

Chapter 6   Review

1. 88305   Pathology and Laboratory, surgical pathology, gross and micro exam

3. 82803   Blood gases— pH, CO_2, HCO_3, pO_2, pCO_2

5. 85055   Platelet assay

7. 86510   Histoplasmosis skin test

9. 80061   Organ- or disease-oriented panel, lipid panel

   80051   Organ- or disease-oriented panel, electrolyte

11. 80402   ACTH, *see* adrenocorticotropic hormone (ACTH), stimulation panel

13. 85730   Thromboplastin, partial time (PTT)

   85610   Prothrombin time

15. 88331   Pathology and Laboratory, surgical pathology, consultation, intraoperative

17. 84585   Vanillylmandelic Acid, urine

19. 86615   Bordetella, antibody

Chapter 7:   Evaluation and Management Services

Exercise 7.1   Exploring Evaluation and Management

1. Preventive Medicine Services

3. Psychiatric Collaborative Care Management Services

5. Nursing Facility Services

Exercise 7.2   New or Established Patient

1. Established
3. Established
5. New

Chapter 7   Evaluation and Management Review

1. 99211
3. 99245
5. 99291, 99292, 99292
7. 99396
9. 99212
11. 99235

Chapter 8:   Evaluation and Management Documentation Requirements

Exercise 8.1.   History of Present Illness Component

1. Location (throat), Duration (3 days ago), Severity (getting worse). 3 elements would be a Brief history of present illness.
3. Location (left knee), Duration (two months), Quality (constant), Modifying factors (not relieved by ibuprofen). 4 elements would be Extended.

Exercise 8.2   Review of Systems Component

1. No fever (Constitutional), No shortness of breath (Respiratory), No chest pain (Cardiovascular), Periumbilical abdominal pain (Gastrointestinal). 4 elements would be Extended.
3. Deep in skin (Integumentary), 1 element, Problem-specific

Exercise 8.3   Past, Family and Social History Component

1. Single and lives alone (Social), Knee replacement (Past Medical). 2 areas document would be Complete.

Exercise 8.4   Evaluation and Management (History)

1. HPI is brief (location, quality, and duration). Review of system(s) is problem specific. No PFSH documented. The history component for this visit would be expanded problem focused (brief HPI, problem-specific ROS, and expanded problem-focused PFSH including past, family, and social history). The history component is equal to the lowest category documented.

3. HPI is brief (location, severity, and duration). Review of system(s) is extended (two to nine systems), and PFSH is pertinent (medications). The history is determined by the lowest level from all three categories; therefore, the history level would be expanded problem focused.

Exercise 8.5   Evaluation and Management (Physical Examination)

1. Comprehensive examination: eight body systems were reviewed.

3. Expanded problem-focused examination: two systems reviewed (constitutional and integumentary).

Exercise 8.6   Evaluation and Management (Medical Decision Making)

1. Moderate complexity		
Category	**Documentation**	**Tabulation**
Number of Diagnosis or Treatment Options	New problem; no additional workup planned	3 points = multiple (moderate complexity)
Amount and/or Complexity of Data Reviewed	Review and order clinical laboratory tests (1 point) Review and order test in radiology section of CPT (1 point)	2 points = limited (low complexity)
Level of Risk	Undiagnosed new problem with uncertain prognosis (presenting problem)	
Documentation of prescription drug management (management options)	Moderate complexity	
Final Tabulation	Note that medical decision making is determined by the highest two of three	Moderate complexity

3. Straightforward		
Category	**Documentation**	**Tabulation**
Number of Diagnosis or Treatment Options	Self-limited or minor	1 point = minimal
Amount and/or Complexity of Data Reviewed	No data	Minimal/low complexity
Risk Factors	Acute uncomplicated injury (presenting problem) and over-the-counter medication (management options)	Low complexity
Final Tabulation	Two out of three from straightforward category	Straightforward

Exercise 8.7 Evaluation and Management Case Study

Abstracting Documentation Elements Worksheet

Chief Complaint: Cough, fever, chills

History Elements	Supporting Documentation	Category
HPI		Extended 4 or more elements
	Location nose, chest Duration (3–4 days) Severity (worse today) Sign/symptoms (shortness of breath)	
Review of Symptoms (ROS)	Constitutional (denies fever and chills) Cardiovascular (chest pain), Gastrointestinal (nausea, vomiting, diarrhea) Respiratory (yellow sputum)	Extended (2 to 9 systems)
Personal, Family, Social History (PFSH)		Complete
	Past medical history of cholecystectomy, no medications, smoker	

→*What is the overall level for the History (based on the lowest documented element)?* Detailed

Physical Examination		
Body Areas and Organ Systems	General appearance, vital signs	Comprehensive*
	Body Areas: Neck, Abdomen Extremities	*Although the physician examined 8 body areas/organ system, the extent of the examination lacked comprehensive documentation. If this a determining factor in the overall level of E/M service, many coding professionals would state that is more Detailed than Comprehensive
	Organ Systems: Eyes, ENT, Respiratory, Cardiovascular, Skin	

→*What is the overall level for the Physical Examination?* Detailed

Medical Decision Making		
Dx or Treatment Options	New problem: No additional workup planned	3 points = multiple
Complexity	Chest x-ray	1 point = minimal/low complexity
Risk	Prescription drug management	Moderate complexity

→*What is the overall level for Medical Decision Making?* Moderate Complexity

Final Results: Detailed History, Detailed Examination, Moderate Complexity

Review the code descriptions for 99211–99215. Need two out of the three key components. The case study revealed a detailed history and detailed examination, and the medical decision making was of moderate complexity. The correct E/M code selection is 99214. Note that there may be controversy for the body areas counted. Even though there were 8, the complexity of the examination would not be considered comprehensive by most professionals.

Chapter 8 Review

1. False
3. False
5. False
7. Expanded problem focused—Systems reviewed: respiratory, integumentary, ENT (ears, nose, throat), cardiovascular, gastrointestinal. Expanded problem focused (two to nine systems)
9. Five key elements (location, quality, duration, context, and modifying factors)

Chapter 9: Medicine

Exercise 9.1 Immunizations

1. 90471 Administration, immunization, one vaccine/toxoid
   90714 Vaccines, tetanus and diphtheria toxoid
3. 90471 Administration, immunization, one vaccine/toxoid
   90691 Vaccines, typhoid (*Note:* The index only provides a code for oral vaccine, the IM injection code is listed below.)
   90658 Vaccines, influenza, for intramuscular use
5. 90471 Administration, immunization, one vaccine/toxoid
   90748 Vaccines, hepatitis B and *Haemophilus influenzae B*

Exercise 9.2 Psychiatry

1. 90885 Psychiatric diagnosis, evaluation of records or reports
3. 90847 Psychotherapy, family of patient

Exercise 9.3 Dialysis

1. 90962 Dialysis, end-stage renal disease *see* End-stage renal disease
3. 90945 Dialysis, peritoneal

Exercise 9.4 Ophthalmology

1. 92018 Gonioscopy (See note under code 92020)

Exercise 9.5 Cardiovascular Services

1. 93025 Electrocardiography, Rhythm, Microvolt T-wave Alternans
3. 92977 Thrombolysis, coronary vessels, infusion
5. 92924–LC Artery, coronary, atherectomy
7. 93000 Electrocardiogram, 12 lead

Exercise 9.6 Pulmonary Services

1. 94660 CPAP, *see* Continuous Positive Airway Pressure
3. 94450 Hypoxia, breathing response

Exercise 9.7 Allergy and Clinical Immunology

1. 95017 Allergy Tests, skin tests, venoms

Exercise 9.8 Injections and Infusions

1. 96372 Injection, intramuscular, therapeutic (Also, J3420 would be assigned for specific substance- B12.)
3. 96360 Infusion, Intravenous, Hydration
5. 96420 Chemotherapy, intra-arterial, push

Exercise 9.9 Physical Medicine and Rehabilitation

1. 97032 x 2 TENS, *see* Physical Medicine/Therapy/Occupational Therapy—Modalities, Electric stimulation, attended, manual
3. 97602 Wound, care, debridement, nonselective
5. 97597 Debridement, wound, selective

Chapter 9   Review

1.	90966	End-stage renal disease services
3.	93590	Mitral Valve, closure, paravalvular leak
5.	93600	Electrophysiology Procedure
7.	99502	Home Services, newborn care
9.	92924	Artery, atherectomy, coronary
	92925	(additional branch)
11.	92928-LC	Coronary Artery, angioplasty, with stent placement
	92973-RC	Thrombectomy, percutaneous, coronary artery
13.	95863	EMG, *see* electromyography, needle, extremities
15.	99050	Special services, after-hours medical services

Note: An E/M code would also be assigned in addition to this service.

17.	98926	Osteopathic Manipulation
19.	91034	Acid Reflux Test, esophagus
21.	95807	Sleep Study

Chapter 10:   Anesthesia

Chapter 10   Review

1.	00406–P2	Anesthesia, breast
3.	00567–P4	Anesthesia, heart, coronary artery bypass grafting
5.	00914–P1	Anesthesia, prostate
7.	00580–P5	Anesthesia, Heart, transplant
	99100	Anesthesia, special circumstances, extreme age
	99140	Anesthesia, special circumstances, emergency
9.	00350–P3	Anesthesia, neck
	99100	Anesthesia, special circumstances, extreme age
11.	00732	Anesthesia, gastrointestinal endoscopy

Chapter 11: HCPCS Level II

Exercise 11.1 Auditing HCPCS Level II Codes

1. The answer provided is correct.

3. The answer is correct.

5. The answer is incorrect. The correct code is E0310.

Exercise 11.2 HCPCS Level II Codes

1. A4611 Battery, heavy duty; ventilator; or ventilator, battery

3. P3001 Papanicolaou (Pap) screening smear

5. V5362 Assessment, speech

7. J9209 Mesna

9. L0170 Cervical, orthosis

Chapter 11 Review

1. E0186 Mattress, air pressure

3. J3420 Vitamin, B_{12}

5. J1710 Hydrocortisone-sodium phosphate

7. 51702 Insertion, catheter, urethra

   A4355 Catheter, irrigation supplies

9. 67938-E1 Removal, foreign body, eyelid

11. 26055–F8 Trigger finger repair

Chapter 12:   CPT and Reimbursement

Chapter 12   CPT and Reimbursement Exercise: Cost of Errors

1. Incorrect. The documentation supports a code for abdominal hysterectomy, not vaginal hysterectomy. Correct code should be 58150.
   Facility Price for CPT Code 58262: $934.91
   Correct CPT Code Assignment: 58150
   Facility Price for CPT Code 58150: $1,042.19

3. Incorrect. The excised diameter is the size of the lesion plus the margins. 2.0 + 0.5 + 0.5 = 3.0 is correct but it the lesion is malignant, not benign. The correct code is 11603
   Facility Price for CPT Code 11403: $152.64
   Correct CPT Coding Assignment: 11603
   Facility Price for CPT Code 11603: $203.40

5. Incorrect. Because all repairs were of the same type (simple) and same site classification, the lacerations may be added together. However, the code of 12053 is for intermediate wound repair, not simple. The correct CPT code is 12014.
   Facility Price for CPT Code 12053: $226.44
   Correct CPT Coding Assignment: 12014
   Facility Price for CPT Code 12041: $77.04

7. Incorrect. The benign tumor extended beyond the skin and would be assigned code 28041 for Excision, tumor, soft tissue.
   Facility Price for CPT Code 11402: $118.44
   Correct CPT Coding Assignment: 28041
   Facility Price for CPT Code 28041: $472.67

9. Incorrect. The CPT incorrectly identifies a ureteral stent. The correct code 52282 is for urethral stent.
   Facility Price for CPT Code 52332: $162.72
   Correct CPT Coding Assignment: 52282
   Facility Price for CPT Code 52282: $352.08

Chapter 13:   Computer-Assisted Coding

Chapter 13   CAC Simulation for CPT Coding Exercise

1. The correct answer is 11042 Debridement, subcutaneous tissue. The use of 15930 would require documentation of "excision."

3. The correct answer is 31534 Direct laryngoscopy with biopsy.

5. 58150 Hysterectomy, abdominal, total. *Note:* The National Correct Coding Initiative states that if an endoscopic procedure is converted to an open procedure, only the open procedure may be reported. Neither a surgical endoscopy nor a diagnostic endoscopy code should be reported with the open procedure code when an endoscopic procedure is converted to an open procedure. (Chapter 7 of NCCI Policy Manual for Medicare Services, Effective January 1, 2013).

Index